MEN'S HEALTH TODAY 2000

The World's Best New Advice on Living
Longer, Stronger, Healthier, Better

Edited by Kenneth Winston Caine, **Men'sHealth** Books

RODALE

© 2000 by Rodale Inc.

Illustrations © 1998 by Chris Gall

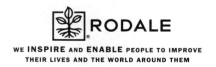

WE **INSPIRE** AND **ENABLE** PEOPLE TO IMPROVE
THEIR LIVES AND THE WORLD AROUND THEM

Men's Health Today 2000 Staff

EDITOR, *MEN'S HEALTH* MAGAZINE: Greg Gutfeld

MANAGING EDITOR, *MEN'S HEALTH* BOOKS: Kenneth Winston Caine

EDITOR: John D. Reeser

WRITERS: Colin Beavan; Debra Birnbaum; Ethan Boldt; Rick Chillot; JoAnne Czarnecki; Grant S. Davis; Bridget Doherty; Amy Donohue; Kelly Garrett; Stephen C. George; Ron Geraci; Brian Good; Melissa Gotthardt; Bill Gottlieb; Dave Gould; Teesha Graf; Greg Gutfeld; Doug Hill; Robert Huber; Kirk Johnson; Joe Kita; Richard Laliberte; Michelle Lee; Noah Liberman; Julie Liebowitz; Jennifer Lynch; Jordan Matus; Holly McCord; Christian Millman; Virginia Leoni Moles; P. Myatt Murphy; Roberta Naas; Martin Padgett Jr.; Joseph Mark Passov; Joan Price; Lou Schuler; Carol Ann Shaheen; Sarah Bowen Shea; Ted Spiker; Jeff Stevenson; Bill Stump; Zachary Veilleux; Dan Vergano; Wayne L. Westcott, Ph.D.; Janet Wright; Selene Yeager

ASSOCIATE ART DIRECTOR: Charles Beasley

COVER DESIGNER: Christopher Rhoads

PHOTOGRAPHER: Mitch Mandel/Rodale Images

ILLUSTRATOR: Chris Gall

ASSOCIATE RESEARCH MANAGER: Jane Unger Hahn

PERMISSIONS: Lois Guarino Hazel, Elizabeth B. Price

EDITORIAL RESEARCHER: Lois Guarino Hazel

SENIOR COPY EDITORS: Susannah Hogendorn, Amy K. Kovalski

COPY EDITOR: Kathryn A. Cressman

PRODUCTION MANAGER: Marilyn Hauptly

LAYOUT DESIGNER: Pat Mast

STUDIO MANAGER: Leslie M. Keefe

MANUFACTURING COORDINATORS: Brenda Miller, Jodi Schaffer, Patrick T. Smith

Rodale Active Living Books

VICE PRESIDENT AND PUBLISHER: Neil Wertheimer

EXECUTIVE EDITOR: Susan Clarey

EDITORIAL DIRECTOR: Michael Ward

MARKETING DIRECTOR: Janine Slaughter

PRODUCT MARKETING MANAGER: Kris Siessmayer

BOOK MANUFACTURING DIRECTOR: Helen Clogston

MANUFACTURING MANAGERS: Eileen Bauder, Mark Krahforst

RESEARCH MANAGER: Ann Gossy Yermish

COPY MANAGER: Lisa D. Andruscavage

PRODUCTION MANAGER: Robert V. Anderson Jr.

OFFICE MANAGER: Jacqueline Dornblaser

OFFICE STAFF: Suzanne Lynch Holderman, Julie Kehs, Mary Lou Stephen, Catherine E. Strouse

Contents

Introduction

Be Prepared

By now, you've probably gotten tired of hearing about the millennium. Whether it's a marketer touting the deal of the millennium or a computer wiz warning of total darkness at the stroke of midnight on January 1, we've been inundated with references to Y2K and the new century. Well, we're going to throw one more mention your way. But this time, it involves something that you really need. With *Men's Health Today 2000*, you'll be able to face any challenge that the new century brings you.

You can make intelligent decisions about your health and life for 2000 and beyond. Decisions that translate into getting the most out of every minute that you spend exercising. Eating the right foods at precisely the right times to fuel muscle growth and boost energy and stamina. Finding creative new ways to keep sex satisfying for you and your partner. Staying healthy while others around you get sick. Keeping mentally sharp. Even dressing in style for every occasion.

We realize that, in today's hectic world, men don't exactly perk up at the thought of diving through murky studies to recover the pearls of wisdom. That's where we come in. We tracked down the latest health studies and findings. We read the dense books. We talked to the top health profes-

sionals. We checked into exciting developments that are on the horizon.

The result is a powerful collection of the most up-to-date, actionable health information that you'll find anywhere. And we've packaged it so that you can tap into this amazing source quickly. No false prophets allowed in this book.

Here's some more of what you can expect to find inside.

"Benchmarks" is a feature that appeals to men's innate curiosity about seeing how they measure up to other men. Each one is a list of averages and oddball facts that provide an intriguing look into what men do. Want to know how many times per month men have sex? Or the average American man's body-fat percentage? Or what the most popular piece of exercise equipment is? Then you need to check these out.

In "Vital Reading," we present the very best advice from a variety of publications. There also is a growing field of books that address the health concerns of men. We culled the best parts of the best books, and you can read them in "Best Reads." Find out how to sidestep the seven roadblocks to weight loss, ward off the effects of aging with simple memory tricks, and spruce up your wardrobe with 10 style fundamentals.

One of the biggest services that we can do for readers is provide timely, breaking news about what's going on in men's-health research. Check out "News Flashes" to discover the latest findings on the common food that is loaded with antioxidants, and how you can build more strength by working out less.

Even more exciting than the latest findings are what researchers and doctors are in the process of cooking up in their laboratories. "Soon to Be News" reveals fascinating studies and research that are in the works. In the near future, you can expect to see such amazing discoveries as shock-wave treatment instead of surgery for some bone, tendon, and tissue injuries; genetically altered tomatoes that can provide 10 to 25 times as much beta-carotene as regular tomatoes; a speedier Viagra that takes effect in minutes instead of an hour; an antioxidant that may prevent hearing loss; and a drug that could be the key to stopping many addictions.

For a look at the latest trends, how they got started, and whether they are legitimate, check out "Fad Alerts." You'll get the real scoop on supplements like DHEA, chromium picolinate, and pyruvate; find out if the latest herbal superstar, ginseng, can really improve stamina, increase libido, and lessen fatigue; and get the lowdown on whether the best-selling book *Sugar Busters!* can lead to healthy weight loss.

"New Tools" is one of our favorite features. Why? Because we love gadgets and gizmos. And that's exactly what this section showcases. Some of the cool stuff that we found includes a drug to blunt flu symptoms and help you recover a few days sooner, a Web site to help you calculate your ideal weight, a simple equation to predict heart disease risk, and a nasal spray to end migraines.

Between periodic surveys and letters to the editor, a large number of questions roll into our office. We love to read them because they give us great insights into what's on our readers' minds. We collected the best of the bunch and present them in "The Answer Man" section of each part.

Topping off each part is a very useful section called "Actions." Here, you'll find great tips to help you change your lifestyle for the better— right now. From 20 things that you can do to shed those extra pounds to a list of some of the best stress relievers to the style secrets that ever guy should know, you get your money's worth with this feature.

So there's a taste of what's inside. The book is arranged so that you can access the information quickly and easily. Whether you read it for a few minutes before you hit the sack or crack it open on a lazy Sunday afternoon, there will always be entertaining reading ahead and interesting information to start you on the road to success and good health in the new millennium.

Kenneth Winston Caine
Managing Editor, *Men's Health* Books

1

FITNESS

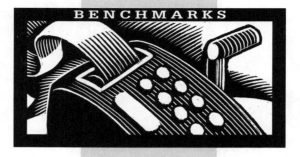

BENCHMARKS

- Girth of the largest biceps in the world: 30¾ inches

- Ounces of body fluid lost through perspiration per hour of exercise in hot weather: 54

- Percentage of Americans between the ages of 6 and 17 who cannot pass a basic fitness test: 64

- Number of men who do aerobics: 4 million

- Number of women who do aerobics: 18 million

- Number of Americans who used a treadmill in 1997: 36.1 million

- Percentage increase over 1987: 772

- Average number of steps it takes to hike the entire Appalachian Trail from Maine to Georgia: 5 million

- Number of deaths in the United States each year attributed to lack of regular exercise: 250,000

- Average number of minutes a sedentary person can add to his life with each mile he walks or runs: 21

- Average percentage by which a male sports fan's testosterone level rises when his team wins: 20

- Average points by which it falls when they lose: 20

- Number of injuries from using trampolines that occurred between 1990 and 1995: 250,000

- Number of people injured in boating accidents in 1996: 4,400

- Cost of calf-implant plastic surgery to make legs look stronger and fuller: $6,500 to $8,000 per pair

- Cost of a pair of pectoral implants for men: $6,500

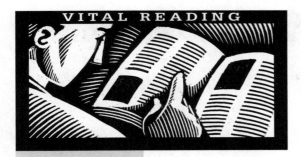

No More Waiting to Work Out

Train with these alternatives when your regular workout stations are jammed up.

You suck rush-hour exhaust fumes on your way to work in the morning, you flail around in the corporate trenches all day, then when you go to the gym to kick out the carbon, what do you find? More idling in neutral, with a crowd at each workout station.

We polled six of the nation's busiest trainers and asked them what their clients do when long lines preclude successful workouts. They suggested seven exercises to help you break away from the pack. When everyone else in the gym is stalled, you'll be pumping on all cylinders. You'll save time and eliminate frustration, plus you'll get better results from your regular workouts.

"You'll see more muscle gains in a shorter period of time because you'll utilize different muscle fibers instead of working the same ones again and again," says Jeff Cherubini of Frog's Athletic Club in Solana Beach, California. The other trainers we consulted—Doug Brignole of Venice, California; Phil Pfeifer of the East Bank Club in Chicago; Michael George of Santa Monica, California; Kurt Brungardt, coauthor of *The Complete Book of Shoulders and Arms;* and Jon Watt of Crunch in New York City—concur. Here's your ticket to the front of the line—and to a better body.

BODY-WEIGHT PUSHBACK
(works your triceps)

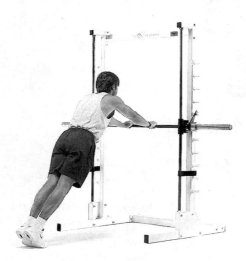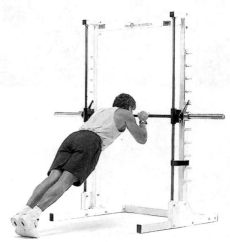

This is an alternative to a cable pushdown. Set the bar of a Smith machine (a rack with a barbell that slides up and down on rails) at waist level. Using an overhand grip, grasp the bar in the center, with your hands 4 inches apart. Step back from the bar until your arms are extended. Your weight should be on your toes.

Lean into the bar, stopping when your elbows are bent 90 degrees. At this point, your chin and elbows should point toward the floor, with your forehead at bar level. Push yourself up and back until your arms are extended again. The farther back you stand from the bar, the more difficult the exercise will be. Do 3 sets of 10 to 12 repetitions.

CABLE LEG CURL
(works your hamstrings)

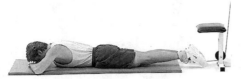

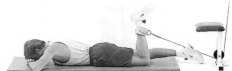

This exercise is an alternative to a lying leg curl. Attach an ankle strap to a low cable and slide it onto your right ankle. Lie on your stomach with both legs extending straight out from the machine, and rest your head on your forearms.

Slowly bend your right knee and pull your right foot as close as you can to your butt. Pause, then slowly lower your leg back to the starting position. Throughout the movement, press your pelvis to the floor to prevent lower-back strain, and keep your left leg as straight as possible. Complete 8 to 10 repetitions, then repeat with your left leg. Do 3 sets with each leg.

STEP PUSHUP
(works your chest, front shoulders, and triceps)

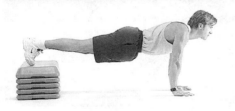

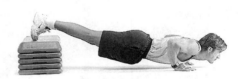

You can do this exercise instead of a bench press. Get on your hands and knees with no more than four step platforms stacked on top of each other and positioned behind you. With your hands shoulder-width apart, use your arms to support yourself as you lift both feet onto the steps. Keep your knees straight and your back in line with your legs (in other words, don't bend at your hips).

Slowly lower your chest to the floor. Then push up until your arms are extended, but keep your elbows unlocked. Repeat until you reach exhaustion.

For your second set, remove some of the step platforms. Do another set of pushups to exhaustion. Then remove the remaining steps, place your toes on the floor, and perform your last set to exhaustion. You can also do this exercise with your feet on one or two stairs.

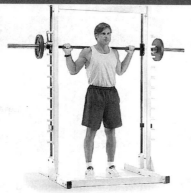 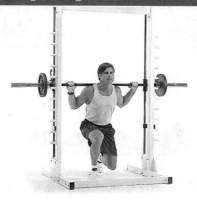

This exercise can stand in for a leg press. Position the bar of a Smith machine at shoulder height. Duck under the bar, unhooking it as you grasp it with an overhand grip that's just wider than shoulder width. Rest the bar on your trapezius. Set your feet hip-width apart.

Take a large backward step with your left foot, bending both knees until your right leg forms a 90-degree angle. (The lower part of your right leg should stay perpendicular to the floor.) Make sure your back remains in its natural alignment. Step back to the starting position, then take a backward step with your right foot. That completes the repetition. Do 3 sets of 8 to 10 repetitions.

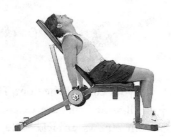 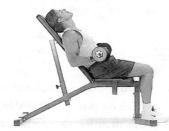

This is an alternative to a cable or barbell biceps curl. Set an incline bench at about 45 degrees. Grab a relatively light dumbbell in each hand (15 or 20 pounds is adequate for most guys) and lie back, with your feet flat on the floor in front of you and your knees together. Let your arms hang straight down from your shoulders, your palms turned forward.

Curl both dumbbells upward, keeping your upper arms stationary. Once you've curled the weight as high as you can without moving your elbows forward, stop and count to two. Slowly lower the dumbbells to the starting position, and repeat. Do 3 sets of 10 to 12 repetitions.

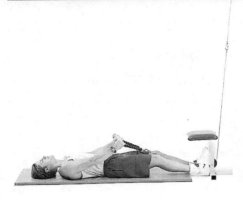 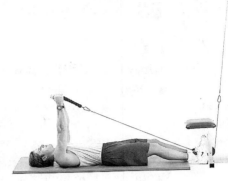

You can do this exercise instead of a dumbbell front raise. Attach a rope handle to a low cable and grasp the rope's ends with your hands facing each other. Lie on your back on the floor with your feet hip-width apart, one foot on each side of the cable's pulley. Hold the rope over your hips; your arms should be straight, with just a slight bend in your elbows.

Without bending your elbows any farther, slowly pull the rope up until your hands are over your face. You'll feel the squeeze in your front shoulder muscles. Slowly return to the starting position and repeat. Do 3 sets of 10 to 12 repetitions.

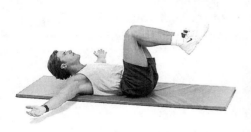

This is an alternative to a slant-board crunch. Lie on your back on a mat with your feet up, your knees bent, and your thighs perpendicular to the floor. Extend both arms straight out from your sides. Slowly lift your head and shoulders off the floor and curl your rib cage toward your pelvis. Pause, then lower your body, stopping just before your shoulders touch the floor, and repeat. Do 3 sets of as many repetitions as you can. To shift the emphasis to your lower-abdominal muscles, drop your thighs to a 50-degree angle and hold this position throughout the exercise.

A Strong Body Right Now

All you need are these four moves for a total-body workout.

At the gym, you probably treat your muscles like cuts of meat: two exercises for the rump roast, three for the tenderloin, one for the beef tips. You isolate muscles instead of making them work together. This type of training, popularized by bodybuilders, has two problems. First, it's a very slow way to build muscle. Second, it teaches your body to work as a bunch of separate pieces, not as an integrated whole.

There's another way to build a body: complex combination lifts. These odd-looking exercises combine several movements that you're not used to doing in sequence. In one move, for example, you lift a bar to your shoulders, then squat down and rise back up, then press the bar over your head. "All your muscles are involved—they're either lifting the weight or stabilizing your body," says Eric Ludlow, senior trainer at World Gym in New York City, who learned these moves from Olympic strength coaches. "That's why these exercises will stimulate real changes in the way you look." What's more, you need only four of these exercises to achieve a total-body workout.

Ludlow recommends doing one set of each of the four exercises shown here. Start with really light weights for 10 to 12 repetitions. As you become more comfortable with the moves, you can use heavier weights and work your way up to 3 sets of each exercise.

Three caveats: One, these movements are not for beginners. Two, they're definitely not for anyone with a history of back injuries. And three, they look weird. But if you've spent some time in the weight room, if your back is strong and healthy, and if your ego can handle the stares of disbelief, give this workout a try.

You have everything to gain.

CLEAN/SQUAT/PRESS
(works your back, shoulders, arms, quadriceps, hamstrings, glutes, and calves)

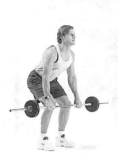

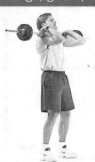

Stand holding a barbell against your thighs, your feet spread a few inches wider than hip width. Use an overhand grip, with your hands shoulder-width apart. Bend your knees slightly and lean forward from the hips until your back is at a 45-degree angle to the floor. The bar should hang just below your knees.

In one continuous movement, stand straight and pull the bar up until it rests on the fronts of your shoulders, with your palms facing the ceiling.

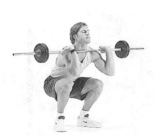

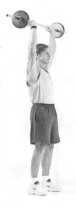

With the bar in this position, perform a squat: Shift your hips backward and bend your knees, as if you were sitting back in a chair, lowering yourself until your thighs are parallel to the floor.

Return to standing, and finish the movement by pressing the bar overhead.
To prepare for the next repetition, slowly and carefully lower the weight back to your shoulders, then to your thighs; then bend forward from your hips. Keep your back in its natural alignment throughout the exercise.

TRANSVERSE-PLANE PUSHDOWN
(works your back, triceps, and abdominals)

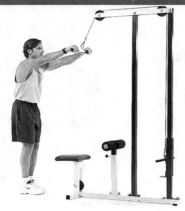

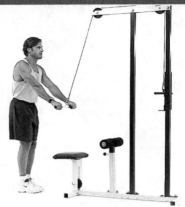

Attach a V-shaped bar to an overhead cable and stand in front of it. (You can use either a triceps-pushdown station or a lat-pulldown station.) Grasp the bar with your hands facing each other and your arms straight out in front of you.

In one fluid motion, pull the bar down until your elbows are at about waist level, and continue pulling the bar down and off to your right, just outside your hip.

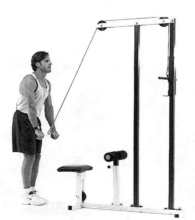

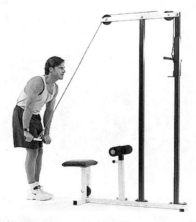

Keep your shoulders square to the weight stack; you don't want to twist your lower back.

Finish the move by pulling your ribs down toward your pelvis and crunching your abdominal muscles. Reverse the motion until the bar is back at shoulder level, then repeat the exercise on your left side. That's 1 repetition.

SINGLE-LEG BENT-OVER ROW
(works your upper and lower back, quadriceps, glutes, calves, and abdominals)

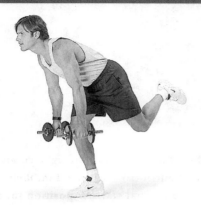

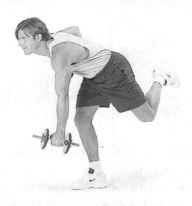

Stand holding a light dumbbell in each hand. Raise your left foot toward your butt, keeping your right knee slightly bent. Carefully bend forward at your hips until your back is almost parallel to the floor, letting your arms hang straight down.

Pull the weight in your right hand up to the right side of your chest.

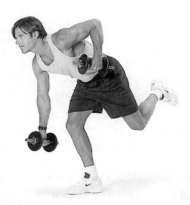

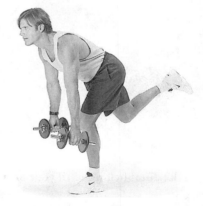

Lower the weight in your right hand as you begin to raise the weight in your left hand to the left side of your chest. That's 1 repetition.

Continue to alternate arms for a total of 5 repetitions, then switch legs and do 5 more, for a set of 10.

SINGLE-ARM ROTATIONAL CHEST PRESS
(works your chest, serratus, abdominals, and legs)

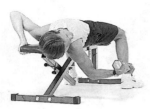

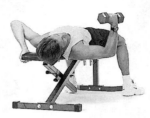

Lie on a bench with a light dumbbell in your right hand and both feet flat on the floor. Slide over until your right side is hanging off the bench. (Your spine will be on the right edge of the bench.) You can hold on to the bench with your left arm, but your right foot should support most of your body weight. Hold the weight close to the right edge of your chest, using whatever grip is comfortable. Drop your right side until your right forearm is parallel to the floor.

Tighten the muscles in your right leg, and rotate your torso until the dumbbell is near the normal starting position for a chest press.

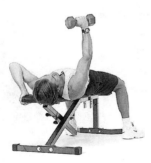

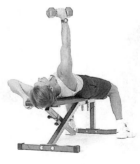

Press the dumbbell up until your arm is straight.

Continue pushing up as you lift your right shoulder as high as you can. The weight should rise about 6 inches higher than it would during a regular chest press. This final action works your serratus muscle. Lower the weight to the starting position and finish the set on that side of your body, then repeat on your left side.

An Eye toward Better Performance

Improve your athletic prowess with better eyesight.

If Michael Jordan had the eyes of the average man, he'd be a Division II college player, at best. So says Barry L. Seiller, M.D., an ophthalmologist and founder of the Visual Fitness Institute in Vernon Hills, Illinois. Dr. Seiller has been a sports-vision trainer since 1989, and he's convinced that the athlete's eyes are a window to peak performance. As he puts it, "your entire visual system must be trained along with your body."

Dr. Seiller has worked with pro athletes—NFL quarterback Jim Harbaugh among them—but increasingly, he and others in the sports-vision field are helping serious recreational athletes, too. "For a pro or a developing high school athlete, we can definitely make a significant difference," he says. "For a weekend warrior, it depends on his motivation."

When you visit a sports-vision trainer, you receive a specialized vision assessment that usually includes standard tests for visual acuity and eye health as well as tests for more subtle assessments of visual agility, such as depth perception, binocularity (the ability to use both eyes together), contrast sensitivity, accommodative amplitude (the ability to focus quickly on shifting targets), near/far focusing ability, and ocular alignment.

The vision training can involve sitting in front of a computer wearing special sunglasses (one lens is red, one green) and clicking a joystick in chase of floating objects. This improves smooth eye movements, or pursuits. Picking out random objects on the computer trains rapid eye movements, known as saccades (pronounced suck-AIDES). To increase eye-hand coordination, you stand before a 3-foot-square, wall-mounted apparatus with lights arranged in concentric circles and smack whichever light flashes.

The science of sports-vision training is still fairly speculative. While roughly 1,000 ophthalmologists and optometrists make it a part of their practices, much of the medical world views it with indifference or even skepticism. This is partly because it appears dilettantish compared with traditional vision medicine, and partly because it's not a guaranteed moneymaker. Medical insurance rarely covers the specialized vision assessment, which can cost up to $225, or the 4 to 20 recommended training sessions, which can cost up to $75 each.

According to Paul Berman, O.D., chairman of the American Optometric Association's sports-vision section, 1980s sports-vision research confirmed that athletes score better than nonathletes on numerous vision tests, and elite athletes score even better than average athletes. Furthermore, repeated drills, such as the ones Dr. Seiller prescribes, can improve an athlete's visual test scores. But it is still not known for certain whether mastering the joystick and the flashing lights translates to better performance on the court—or just the ability to kick major-league butt in video games like Tomb Raider II.

Also, visual training may not help everyone. Harold Koller, M.D., clinical professor of ophthalmology at Thomas Jefferson University in Philadelphia, notes that "the training doesn't alter eye function or brain function; it alters your ability to learn by developing the skills that boost visual efficiency. Sports-vision training may improve your eye-hand coordination but there's no guarantee that it will improve your athletic prowess."

Still, sports-vision professionals have attracted legions of believers, professional and amateur alike. Dr. Seiller's clients include the U.S. Ski and Snowboard Association and the U.S. Luge Association. (According to Dr. Seiller's tests, bobsled drivers have the best visual performance of any athletes in the world. Try interpreting the contours of a sheer ice run at 100 mph.) And university training rooms across the country are installing the eye/hand/body training machines favored by sports-vision specialists.

That's fine for elite athletes. But the real question is, will visual training work for average or below-average athletes? Or does improved performance (if there is any) occur because of increased concentration and confidence, with no clinical foundation? Dr. Seiller is, frankly, unconcerned with the answer to these questions. "When I started exploring this 9 years ago, I was skeptical, too," he notes. "Academics want to see cause and effect established in double-blind studies, and I understand that. I also wonder sometimes: Does the therapy work, or does performance improve merely because of the relationship with the therapist—the support? Actually, as long as someone feels that the results are positive, I don't think it really matters how it works. I think athletics is more a case of the end justifying the means."

Focal Points for Five Games

Anyone who has played Little League knows that you should always "keep your eye on the ball." But what exactly does that mean? "Even on the major-league level, players aren't taught where to watch," says Don Teig, O.D., founder of Sports Performance Centers of America in Ridgefield, Connecticut. "To increase accuracy, athletes need to zero in on the smallest area possible." Here's where to look.

Returning a serve: Follow the leading edge of the ball instead of reactively "watching" it. Put different-colored dots on a bunch of balls and have someone serve them to you, recommends Paul Planer, O.D., an Atlanta-based optometrist and former president of the International Academy of Sports Vision. "After you hit each one, call out the color. This will keep you concentrating on the ball."

Catching a long touchdown pass: Follow the forward end of the football all the way into your hands. "An athlete with bad hands is a misnomer," says Dr. Teig. "It's just bad eye-hand coordination."

"Believe it or not, video games are an excellent way to improve eye-hand coordination," says Dr. Planer. "But it's better to involve body motion, too." For that, he recommends having a friend uncover numbered flash cards. Each number requires a different body movement (for example, when he flashes 1, you jump left; on 2, you crouch; on 3, you jump right; and so on).

Hitting a green: Concentrate on the part of the ball you want to hit. "A lot of people look down at a golf ball and top it because that's where they're looking," says Dr. Planer. Put dots on golf balls where you want to make contact, and practice hitting them while focusing on the dots. To improve directional skills, put a ball marker on the green along the path that you want the ball to follow. Then work on making the ball follow that path.

Sinking the eight ball: Look at the point you want the cue ball to strike, either on the rail or on another ball. Fix a visual line between the cue ball and that point. Now aim for a spot on that line that's just a few inches in front of the cue ball. "It's much easier to aim at a spot just in front of the cue ball than to aim at a spot on the other end of the table," says Dr. Planer. Practice hitting balls right on the numbers. If your aim is off, adjust your close-up target.

Bowling a strike: Bowlers aren't expected to look 60 feet down an alley and aim for a single 15-inch pin; most lanes are set up with a series of dots a few feet in front of the foul line that you can use to guide your throws. (Which dot you aim for depends on how much spin you give the ball, and on where you choose to stand when you release it.) The real problem for experienced bowlers is drowning out the distractions that come from adjoining lanes.

If the alley allows it, have friends set up on adjoining lanes and cheer like crazed soccer fans. Have them hoot and holler, creating as many visual and aural distractions as possible. Practice maintaining your focus on the spot through which you want to roll your ball.

Weight Lifting for Your Eyes

Here are some drills to improve your general vision skills.

Visual concentration (ability to focus while filtering out distractions): Practice an activity (such as putting golf balls) with plenty of visual interference, recommends Dr. Planer. Practice your sand shots at the beach, or have a friend try to distract you as you putt.

Eye tracking (ability to smoothly follow a moving object with as little head movement as possible): Track a baseball as it rolls around the inside of a Frisbee, but keep your head motionless.

Eye-hand-body coordination: Paste a target on an old record album, and practice sticking a Post-it note on the target as the record revolves at 33, 45, and 78 rpm.

Accommodative skills (ability to rapidly switch the distance of your focus): Stare at the words on a page that you've set up 1 foot away; then quickly focus on the words on a poster across the room. Or do this exercise with two identical eye charts at different distances, finding a letter on one and then the other.

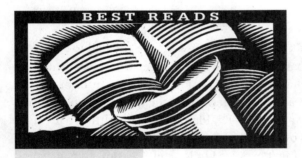

BEST READS

Use It or Lose It

Continuing to exercise as we age is one of the most influential things we can do in terms of living a long and healthy life. The intensity, duration, and activity don't have to remain the same as what you did in your twenties. The important thing is that you get out there and do something. Amby Burfoot spells this out clearly for runners in The Principles of Running: Practical Lessons from My First 100,000 Miles *(Rodale Press, 1999), yet what he has to say applies to all exercisers, not just runners.*

Life is about choosing. We can't influence everything we might like to, but we still face an endless array of decisions. And living with an aging body certainly presents its share of tough ones.

In the end, though, the biggest choice is a simple one: Do we give up or do we fight? Do we acknowledge that we reached our physical peak in our midtwenties and that it's all downhill from there? Or do we fight for all the fitness and vitality we can muster at every age?

Of course, no one can deny the biological process. You can't live forever. Some diseases seem horribly random, and others appear to have a strong genetic influence. Doing something, though, is far better than doing nothing at all. A positive, proactive attitude is the most important health attribute you can have. I'd take it over a good cholesterol ratio any day.

Too many runners give up on their training when they reach an age where they start slowing down noticeably. The stopwatch is a cruel master, and it can rob your motivation. But this is precisely the time when, because of the illnesses associated with aging, you most need to maintain a high level of fitness. Here's why (and all these reasons are taken directly from a medical journal resting on my desktop right now).

- Exercise lowers the risk of depression, heart disease, high blood pressure, diabetes, osteoporosis, and some cancers.
- Exercise controls obesity, a major risk factor for all of the above (and other) diseases.
- Exercise improves endurance, strength, flexibility, and joint range-of-motion in people with arthritis.

I'd like to add two more points to this already impressive list. First, exercise simply makes you feel better and more alive every day. Second, exercise gives you more energy.

Because this second point is counterintuitive, many people simply refuse to believe it. They reason that 30 to 60 minutes of exercise a day has to make you more tired. They visualize runners collapsing at the end of a marathon. "So where's all this energy?" they ask sarcastically. Ha, ha. Very funny. But the fact remains that physical fitness improves energy levels all day, every day.

Last, a simple point about running. All of the above medical benefits accrue to those who exercise. You don't have to run. It's just that running, or a mixture of running and walking, is the quickest, easiest, most effective, and most all-weather method of vigorous exercise. When your goal is lifelong health and fitness, it pays to keep things simple and effective.

Principles

1. The most important thing you'll ever do with your running is to continue running . . . for the rest of your life. You'll run slower during these years, maybe even mixing together running and walking, but you'll also gain more physical and emotional benefits than ever before.
2. The list of medical benefits that exercise provides is almost endless, and running is the best lifelong exercise simply because it's the simplest, most time-efficient, and most effective.

3. Naturally, you'll have to adapt your training as you age. You should think less about performance and more about maintenance and injury prevention. When you feel the need for a rest day or a recovery day, take it.

4. You might switch to running every other day or every third day. You should definitely do more strength training, more cross-training, and more flexibility exercises.

5. By all means, keep running at the pace and level that seem appropriate to you. The energy you derive from your fitness program will spill over into other areas of your life, allowing you to stay active and involved in all the activities that are most important to you.

Dayhiking: Wonderful Walking

Walking is one of the most popular forms of exercise in the United States. Millions take daily walks for their health or for the sheer enjoyment of it. In The Ragged Mountain Press Guide to Outdoor Sports *(Ragged Mountain Press, 1997), Jonathan and Roseann Hanson describe the benefits and ease of what could be called advanced walking. What they call dayhiking is just hiking without staying in the outdoors overnight. If you're a walker, or even if you aren't, taking up hiking is not only healthy but invigorating and scenic.*

Of all the outdoor pursuits profiled in this book, hiking is perhaps the only one that comes naturally to just about everyone. In the mists of prehistory, before we made planes and cars and bikes and canoes and kayaks, when we wanted to go somewhere, we walked. Some atavistic hiking gene must hang on in most modern humans, because for so many of us, hiking triggers feelings of belonging and well-being. The mountains, deserts, forests, canyons, and jungles of long ago were all just the background of our comings and goings as we foraged and hunted for our families, but when we enter those landscapes today, many of us feel like we've really come home—we've not forgotten our roots.

Fortunately, today we forage in supermarkets and our time hiking in the wilds can be devoted to full enjoyment of the place itself, instead of finding dinner for six mouths back at the cave. Hence we have witnessed the evolution of hiking as a "sport"—one that can take many forms.

Basic. The most basic dayhiking involves throwing food, water, and a first-aid kit into a simple pack and exploring any place that interests you for however long you like.

Intermediate. Moderate, or intermediate, dayhiking involves a little more planning, over distances of a few miles or more, probably with a specific goal in mind. The pack will be a little more substantial in design and will contain more food and accessories to cope with being outside all day.

Advanced. Hiking more than 10 miles in a day, over steep or rugged terrain, and carrying a well-honed backcountry dayhiking kit in a contoured daypack constitute advanced dayhiking.

If you've never hiked before, the best way to start is to find a like-minded friend or two, read the tips in this chapter for starting out, and then go for it. (Until you're an experienced hiker, it's best not to hike alone.) Hiking with others will expose you to lots of different gear and technique preferences, which is invaluable to any beginner. If none of your friends is game, see if there are any hiking clubs or informal hiking groups at your local recreation center.

As your hiking experience grows, you will probably meet others with whom you can gradually explore more and more adventurous endeavors—topping your first 14,000-foot peak in Colorado (called a fourteener), wading chest-deep down a slot canyon in Utah, or traversing a cliff-wrapped beach on the Olympic Peninsula, for example. You can also opt for a trip with an adventure travel company; the price can be a little high, but if you think of it as tuition, it's a bargain indeed.

Or you may be perfectly happy ambling down a trail for a few miles and enjoying lunch under a gently spreading oak before taking an afternoon snooze.

Whatever type of hiking you do, it will be tremendously good for you. Studies show that people who walk regularly have stronger immune systems than do people who jog regularly. And the wonderful thing is that hiking is not a sport you outgrow as you age. Hiking improves with age—or perhaps it's age that improves with hiking.

First Time Out

How far can I hike in a day? How long will it take me? What is the definition of *steep*? Each hiker will have a different answer to these questions, but there are some good general rules for beginners.

- If you're hiking on level ground with a light load, with moderate elevation gain, expect to cover 2 to 4 miles per hour at a steady pace.
- If you're hiking on uneven, steep ground (ridges and mountainsides), expect to cover ½ to 1 mile per hour.
- If you're hiking cross-country (bushwacking), expect to cover ½ to 2 miles per hour depending on terrain.

- Add approximately 1 hour for every 1,000 feet of elevation change. For example, if you hike 4 miles per hour, a 4-mile hike with 2,000 feet of elevation change might take you as long as 3 hours.
- Take note of elevation gain in relation to distance traveled. A trail that climbs 1,000 to 1,500 feet in over a mile may be considered moderate, while one that zooms up 1,500 feet in half a mile may be considered steep.
- Don't overdo it. Turn around when you begin to feel fatigued (or preferably before), since at that point you're only halfway into your hike.
- All beginners should stay on trails and use maps. Don't venture off-trail on your first hikes: That's the way most people get lost.

What You'll Need

The beauty of dayhiking as a sport lies in its simplicity: You don't need much to get out there. In fact, a good rule to remember is to keep it simple—your gear, your hikes—until you're pursuing advanced dayhiking goals such as canyoneering or alpine trekking.

All you need for your essential starter kit is footwear, water bottles, a first-aid kit, a map and compass, and a pack to put them in. Of course, in theory you can do without all those things, but think of this: Early people had callused feet, drank water they found (no matter what condition it was in), knew how to administer first-aid with natural resources, could navigate by memory and constellations, and used an animal hide to carry jerky and a flint fire starter. If you can do all that, then happy hiking, and the outdoor retail industry mourns your loss. The rest of us need a little help, however.

Walking Lessons

You really don't need any special instructions to hike: Just point yourself down the trail and put one foot in front of the other. The rest comes naturally. Following are some tips to make your hiking more enjoyable.

Basics

- Warm up. Warming up for hiking can help you avoid stress injuries. The best kind of warmup for all activities is simply performing very low level repetitions of what you will be doing during your activity. Stretching alone should not be considered a warmup. It can be part of a warmup, but take care—many people stretch too far and aggressively and end up injuring themselves.

- The best warmup for hiking is to start out hiking very slowly; if you know the trail is going to climb very soon after the trailhead, do some gentle step-ups on rocks or logs before you start. Windmill your arms a little. Walk around the trailhead area with exaggerated, long steps and then tiny steps. Relax, take it easy, and your body will do the rest.
- Walk balanced. Stand tall, swing your arms naturally at your sides, and make sure you're not bending forward too much at the waist. Take care not to lock your knees. Use common sense, and you'll do fine.
- Use your upper body. When ascending, use your upper body to help your knees. As you step up, press down on the uphill thigh with your hands and use your arms and legs in tandem to lift your weight.
- Take small steps. In general, remember that small steps are easier on your body than big strides. This is especially true when going downhill, when you should take care to keep your knees bent.

Advanced Techniques

- Poling. Trekking-pole manufacturers claim that poling reduces impact to the body from walking by up to 250 tons per day. To get the most from trekking poles, use them like you would when cross-country skiing—alternating arms (the forward pole is on the opposite side of your forward leg), swinging, planting, and pulling forward as you hike swiftly. For hikers who want to make time and distance, trekking poles provide an excellent tool. Use downhill ski poles (trekking poles should be a little higher than your elbow) or look at adjustable models just for hiking at outdoor retailers.
- Speed and endurance hiking. Called fastpacking or power hiking by some, this combination of hiking and trail running is an extremely efficient, challenging, low-impact way to cover a lot of backcountry ground. Experienced fastpackers can cover 20 to 35 miles in a day. Sometimes the trips are overnight, sometimes in-and-out. Experts recommend carrying no more than 10 percent of your body weight while fastpacking, so you really need to think hard about what to carry. Most fastpackers carry their essentials in specialty fanny packs, such as those made by Ultimate Direction, a pioneer in fastpacking gear. If you want to get into it, check around with your local hiking club, Sierra Club, and running clubs to see if there are any groups specializing in fastpacking.

A number of tips and some of the information in this chapter were adapted from *The Dayhiker's Handbook*, by John Long and Michael Hodgson.

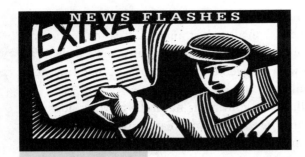

Less Rest Means More Strength

STILLWATER, Okla.—Now there's a way to cut the length of your workout and gain strength at the same time. A study at Oklahoma State University found that shorter rest intervals during weight training produce greater strength gains. Researchers measured the strength of 55 people before and after they completed a 12-week resistance-training program. The men who took 30-second breaks between sets gained 6 percent more strength than those who rested for 90 seconds. "Less rest may force different muscle fibers into action, resulting in improved overall strength," says Frank Kulling, Ph.D., the study author. Take a few weeks to gradually decrease your resting time.

Bail Out when Jumping Waves

JACKSONVILLE, Fla.—Before you ride a personal watercraft, make sure your medical insurance is paid. The impact of landing after jumping a wave can injure your spine. The trauma unit of the University of Florida Health Sciences Center recently treated several spinal fractures that occurred after riders jumped waves and then landed too hard. If you can't resist renting or buying a personal watercraft, at least avoid shallow water, and consider jumping off the craft if a wave catapults you high above the surf, advises Gregory Solis, M.D., chief resident of orthopedic surgery.

Running Can Stop Gallstone Formation

CAMBRIDGE, Mass.—Here's another reason to dust off those running shoes: Researchers at the Harvard Graduate School of Public Health found that aerobic exercise can stop gallstone formation in men. After tracking 45,813 men for 8 years, researchers determined that 2 to 3 hours of running each week can lower your risk of producing a gallstone by as much as 40 percent. "All types of aerobic exercise are associated with reduced risk for gallstones," says Michael Leitzmann, M.D., the study author. Exercise may affect gallstones by lowering triglyceride levels, a gallstone risk factor.

Vitamin C May Give a Boost to Muscles

FULLERTON, Calif.—Vitamin C has long been touted as a way to ward off colds, but one study suggests that it can do even more for your body. A study from California State University suggests that vitamin C can increase muscle strength. Thirty-seven students in a strength-training program took either 1,000 milligrams of vitamin C or a placebo every day. Eight weeks later, the vitamin-C group showed a 15 percent increase in the strength of their knee extensor muscles. The other group posted a 3 percent gain. "Vitamin C helps muscles recover after intense exercise," says William Beam, Ph.D., the study coauthor. If you train frequently, up to 1,000 milligrams of supplemental C per day may help other muscles, too.

Weight Training Builds Muscle Faster Than You Thought

ATHENS, Ohio—When you start (or restart) your weight-lifting regimen, it's natural to assume that months will pass before you reap any benefits except stiff, sore muscles. Wrong. A study done jointly by Ohio University and Pennsylvania State University found that you start building new muscle almost immediately. Researchers had 13 men and 8 women perform 5 sets (2 light, 3 heavy) of leg squats and leg presses two times a week. After just 12 workouts, their testosterone levels had risen roughly 10 percent. "We were astounded by how quickly these beneficial changes occurred," says Robert S. Staron, Ph.D., an exercise physiologist at Ohio University and coauthor of the study. At the end of the 2-month study, the subjects had increased the size of their muscle fibers by roughly 20 percent.

But you won't see these results by lifting casually. "It's important to continually work harder," says Dr. Staron. The researchers steadily increased the weight resistance, and the trainees performed repetitions to the point of exhaustion. Trainees also tried to complete a few more repetitions each time out than they had during the previous workout, forcing their muscles to work harder.

Yoga Reduces Carpal-Tunnel Pain

PHILADELPHIA—Yoga can do more than bring harmony to your life. A study at the University of Pennsylvania found that yoga may help relieve the pain associated with carpal tunnel syndrome (CTS). Researchers studied 42 patients with CTS: 22 who practiced Iyengar yoga (a form of yoga that uses progressive stretching) twice a week, and 20 who used a wrist splint or nothing at all. After 8 weeks, the patients who did yoga reported 42 percent less joint pain (the other group reported 17 percent less), and they also showed improved grip and muscle coordination. "Yoga improves a person's awareness of proper posture and his use of upper-body muscles, which can lead to a reduction in CTS symptoms," says Marian S. Garfinkel, Ed.D., the study's lead author.

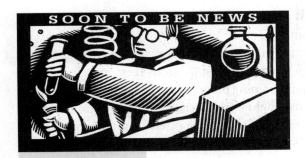

A Better Alternative to Surgery?

Shock waves may treat some bone, tendon, and tissue injuries better than surgery can. Instead of cutting away damaged tissue, physicians can use shock waves to blast away the calcification (extra bone growth) and scar tissue that can interfere with healing. Surgery can require days in the hospital and months of recuperation, but shock-wave therapy is a 1-day outpatient procedure. The waves may also trigger a release of chemicals that encourage healing, says John A. Ogden, M.D., of the Atlanta Medical Group.

National shock-wave trials show healing and restored function in more than 80 percent of all patients for whom prior treatments have failed. The FDA may approve the procedure within the next year.

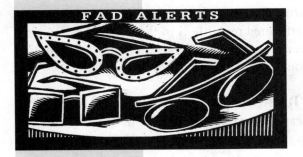

Wobble Boards

Spending around 15 minutes a day on a wobble board—a rocking platform that makes you teeter like Boris Yeltsin after lunch—can help an injured ankle heal faster. But it can also prevent ankle sprains, says John Cianca, M.D., assistant professor of physical medicine and rehabilitation at Baylor College of Medicine in Houston. Using a wobble board strengthens your peroneal muscles, which brace your ankles during side-to-side movements. "These muscles prevent your ankles from rolling inward, the most common cause of sprains," says Dr. Cianca. The exercise also improves your balance for running, inline skating, skiing, and golf.

Wobble boards offer upper-body benefits, too. Doing pushups on a round wobble board or a rectangular balance board forces you to push equally hard with both arms, says Kyle Pierce, Ed.D., an Olympic weight-lifting coach and director of the USA Weight-Lifting Development Center in Shreveport, Louisiana. That's useful because many men have uneven muscle development. Wobble and balance boards sell for less than $100. To order both models, call Fitter International at (800) 348-8371.

Supplements

 Walk into any muscle mart, and you'll see thousands of pills, powders, and potions—many of them purported to give you biceps like VW Beetles or a gut as rippled as a washboard. And pick up any of those muscle magazines at the counter, and you'll find even more pretty persuasion—articles that push the latest brawn-building elixir. (Some of those muscle magazines are either owned by or affiliated with supplement companies.) Do they really work? Right now, the research isn't there—even if the marketing plans are.

In 1994, Congress bowed to public will and relaxed stringent regulations governing the FDA's control over supplements. Today, supplement manufacturers aren't allowed to make explicit medical claims (like "controls hypertension"), but they can say that a product affects the body's structure or function ("aids metabolism") as long as they back up their claims with research. If a supplement maker does make unsupported or unauthorized claims, the penalty is a letter of reprimand and, if changes are not made, a referral to the Justice Department. The burden of compliance is on the manufacturers' shoulders, not the government's.

"I could fill capsules with sugar and sell them as a new miracle supplement," says Owen Anderson, Ph.D., editor of *Running Research News*, a newsletter written by exercise physiologists. "Unless someone died from them, I could market them with no problem."

Here's a look at some of the specific products that you'll see being pitched.

Protein supplements. Everyone agrees that a guy who's lifting weights needs more protein than a guy who isn't. There's even a formula for it: The Recommended Dietary Allowance for an average (nonexercising) adult is 0.8 gram of protein per 2.2 pounds of body weight per day. If you're pumping serious iron, you need 1.6 to 1.8 grams per 2.2 pounds, or up to 143 grams of protein per day for a 175-pound man.

"But I have yet to see a strength-training athlete who's not already eating enough protein," says Susan M. Kleiner, R.D., Ph.D., a nutritionist and coauthor of *Power Eating*. "They're already focusing on it," having an extra chicken breast here, a glass of skim milk there. And that's fine. "There's no advantage to taking protein as a supplement," Dr. Kleiner says. "It's not absorbed better. It's not utilized better." In fact, extra protein may put undue stress on your kidneys over time.

More important than where your nutrients come from—food or a powder—is when you eat them. If you want to build serious muscle, you have to eat or drink carbohydrates and protein after a workout, and the sooner, the better. If you do, you'll stimulate the hormones responsible for building muscle.

DHEA. Short for dehydroepiandrosterone, DHEA is long on hype. DHEA is a hormone produced in your adrenal glands. Your body converts it to testosterone, the manliest hormone. Supplement makers claim that taking supplemental DHEA will increase your body's supply of testosterone, giving you all the benefits that that implies. But creatine researcher Richard B. Kreider, Ph.D., of the University of Memphis, says that not a single published study has shown that DHEA can have this testosterone-boosting, muscle-building, strength-increasing effect in guys who lift weights. So forget it.

Chromium picolinate. Chromium is a lot like Jerry Springer—everyone privately agrees that it offers no benefit, but some people still lap it up. The notion that this supplement builds muscles and burns fat was debunked long ago, but every now and then a new study comes out to renew interest in the mineral. One study, presented at the 1996 meeting of the American College of Sports Medicine, found that swimmers on chromium picolinate gained 3.3 percent more muscle on average and lost 4.6 percent more fat than swimmers taking a placebo. Those are tiny differences over 24 weeks, and women had better results than men. "One study does not support a hypothesis," says Melvin Williams, Ph.D., an exercise physiologist at Old Dominion University in Norfolk, Virginia, and author of *The Ergogenics Edge*.

Fat-burning supplements. A lot of these fat-burner formulas contain ephedra (also known as ma huang), a stimulant usually used as a decongestant but also employed in medically supervised weight-loss plans (often in combination with caffeine) to increase patients' metabolisms. Unfortunately, it can do more than just clear up noses and crank up fat burners.

For some people, ephedra-based supplements may cause increased blood pressure and heart palpitations, and perhaps even catastrophic events such as seizures, strokes, and heart attacks. In the United States, 22 deaths have been linked to ephedra.

And even healthy men may be at risk. Some of these supplements may actually contain more ephedra or caffeine than their labels claim, which could make using these pills even riskier than you might think.

Pyruvate. According to the ads in the muscle magazines, this naturally occurring acid can reduce weight by 37 percent and fat by 48 percent. These spectacular claims rest on some pretty skimpy evidence. The ads are based on a few small studies conducted on regular guys, not trained athletes. When you use untrained people in research, you can't prove that any improvement is due to a supplement, rather than to exposure to a resistance program, says Kristine Clark, Ph.D., R.D., director of sports nutrition at Pennsylvania State University in University Park.

Studies touting pyruvate as a master fat blaster were also poorly designed, Dr. Clark adds. They were conducted on obese folks who, along with taking pyruvate, were confined to a hospital and fed extremely low calorie diets. "Under those conditions, anyone would lose weight," says Dr. Clark. "There's no evidence that pyruvate is responsible."

Weight-Lifting Belts

Those ultra-wide leather belts favored by weight lifters and UPS deliverymen are unnecessary. Research suggests that they can actually hinder the development of abdominal and lower-back muscles. In a study at the Albany Medical Center in New York, 50 men (all novice lifters) performed identical workouts, but 25 wore belts and 25 didn't. After 2 years, all 50 men had similar strength gains and injury tallies—but an exercise test proved that the beltless group had stronger abs and lower backs.

Weight-lifting belts increase your abdominal pressure, says Sohail Ahmad, M.D., the lead researcher. "This helps you thrust a heavy weight above your head," he explains, "but if you're working out for conditioning purposes, you don't need to lift heavy weights." If you feel the need to buttress your midriff, it's a clue that you're trying to hoist too much iron. Scale back the tonnage. Without a belt, your abs and lower back will contract naturally to generate this pressure, and you'll build a stronger torso.

Androstenedione

Androstenedione, or andro, is the muscle pill that Mark McGwire took while pummeling Roger Maris's home-run record in 1998. It's the synthetic version of a steroid that our bodies convert to testosterone. A bottle of 60 to 100 pills, containing up to 100 milligrams apiece, costs $19 to $30. The NFL, the NCAA, and the International Olympic Committee have all banned this supplement.

Manufacturers say that taking 50 milligrams to 300 milligrams of andro every day will increase your testosterone levels. One manufacturer goes so far as to claim that it can increase your energy, sex drive, and muscle mass.

The only human experiments took place in the 1960s. A group of women took 100 milligrams daily and increased their testosterone levels. (Women have little testosterone, so that's no big deal.) "It's a big assumption that the pill will be absorbed and converted into testosterone in normal men," says David Pearson, Ph.D., an exercise physiologist and associate professor at the Ball State University human performance laboratory in Muncie, Indiana.

Even if your body absorbs it, a measly 300 milligrams will probably have no effect on men, says Dr. Pearson. And if andro does increase testosterone levels, there might be side effects.

"Anything that artificially increases testosterone is an anabolic steroid," says Charles Yesalis, Ph.D., of Pennsylvania State University in University Park, author of *The Steroids Game*. "Steroids can cause heart disease, liver tumors, and temporary infertility."

Bodyblade

 A little more than 10 years ago, Bruce Hymanson, a physical therapist in Playa del Rey, California, came up with an unusual exercise: shaking a 4-foot, 1½-pound, flexible bow. Now he sells the Bodyblade on infomercials and the Internet as a muscle-strengthening and rehabilitating tool. Don't snicker; he's sold at least 100,000 at $99 each.

When you shake it by its center, it oscillates steadily, making it tough to hold. The promotional literature claims that the Bodyblade's motion "replaces weight training forever" and can "develop strength, quickness, coordination, and stamina in as little as 6 minutes a day." Hymanson says that he has studies under way to prove this, but some experts are skeptical about the device's effectiveness.

Rafael Bahamonde, Ph.D., a biomechanics expert at Indiana University in Bloomington, says strength or endurance gains would be minimal. "The resistance provided by the Bodyblade is relatively small compared with other methods of strength training, such as weights or elastic bands. I would not recommend this product as a chief means of gaining strength, endurance, or flexibility."

Some rehabilitation experts, however, say that the Bodyblade is useful for working with injuries. "Since the blade is moving, it challenges the muscles and forces them to react to the movement," says Edward Laskowski, M.D., codirector of the Mayo Sports Medicine Center in Rochester, Minnesota. If the Bodyblade helps you come back from an injury, great.

Pycnogenol

Pycnogenol, a supplement derived from a French pine tree, is said to improve athletic endurance. In a study at California State University, 24 athletes who took 200 milligrams of pycnogenol daily for a month increased their running endurance by 21 percent. Such a bump in stamina could shave more than a minute off your 5-K time, says David Swanson, Ph.D., coauthor of the study. (The research was funded by a company that sells pycnogenol, but Dr. Swanson has no association with the company.)

Pycnogenol seems to work because it contains antioxidants that fight free radicals (potentially harmful particles produced during exercise). Dr. Swanson's study suggests that free radicals may not only damage muscle cells but also slow recovery. "Boosting your antioxidant levels to reduce free radicals may be critical if you exercise strenuously," he says.

If you're training for a race, taking 200 milligrams of pycnogenol every day may help speed your recovery between runs. But that can cost up to $3 a day. "Pycnogenol has multiple antioxidant compounds common to many fruits and vegetables," says Lester Packer, Ph.D., a pycnogenol expert at the University of California, Berkeley. Five daily half-cup servings of blueberries, strawberries, cantaloupe, spinach, peas, grapes, or corn will provide enough antioxidants.

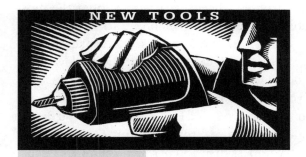

NEW TOOLS

Tighter Stomach

Negative Situps

Many men have put themselves through holy hell trying to build abdominals like Holyfield's. And then some bad news came out: Even 100 crunches a day won't give you heavyweight abs. "Over time, your abdominal muscles adapt to the crunch motion, so the exercise grows less effective," says Karen Branick-Martinez, strength and conditioning coach at Stanford University. "To continue to build definition, you need to constantly shock and fatigue your stomach muscles in new ways." She recommends negative situps, in which you stress the downward phase of the movement. Done very slowly, negative situps fatigue your abdominal muscles faster than crunches by keeping them tensed longer.

To do a negative situp, lie faceup on a mat with your knees bent, your feet flat on the floor, and your hands behind your ears. Curl your body up until your torso is at a 45-degree angle to the floor. Now, clasp your fingers together facing your knees, and turn your palms out so you see the backs of your hands. Keep your hands clasped throughout the movement; they serve as a counterweight to ease the strain on your lower back. Keep your abdominal muscles tight, and slowly lower your torso while counting to 10; don't let your head touch the floor. Your shoulders should touch the mat by the time you say "10." Then raise your torso back to the 45-degree starting position and repeat the exercise. Go for 10 repetitions first, then 15 when you can handle the burn.

Better Water Workout

Hydro-Bronc

Imagine that you're a hamster running in a plastic wheel. Now, imagine that wheel being tossed in a washing machine. That's an idea of what it's like to climb into a Hydro-Bronc—a giant, inflatable wheel that lets you shoot the most treacherous rapids with laughable ease. You simply run on a track of rubberized netting to propel yourself forward, and lean on one of the seven "spokes" to steer the monster. You'll get a vantage point no raft can provide, and a cardiovascular workout that makes paddling look one-dimensional. "It's like running on sand, and the constant movement of your upper body helps you steer," says co-inventor Philip Chauvet. When you tire out, you can rest and let the water wash you downstream in perfect safety. You can rent a Hydro-Bronc at rafting companies and surfside resorts across the country for less than $30 per half-hour. Call Virtual Sports at (503) 363-0013 to find the closest rental location.

More Enjoyable Golf

Taylor Made Durango

This golf bag ($170) has more options than Leonardo DiCaprio at his high school reunion. It has an Aqua-Flo hydration system with a 1-liter bladder, so you can suck water hands-free on the fairway. Dual shoulder straps let you carry the bag like a backpack, which can help prevent painful end-of-the-day golfer's stoop. The brainiest feature is the elliptical shape; the bag's sides are flat, not round, so it rests comfortably against your back. The Durango also includes the requisite built-in stand and umbrella straps.

Easier Stretching

SportStretch Cord

To avoid muscle pulls and backaches, runners should stretch daily. One of the best ways to do this is to complete a series of calf, hamstring, and quad stretches by gently pulling on a belt or rope looped around the arch of your foot. The SportStretch cord from Spydi ($25) makes this awkward move more comfortable. It's a nonslip cord that lets you stretch your legs without extending your arms or bending at the waist, and there's no skinny rope cutting into your foot.

Better Basketball

Spalding NBA Ultimate Indoor ZK Ball

Layups are a lot easier if you can palm the basketball or grip it with one hand like it's a teenager's head. But unless you have mitts the size of manhole covers, this is a tough stunt. For help, try the Spalding NBA Ultimate Indoor ZK Ball ($58). The skin on the Spalding ball is made of a slightly tacky composite material that adheres to your hands better than a regular leather basketball. And better ball friction can give you a crisper game all around. Just don't ask Spalding how they created a ball with adhesive qualities: "The competition will never get their hands on this information!" said a nervous rep.

Lighter Locks

Specialized Wedlock

The typical bike lock is either too heavy or too cumbersome, or it sounds like Jacob Marley exiting the basement. The Specialized Wedlock ($69) is none of the above. The 18-inch-long by 1½-inch-wide hinged steel lock folds up into a 6- by 1½-inch package that easily tucks away into a Velcro-backed rubber case. The case attaches quickly to a tube or seatpost. It may not be thiefproof, but it beats most of the other lock options.

Safer Skiing

CamelBak W.A.R.P.

The CamelBak W.A.R.P. (Water and Radio Pack) is a lightweight, low-profile way to stay safe and hydrated while skiing or snowboarding. Even when filled to capacity with 50 ounces of liquid, the W.A.R.P. ($90) is sleek enough to fit under a waterproof shell. There are plenty of pockets for storage, too: a zippered one for keys, ID, and money; a larger one for an avalanche beacon and radio; and another for a map. The hose and bite valve are even insulated to keep liquid from freezing.

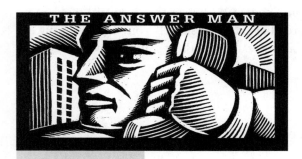

THE ANSWER MAN

Pain-Free Running

After 2 years of sloth, I've started running three times a week. About 15 minutes into my run, I feel pain in both of my shins. What can I do to prevent this?

—M. C., Cedar Rapids, Iowa

"Your best bet is to strengthen the anterior tibialis muscles, which run down the fronts of your shins," says Bill Case, a physical therapist and president of Case Physical Therapy in Houston. These muscles are natural shock absorbers that cushion the impact every time you take a step. If they're weak, the force is absorbed by the shinbone, causing shinsplints. To improve your flexibility, Case recommends doing calf and Achilles tendon stretches every day. Try the following two exercises to build strength in your lower-leg muscles.

Heel walks. Walk on your heels, lifting your toes as high off the floor as possible. "Do this periodically throughout the day, for 5 minutes at a time," says Case. "It'll promote the endurance and stamina in your lower-leg muscles to prevent future shinsplints."

Bucket lifts: Sit on a chair or table that's high enough to keep your feet from touching the ground. Hang an empty bucket or paint can from the toes of one foot, and slowly lift and lower the can by flexing your foot. Add water until you find a weight that allows you to do only 20 repetitions.

Case also recommends replacing worn-out running shoes because using old shoes can lead to shinsplints.

Help for Hamstrings

I do a rigorous free-weight program, but there are no leg machines in my gym. How can I work my hamstrings?
—R. W., Baton Rouge, La.

You can get a great hamstring workout with no more sophisticated equipment than a chair, says Torje Eike, a trainer who works with Mick Jagger and numerous Olympic and professional athletes.

Lie flat on the floor with your arms at your sides, your left heel on the seat of a sturdy chair, and your right leg extended up. Your hips and your left knee should be bent at right angles. Push down with your left heel and lift your pelvis as high as you can off the floor. Return to the starting position without letting your butt touch the floor. Switch legs and repeat.

Do 3 sets of 10 repetitions, and give yourself at least 2 days to recover between hamstring workouts. If you can't finish 10 repetitions, work up to that amount by doing a two-legged version of the exercise, keeping both feet on the seat of the chair. Once this becomes easy, try the one-legged version.

Because this exercise limits your range of motion more than leg curls at a gym would, be sure to stretch your hamstrings after completing each set.

Strong Hands

I've recently started using the indoor climbing wall at my gym. Are there any exercises I can do to improve my grip strength?
—R. T., Binghamton, N.Y.

First, buy some hand-strengthening putty, recommends Jane Fedorczyk, a certified hand therapist and assistant professor of physical therapy at Allegheny University of the Health Sciences in Philadelphia. You can find a brand called Power Putty at many fitness stores. (One container holds 3 ounces; you'll need to buy two.) Then do 20 to 25 repetitions of the following exercises with each hand.

1. Hold the putty in your palm, then grip with your fingers. Squeeze tightly against the resistance of the putty.
2. Roll the putty into a barrel shape, then hold it upright in your palm. Tunnel your thumb into the putty with as much force as you can manage until your thumb has pressed through to your palm.

3. Roll the putty into a 6-inch-long cylinder, and place it in the space between two neighboring fingers. Squeeze your fingers together like scissors. (Start at one end of the cylinder and move across it, so you can do more than one repetition before having to reroll the putty.) Complete a set between each of the neighboring fingers on one hand before you move on to the other hand.

4. Hold two neighboring fingers together, and wrap the putty around the top of them. Now pull your fingers apart. Complete a set with each pair of neighboring fingers on one hand before you move on to the other hand.

5. Roll the putty into a ball, then pinch it between your fingertips and thumb until they meet.

Alternate Pulldown Exercise

When I read about lat pulldowns, it always says to pull the bar to your chest. But what about pulling it down behind your head? Does this do the same thing?
—B. B., Montpelier, Vt.

The exercise that you're describing works the back muscles much the same way that pulling the bar to your chest does, according to Len Kravitz, Ph.D., an exercise physiologist at the University of Mississippi in Oxford. "Many trainers choose not to do behind-the-neck pulldowns because they think there's a higher risk of injury, but I disagree," says Dr. Kravitz. "Done properly, lat pulldowns behind the neck are perfectly safe—and the variation keeps your workout interesting."

The key to avoiding injury with any exercise, of course, is proper form. Sit at the pulldown machine and grip the bar overhead with palms facing away from you, your hands slightly more than shoulder-width apart. Keeping your upper body perpendicular to the floor, slowly pull the bar down behind your head, with your elbows pointing to the ground and slightly outward. (Forcing your head forward or not maintaining an erect posture can lead to injury, warns Dr. Kravitz.) Slowly return to the starting position.

Strong Thighs with Dignity

The fronts and backs of my thighs are pretty hard, but the insides are squishy. I'm not going to use that thigh contraption at the gym, so please give me a more dignified solution.
—M. N., Seattle

A thigh adduction machine is a great way to tone up this area. But, like you, we'd rather not be seen using any apparatus that looks like it ought to have stirrups. Fortunately, you can reap the same results from a wide-stance squat, says David A. Kirsch, owner and head trainer of the Madison Square Club in New York. He recommends moderately light weights—about 12 to 15 pounds—for this exercise. That may not sound like much, but when you're doing many repetitions and multiple sets, it's plenty, he says. Do these three times a week.

Stand with a dumbbell in each hand, your feet slightly wider than shoulder-width apart and pointing out to the sides at 45-degree angles. Make sure that your knees and feet point in precisely the same direction. This is the starting position. Keeping your back straight, slowly lower yourself into a squat position, sticking your butt out as if you were about to sit on a chair. Stop when your thighs are parallel to the floor. Hold for a moment, then raise yourself back to the starting position. Do 3 to 5 sets of 15 to 25 repetitions.

Hard Running

Why does it feel easier to run on the sidewalk than on the road? Is it actually softer?
—T. D., Los Angeles

Concrete is harder than asphalt. So the sidewalk gives you more bounce as you push off, which makes it feel easier. But is bouncier better? No. Over time, running consistently on harder surfaces increases the risk of repetitive injuries of your muscles and joints, says Edward Laskowski, M.D., codirector of the Mayo Sports Medicine Center in Rochester, Minnesota. "Run on grass or cinder surfaces. The more you mix it up, the less risk you'll have of overloading your muscles and bones."

Out of Breath

When I'm really winded, why do I instinctively bend over with my hands on my knees? This seems as if it would be counterproductive—and my high school football coach always used to yell at us to stand up to catch our breaths.
—D. E., Tucson

You bend over in an attempt to maintain adequate bloodflow to your head, according to Robert Gotshall, Ph.D., of Colorado State University's department of exercise and sports science in Fort Collins. "When you're exercising, your muscles are helping your heart fill with blood quickly so you can have a high cardiac output, which helps maintain blood pressure," he says. "If you stop suddenly—which most athletes tend to do—you no longer have the support for that cardiac output." Stopping often results in a rapid drop in blood pressure—so much so that there's barely enough pressure to pump blood up to your head.

You instinctively lower your head to heart level or below to get more blood flowing to your brain.

Your coach was right to tell you to stand up to catch your breath, but "take care of the bloodflow to your head first," Dr. Gotshall says. "Once the nervous system regains control of your blood pressure, you'll be able to stand up and catch your breath." That will be even easier, by the way, with your hands on your head.

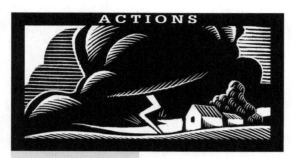

The long-term benefits of exercise should be hardwired into your brain by this time: thinner waist in 4 months, bigger muscles by spring, feel better, look better, live longer. But knowing how the book ends isn't always enough to make you hit the gym or clear the clothes off the ski machine.

Quit thinking about ripped abs. Concentrate instead on what one bout of exercise will do for you immediately. Here are some tips to get you on the road to lifelong fitness and all of the benefits that it brings.

1. Stay in the pool for stronger muscles. If you just finished your laps and want to squeeze in some resistance training, stay in the pool for a few dips. Just by swimming to the edge of the pool and raising your body in and out of the water (like you would with a dip machine) you'll exercise your triceps, chest, and back—and also get in some shoulder and forearm work. "It's a super upper-body exercise," says John McVan, aquatics specialist at Iowa State University in Ames. "After you're done, you won't need dumbbells or a trip to the weight room."

Place your hands palms down and about shoulder-width apart on the deck of the pool. Raise yourself until your arms are extended but not locked. Then bend your knees at a 90-degree angle and pull your elbows in close to your body. This is the starting position. Keeping your back up and your head as straight as possible, slowly lower yourself until the bottom of your chest is even with the deck and your elbows are bent at 90-degree angles. Pause, and then raise yourself back up to the starting position. Hold this position for 3 to 5 seconds, then lower yourself. This is tough, so don't be surprised if at first you can only do 3 or 4 repetitions. Work your way up to 3 sets of 8 to 12 repetitions.

2. **Roll to relief of foot pain.** Plantar fasciitis, a painful strain in the thin band of ligaments running the length of your foot, can hobble you for weeks. Aside from rest, common treatments to speed healing are ice and light stretches. To relieve plantar fasciitis, try rolling a can of frozen fruit juice back and forth under the arch of your foot. Using light pressure, roll for 1 minute, then take a 2- to 3-minute break. Repeat four or five times. This applies ice therapy while stretching your foot, according to a letter published in *The Physician and Sportsmedicine.*

3. **Ask for help in a strange city.** If you're looking to do a workout while on the road, ask the concierge to help. If he's worth his clip-on tie, he'll know all the safe, scenic running routes in the area and have a map at the ready. This often-unadvertised service can be a boon when you want to escape the business district in a strange place. "We offer a map that gives you a choice of running paths through residential areas and around ponds," says John Oliver, a concierge at the Four Seasons Hotel in Dallas. Before your trip, you can also hit the *Runner's World* magazine Web site at www.runnersworld.com for pointers on running routes and other travel information for more than 50 cities.

4. **Analyze your swing.** A post-golf backache may stem from lugging your overweight golf bag. But you might have wrenched your back simply by teeing off. Researchers at Good Samaritan Medical Center in West Palm Beach, Florida, videotaped the swings of golfers with back pain and disk damage. They found that the golfers twisted and bent excessively as they hit the ball. Instead of hunching over the ball, adjust your stance—or your club length—so you'll be upright when you follow through on your swing. "This may eliminate your back pain," says study author Scott Banks, Ph.D.

5. **Use proper form when squatting.** Almost anyone can walk in off the street and squat his body weight. But few guys can rest a stacked bar on the backs of their shoulders and lower it with proper form. That's because proper technique requires them to drop their hips down and back; most guys just bend their knees when they squat. "This improper form shifts the weight of the barbell forward and strains the tendons in your knees," says Rick Huegli, head strength and conditioning coach at the University of Washington in Seattle. To protect your knees, try moving the barbell to the fronts of your shoulders. Repositioning the weight will direct most of the force from the barbell to the right muscles—your quadriceps and, to a lesser degree, your hamstrings.

Place a barbell at about chest height on a squat rack. Position yourself so that the barbell is resting evenly across the fronts of your shoulders. Reach around the barbell with both hands and cross your wrists in front of the center of it. Use your hands to press the bar against your shoulders. Your elbows should be pointing straight ahead. Stand up and take a few steps back until the barbell clears the rack. Next, position your feet shoulder-width apart and point your toes slightly out. With your shoulders back, lower back straight, and knees behind your toes, slowly squat down until your thighs are parallel to the floor. Be sure to keep your feet flat on the floor. Pause, then return to the starting position. Do 6 to 12 repetitions.

6. **Throw a ball farther.** Most guys think that long throws are a matter of arm strength, but your whole body plays a big role in generating power and distance. To throw much harder, you need to strengthen your whole body, including those forgettable body parts such as your hamstrings, hips, and lower back. This isn't something you can accomplish quickly, so in the meantime, try these tips.

1. Position yourself sideways to the target so it's in a straight line with your shoulders. If you're right-handed, your left foot should be forward.
2. Don't be a stiff. Keep your whole body loose as you throw, to enhance the whip effect.
3. Step comfortably forward with your lead foot, plant it firmly, and quickly rotate your hips forward. This rotation is what produces the power.
4. Reach out during your throw. Keep your throwing elbow up and away from your body.
5. As your throwing arm speeds forward, pull your other arm down and back to rotate your torso with greater force.
6. Throw the ball at a 45-degree angle to the ground. Higher or lower throws cut the distance that the ball travels.

7. **Hit out of the sand.** The objective of the sand-trap shot in golf isn't to whack the ball out of the dune with a surgical strike. Assuming you have a clean lie (meaning the ball isn't buried), hit the sand with the club and let the sand move the ball. It's sloppy, blunt force, son, but if you move enough beach, the ball will ride onto the green with the dust storm. Here are the mechanics to get you there safely.

1. Setup: Dig your feet a few inches into the sand for solid footing. Flex your knees and bend slightly forward at the waist. Grip the club loosely so you can really feel the pulling weight of the club head, and relax your arms so that they hang straight down.

2. Backswing: Keeping your lower body still, slowly swing the club back. The farther you swing back, the farther the ball will go. The slower your backswing, the better your control.
3. Impact: Swing the club forward just as slowly as you took it back. In this game, speed kills. Hit the sand solidly about 2 inches behind the golf ball.
4. Follow-through: Swing around until your hands are level with your left ear. Never grind the club to a dead stop in the sand, even if the hole is close by—the ball won't go anywhere if you don't keep the club moving through the sand.

8. **Curve away from injury.** Some guys leave the handlebar ends on their mountain bikes pointing straight up because they're comfortable to grip when you're tearing down a grade. But it's dangerous. Austrian researchers found that 15 percent of riders who fell onto vertical handlebars suffered bruised livers. To keep your handlebars from goring you during a nasty fall, tilt the bar ends forward at 45-degree angles. "Curved bar ends are also safer than the straight, stubby types," notes Ed Burke, Ph.D., former director of sports science for the U.S. Cycling Team.

9. **Grow big triceps.** Before you spend all your sweat doing biceps curls, remember that it's your triceps that really add size to your arms. The California press is one of the most effective exercises for overloading the triceps, says Charles Poliquin, a strength coach for Olympic athletes in Canada. You can lift more weight than you can with other common triceps exercises, so you'll build bigger arms faster. "Power lifters often use this exercise when they hit a plateau," he explains.

To do a California press, lie on your back on a bench, with your feet flat on the floor. Grab a light barbell with your hands about 10 to 12 inches apart. With your elbows slightly bent, position the barbell so that it's directly over the center of your chest. Keeping your elbows close to your sides, lower the barbell to the top of your chest, near your collarbone. (That's right, you'll lower it at a slight angle.) When the barbell touches your chest, your forearms should be flat against your biceps. Pause, then slowly press the bar up and out to begin again. Do 2 to 3 sets of 12 repetitions, and add weight gradually.

10. **Stand up straighter.** Unless chandeliers tickle the top of your head, you're probably grateful for every last inch of height that genetics gave you. To maximize your stature, train your lower-back muscles; they help keep your spine straight. "Kneeling arm flexions are an excellent alternative to back extensions because they strengthen your back in its normal, straight position," says Len Kravitz, Ph.D., an exercise physiologist at the University of Mississippi in Oxford.

To perform kneeling arm flexions, grab a pair of 1- or 2-pound dumbbells and kneel on an exercise mat (or sit on a bench). Let your arms hang at your sides, lean slightly forward (keeping your back straight), and tighten your abdominal muscles. With both arms straight and your palms down, lift the weights slowly in front of you until they're even with your shoulders. Pause, then slowly lower the weights to the starting position. Start with 1 set of 8 to 12 repetitions, and gradually work up to 5-pound dumbbells.

11. **Row like a sailor.** Rowing machines fry more fat than a truck-stop griddle; even at a moderate intensity, a 175-pound man can burn 10 calories a minute. But most guys just plop down on the seat and heave that cable the way they'd try to start a dead lawn mower. "That only strains your back," says Stephen Gladstone, crew coach at the University of California at Berkeley. He gave us the flawless rowing technique described here. To build power, endurance, and tree-size arms and shoulders, pace yourself at about 18 strokes per minute for the first dozen sessions. Then speed up to a sweat-soaking 28 strokes per minute.

1. Prepare for the stroke. Sit on the machine with your legs fully bent and your feet firmly in the platforms. Your chest should be flush against your legs, and your arms should extend in front of you. Be sure to look straight forward. This is your starting position. Hold the handle lightly; don't squeeze it. It's important to stay loose.
2. Start your leg drive. Without moving your arms, push off with your legs, driving your heels (not your toes) into the foot platforms. Use only your leg muscles; the rest of your body should remain relaxed.
3. Pull with your arms. When the cable handle crosses your knees, and not before, lean back at a 30-degree angle and start to draw your elbows behind you. Keep driving with your legs.
4. Touch the handle to your lower chest when your legs are almost straight. Squeeze your shoulder blades together. Now do the entire motion in reverse: Let the cable gently pull you back to the starting position, bending your knees as the handle crosses them. Yell "Stroke!" and start again.

12. **Run fast.** It's healthy to sprint occasionally, and not just when you find yourself at the wrong cash machine after midnight. A study at Hebrew University in Jerusalem, Israel, found that running was the only exercise that strained the shinbones enough to strengthen them—an important factor in fending off stress injuries as you age. Biking, walking, stairclimbing, and doing squats were far less effective bone builders. You don't need to run marathons to reap this benefit. "Running for just 60 seconds will signal the bones to grow stronger," says

Charles Milgrom, M.D., an orthopedic surgeon in Philadelphia. So turn on the speed for 60 seconds during your workout.

13. **Attack those bumps.** Think of moguls—those speed bumps on a ski run—as hurdles on a running track: They're meant to trip losers. Dan Egan, an extreme skier and author of *All-Terrain Skiing*, gave us his technique for slicing over the nubs. This requires practice, so take your first 50 moguls at quarter-speed before trying to impress the snow bunnies.

1. Slow down. As soon as you see the first mogul, put your hands in front of your body and make a few gentle turns. Keep your head up and stay centered over your skis.
2. Hit it. About 15 feet before the mogul, relax your knees to brace for impact, keeping your torso straight. Try to keep your skis shoulder-width apart; bad skiers always close their skis on mogul fields. As you climb the mogul, bend your knees deeper.
3. Plant your pole. When you near the mogul's peak, reach out and plant a pole on its front, downhill slope. Use that as a turning point. Push on the pole with a fast snap of your wrist to turn atop the crest of the mogul.
4. Don't launch. As you pass the mogul's summit, put your entire weight on your toes and use the edges of your skis to control your speed. This will prevent you from flying off the little snow ramp.
5. Recover and watch out. As you ski into the trough, straighten your knees gradually. Be ready to do this again in a few seconds.

14. **Spray away blisters.** A U.S. Army study published in the *Journal of the American Academy of Dermatology* found that applying antiperspirant to your feet before a hike can reduce the chance of blisters. In a study of 667 cadets, only 21 percent of those who had applied antiperspirant to their feet for 3 to 5 days before a 13-mile hike developed blisters, compared with 48 percent of those who had used a placebo. "Antiperspirant helps reduce sweating and keeps your feet dry, so there's less friction to cause blisters," says Colonel Katy Reynolds, M.D., of the Army's Research Institute of Environmental Medicine in Natick, Massachusetts. The tip should work for other activities, too. Use an over-the-counter spray; many roll-ons contain moisturizers, which defeat the purpose. And watch out for skin irritation, which affected more than half the cadets who used antiperspirant.

15. **Protect your lungs.** In a report published in *Occupational and Environmental Medicine*, Dutch researchers found that antioxidant vitamins can protect cyclists' lungs from the harmful effects of ozone. "Air pollutants burn your lungs just as the sun burns your skin," says Gary Hatch, Ph.D., a research pharmacologist with the U.S. Environmental Protection Agency. People who frequently exercise outside in urban areas—cyclists, for instance—face the greatest threat. Because of this, Dr. Hatch urges those who exercise heavily outdoors to eat plenty of fresh fruits and vegetables and to consider taking supplemental vitamin C, vitamin E, and beta-carotene.

16. **Take enough gulps.** To stay well-hydrated, you should drink 4 ounces of water right before your workout and 4 ounces every 20 minutes during your workout, says Felicia Busch, a water-intake advisor for the American Dietetic Association. But if you gulp down H_2O at a water fountain, how can you be sure you're drinking enough? Just swallow at least six times. "An average swallow is about 1 ounce of water," says Busch. "When you're bent over at a fountain, it's a little less." If you think your big mouth is off the chart, count the number of swallows it takes you to empty an 8-ounce glass.

17. **Build a muscular back.** Seated cable rows can add girth to your upper back, making your shoulders appear broader. They also develop tremendous pulling power—a boon when your mower won't start or when your Rottweiler decides that your neighbor is no longer amusing. When you perform two-handed cable rows, though, your two latissimus muscles (the broad bands that connect your shoulders to your spine) brace each other, and each receives less stress than if you trained one alone. That's why the one-armed variation is better. "It requires more coordination and trains more muscle fibers," says Warren Anderson, a sports-training specialist in Phoenix.

Set the machine's resistance to a light weight. With your feet in the foot platforms and your knees slightly bent, grip the edge of the seat with your left hand for support, and grasp the cable handle with your outstretched right hand palm down. Slowly pull the handle inward to your right hip while turning your palm faceup; the twist will also work your biceps. Don't bend at the waist as you pull, and don't rotate your upper body—that can strain your lower back. Hold for 1 second, then return your right arm to the starting position. Perform 10 to 12 repetitions, then switch arms. Work up to 3 sets and gradually increase the weight.

18. **Become fit faster.** To get in shape in a hurry, pick the right exercise. Lower-body exercises, such as running and cycling, can build aerobic fitness more quickly than upper-body activities such as rock climbing and swimming, according to a study at Northern Michigan University in Marquette. Sixteen subjects averaging 26 years old ran on treadmills or climbed for 20 minutes. The groups posted similar heart rates, but the runners used 14 percent more oxygen, indicating that they received better aerobic workouts. To reap the same aerobic benefits from upper-body exercise as you get from running or cycling, you need to keep your heart rate 10 beats per minute higher, says Phillip B. Watts, Ph.D., the study author.

19. **Make a homemade ice pack.** The ice-gel packs you can buy at sporting goods stores are good for chilling sore muscles, because they conform to joints to cool them more thoroughly. But store-bought gel packs can cost up to $20. To make a better and cheaper gel pack at home, mix 1½ cups of water with ½ cup of rubbing alcohol, seal it in a plastic bag, and throw it in your freezer for a few hours. Instead of freezing into a rock-solid brick, the alcohol forms a thick slush that will stay ice-cold for at least 60 minutes. You should apply the pack to your skin for only 15 minutes every hour, however, says David H. Janda, M.D., director of the Institute for Preventive Sports Medicine in Ann Arbor, Michigan. Chilling your skin for longer periods could actually cause frostbite.

20. **Calm down.** Kicking the recycling bin may have stress-reducing benefits, but you might also try some low-intensity aerobics to keep yourself off the window ledge. After 20 minutes of cycling, 10 men and five women at Indiana University were given questionnaires to gauge their anxiety levels. Researchers found a significant decrease in anxiety for at least 2 hours afterward. And it's not only high-intensity exercise that helps; in this study, the benefits were similar for moderate exercise. "You can reap the calming benefits of exercise without running yourself ragged," says Jack Raglin, Ph.D., professor of kinesiology at Indiana University in Bloomington.

Exercise can also dispel the caffeine buzz you've given yourself by downing coffee and cola all day. Between trips to the bathroom, hit the stationary bike for 30 minutes. Cycling at about 60 percent of maximum lung capacity may help reduce the anxiety brought on by a high dose of caffeine. In a study conducted at the University of Georgia in Athens, 11 men in their twenties were given either a placebo or 800 milligrams of caffeine (the amount in 5 to 6 cups of strong drip coffee) 4 days a week for 2 weeks. Then they either exercised or rested. Those who pumped the pedals had three times the reduction in caffeine-related anxiety of those who rested.

2

EATING

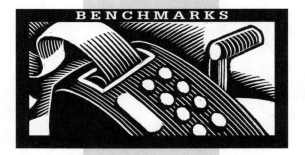

BENCHMARKS

■ Pounds of food consumed by the average American each year: 1,417

■ Pounds of chemical additives consumed: 9

■ Number of Americans who drink Coca-Cola for breakfast: 965,000

■ Amount Americans spend each year on packaged cookies: $3,900,000,000

■ Teaspoons of sugar the average American eats every day: 20

■ Gallons of mint juleps drunk at the Kentucky Derby each year: 1,875

■ Length of the average American business lunch: 67 minutes

■ Factor by which the sweetness of Sucralose, a newly approved sweetener, exceeds that of sugar: 600

■ Percentage of the U.S. potato crop that is french-fried: 22

■ Amount of peanut butter consumed by Americans each year: 700 million pounds (enough to coat the floor of the Grand Canyon)

■ Number of lunches Bill Gates ate on a recent visit to Moscow that were not from McDonald's: zero

■ Percentage of firefighters' meals that are interrupted: 60

■ Percentage of Kellogg's Frosted Flakes eaters who are adults: 46

■ Number of times Fred Magel, a Chicago restaurant reviewer, dined out during his 50-year career: 46,000 (in 60 countries)

■ Amount of soda an average American consumes every year: 45 gallons

■ Number of Americans who are some type of vegetarian: 12 million

■ Number of pounds of peanuts Delta Airlines uses in the average day: 6,000

■ Pounds of butter the average American eats per year: 4

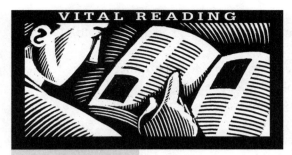

Eat Smart Forever

Good habits are the key to effortless health.

Listening to some experts talk, you'd think healthy eating was more complicated than the arterial map of Larry King's chest. Carbohydrate-to-protein ratios. Phytochemicals. Antioxidants. It's enough to make you nostalgic for high-school trigonometry class.

But don't get out the slide rule just yet. Here's an easier way to improve what you eat: Adopt some of the following smart habits. These simple tactics—if you stick to them regularly—will help you get more of the stuff you need into your diet while eliminating the stuff you don't. The best part? Before long, you'll be dining like a nutrition expert, without even thinking about it.

At breakfast, put coffee in your milk instead of milk in your coffee. Fill your mug to the rim with skim milk first thing in the morning. Drink it down until all that's left is the amount you'd normally add to your coffee; then pour your java on top. You just took in 25 percent of the vitamin D you need every day, and 30 percent of the calcium.

Take your vitamins every morning. Study by study, evidence is mounting that a standard multivitamin fills enough of the gaps in your diet to make a real difference. For example, a study at the Fred Hutchinson Cancer Research Institute in Seattle showed that people who took a multivitamin supplement and 200 international units of vitamin E for 10 years were half as likely to get colon cancer.

Drink two glasses of water before every meal. This will do two things: keep you hydrated and make you eat a little less. A Dutch study showed that drinking two glasses of water can make you feel less hungry, possibly reducing your food intake and aiding weight loss.

Always order your pizza with double tomato sauce and light cheese. Men who eat a lot of tomato products tend to have less prostate cancer—probably because tomatoes are a rich source of lycopene, a type of carotenoid that's believed to cut your risk of cancer. If you double the sauce on your pizza, you get double the lycopene. Reducing the mozzarella by just one-third (you won't miss it) will save you 20 grams of fat. That's as much as in a McDonald's Quarter-Pounder.

Always order your sandwiches with double the number of tomato slices. Another chance for a healthy dose of lycopene.

Pile onions on everything. Research has revealed that onions are so healthful—they're a top source of heart savers called flavonoids—that it's practically your duty to eat them lavishly on hot dogs, pizza, burgers, and sandwiches.

Whenever you eat fast food, drink two glasses of water afterward. Big Macs, subs, fries, and pepperoni pizza are all loaded with fat and sodium, which can be hellish for your heart. You can't do much about the fat once you've eaten it, but you can flush away some of the excess sodium by drinking plenty of fluid afterward, says Tina Ruggiero, R.D., a registered dietitian in New York City.

When the waitress asks what you want to drink, always say iced tea. The more we learn about tea, the more healthful it looks. A recent U.S. Department of Agriculture study found that a serving of black tea had more antioxidants—crucial to your body's defense against heart disease, cancer, and even wrinkles—than a serving of broccoli or carrots.

Have an afternoon snack every day at 3:00. A nutritional boost between lunch and dinner wards off fatigue and keeps you from overindulging later, says Keith Ayoob, R.D., Ed.D., director of the nutrition clinic at the Albert Einstein College of Medicine's Rose F. Kennedy Center in New York City. Just don't scarf down a candy bar. Try yogurt and fruit, crackers and cheese, a hard-boiled egg, an apple, and a thirst-quencher like bottled water. All of these foods will give you long-lasting energy.

Always leave the skin on your fruit. If you peel apples or pears, you're throwing away heavy-duty nutrients and fiber. Same goes for potatoes. Go ahead and peel oranges, but leave as much of the fibrous white skin under the rind as you care to eat—it's loaded with flavonoids. Ditto for the white stem that runs up the middle.

Put a bottle of water in the office freezer every night before you leave work. You already know that you should drink eight glasses of water a day, but how are you supposed to do it? Fill a ½-gallon bottle in the morning, and make sure you've downed it all by the time you go home. If you like your water cold and you have access to a refrigerator, fill the bottle partially the night before and stick it in the freezer. Next morning, fill it the rest of the way. You'll have ice-cold water all day.

Whenever you buy grapefruit, go for red instead of white. Remember lycopene, that stuff in tomatoes that may fight prostate cancer? It's what makes tomatoes red. And it's also responsible for the color in ruby-red grapefruit. (Watermelon and guava also have some.)

Eat salmon every Wednesday. Actually, the day doesn't matter; the important thing is to have it once a week. Salmon is a rich source of omega-3 fatty acids, a type of fat most experts say we don't get enough of. Omega-3's seem to keep the heart from going into failure from arrhythmia—men who eat fish once a week have fewer heart attacks—and they may even ward off depression. A weekly serving of salmon should supply the amount of omega-3 fats you need.

Always wash your meat. Here's an easy way to cut the fat content of your secret chili recipe: As soon as you finish browning the ground beef, pour it into a dish covered with a double thickness of paper towels. Then put another paper towel on top and blot the grease. If you want to remove even more fat, dump the beef into a colander and rinse it with hot (but not boiling) water. The water will wash away fat and cholesterol. Using these methods together can cut 50 percent of the meat's fat content.

Whenever you have salad, keep the dressing on the side. Here's the drill: Dip your fork in the dressing first, then spear a piece of lettuce, then eat it. Sound dumb? In fact, it's one of the smartest habits you can have. Four tablespoons of, say, honey-mustard dressing can have 60 grams of fat—nearly an entire day's worth for an average guy.

Whenever you eat broccoli, put a little margarine, olive oil, or cheese sauce on it. This is our kind of nutrition advice. Broccoli is a rich source of beta-carotene—one of the major antioxidants your body needs. But beta-carotene is fat-soluble, which means it has to hitch a ride on fat molecules to make the trip through your intestinal wall. Without a little fat in the mix, your body won't absorb nearly as much beta-carotene.

Always have seconds on vegetables. If we had to pick one food that represents the best insurance for long-term good health, vegetables would be it. Your daily goal: three servings minimum. A serving, by the way, is ½ cup. Think of a tennis ball—it's about ½ cup in volume.

Do a fat analysis before every meal. It's tempting to go fat-free at breakfast and lunch so you can indulge in a high-fat dinner. Wrong. Studies show that for several hours after you eat a meal with 50 to 80 grams of fat, your blood vessels are less elastic and your blood-clotting factors rise dramatically. "The immediate cause of most heart attacks is the last fatty meal," notes William Castelli, M.D., director of the Framingham Cardiovascular Institute in Massachusetts. Spread your fat intake over the whole day.

Always eat (a little) dessert. Here's why: Sweets such as cookies and low-fat ice-cream bars signal your brain that the meal is over. Without them, you might not feel satiated—which might leave you prowling the kitchen all night for something to satisfy your sugar cravings.

Eat a bowl of dry cereal every night before you go to bed. A low-fat, low-calorie carbohydrate snack eaten 30 minutes before bed will help make you sleepy, says Judith Wurtman, Ph.D., of the Massachusetts Institute of Technology in Cambridge. The nutrition bonus? Cereal is one of the easiest ways to reduce your fiber deficit. (Most men eat only half the 25 grams of fiber they need daily.) So pick a cereal that has at least 5 grams of fiber per serving.

When the Grocer Does the Cooking

There are plenty of good prepared meals to be had at the supermarket.

You put in a few extra hours at the office, and on the drive home you realize that the grinding noise isn't your muffler dragging on the asphalt—it's your stomach demanding tribute. You need dinner, fast. But you've gone the drive-thru route four times already this week, and your kitchen has less food in it than Gandhi's did.

Keep driving till you reach your local supermarket, and don't worry: You won't be cooking tonight. Your destination is the deli section, where, chances are, you can find a tasty selection of precooked entrées, side dishes, and sloppy desserts. But just how healthy are these meals? As healthy as you make them. Here's what you should—and shouldn't—take home with you.

The Best

Just like Mom used to make, if Mom was a registered dietitian and used those little plastic trays.

- **Chicken (grilled, baked, or rotisserie).** You already know that fried chicken has more fat than your heart can handle, so if you're in a poultry state of mind, go for baked bird. Rotisserie is essentially the same thing. Keep your calories down by eating only one breast and no skin. Save the extra meat for lunch tomorrow.
- **Roast beef.** Go ahead—satisfy your lust for red meat. Just keep the serving size at about 4 ounces. That's a little bigger than a deck of cards, or about the size of a woman's palm. See some fat around the edges? Trim it off. If gravy comes with it, apply only a thin layer.
- **Pork tenderloin.** That's right, we said pork. "Meats with 'loin' in the title tend to be lower in fat," says Toni Bloom, R.D., owner of the Food for

Thought nutrition-consulting firm in Burlingame, California. Compare for yourself: A 3-ounce serving of spareribs will bring you about 26 grams of fat. The same amount of pork tenderloin has only 5 grams.

- **Sushi.** This is where to go for fast fish, since fish sticks are the seafaring equivalent of hot dogs. Sushi requires no cooking time, and it's low in fat and cholesterol and high in heart-protecting omega-3 fatty acids. Add vegetables to your meal by choosing sushi with avocados, carrots, or cucumbers. Just go easy on the soy sauce: It's high in sodium.

   One other thing: If you're new to sushi, start out slowly. It could cause such symptoms as diarrhea and nausea, even if the fish is perfectly fine, according to Kristin Reimers, R.D., associate director of the Center for Human Nutrition in Omaha, Nebraska. "In reality, it's just that your body hasn't adapted to eating a new food," she says.

- **Mashed potatoes.** A satisfying choice that's not too high in fat. "Chances are, they're not using a lot of cream or butter in the potatoes, since they want to do it on the cheap," says Bloom. Potatoes supply enough carbohydrates, so be sure to pair your spuds with a dark-green or orange vegetable. Starchy vegetables, such as corn, contain fewer nutrients, calorie for calorie.

- **Glazed carrots.** Grab the carrots, even though the glaze may add a little butter and sugar to the meal. A little fat will help your body absorb the beta-carotene that carrots are loaded with, says John Erdman, Ph.D., professor of nutrition at the University of Illinois at Urbana-Champaign.

- **Green beans.** These were just about the only vegetable we found that didn't come drenched in a fatty sauce of some kind. Green beans also scored points with our experts for their nutrient content. "At just 44 calories per cup, green beans are a good source of folate, beta-carotene, and vitamin C," says Reimers.

The Acceptable

Just like Dad used to make. The spirit was willing, but the nutrition was weak.

- **Spaghetti and meatballs in tomato sauce.** Two meatballs won't hurt you—it's the rare supermarket that doles out more—and there probably isn't enough Parmesan to set off the fat alarms. What's more, the tomato sauce is rich in lycopene, a nutrient that has been linked to a lower risk of prostate cancer. Our only criticism: There are no vegetables here, except those that went into the sauce. Remedy that by scooping up some greens at the salad bar. Or grab some frozen spinach, thaw it in the microwave, and toss it in with the pasta.

- **Meat loaf.** Most supermarket meat-loaf dinners give you about 4 ounces of meat, which isn't unreasonable from a dietary point of view. But meat loaf has an inherent uncertainty to it, as many a suspicious 4-year-old will tell you. "I advise people to buy dinners that have ingredients they can identify," says Bloom. That reduces the chances of getting sucker punched by hidden calories. If you're set on meat loaf for some reason, balance it with a hefty serving of a low-calorie vegetable—preferably carrots, green beans, or broccoli.
- **Chicken marsala.** It's okay, but there are better chicken choices. Marsala sauce is comparable to gravy with an oil or butter base. And that's more fat than you need. So remove sauce until you can see the chicken. Keep the rest of the meal low-fat by pairing it with mashed potatoes and some chopped fresh red or green bell peppers.
- **White rice.** "It's healthy, but most people don't realize it's high in calories," says Bloom. On the plus side, white rice is enriched with B vitamins. Keep your serving size to a cup—about a handful—or less. If possible, choose brown rice instead; it'll give you extra fiber.
- **Peas.** Peas are higher in calories and lower in antioxidant vitamins than many other vegetables. But they're a great source of fiber, Reimers says. They also contain folate, which some studies say may lower your levels of homocysteine—a blood component that, like cholesterol, has been linked to heart disease.
- **Corn.** Another relatively high-calorie choice, but not a nutritional dud. "Like peas, corn offers fiber and folate," Reimers says. That means it's okay to put the kernels on your plate, but watch your portions.

The Worst

Just like you used to make—and probably still do, given half a chance. Bad stuff.

- **Pot pie.** You know what's in pot pie? Calories. Lots of 'em. "Some pot pies can have over 1,200 calories," says Bloom. Most guys need only 600 to 800 calories in an entire dinner, so stay away unless you're a professional wrestler.
- **Lasagna with meat sauce.** Lasagna is hard to walk away from, but save it for dinner at your aunt's. At least she'll dial 911 if you start feeling chest pains. "The meat-and-cheese combination makes this a double whammy," says Bloom. "And though you might find a few mushrooms or onions in the sauce, there aren't enough vegetables to make it worth all that fat."

- **Vegetable fried rice.** So you're taking that calorie-dense rice and frying it? Haven't you been listening? There are probably three little pieces of vegetables. The rest is rice. And oil.
- **Macaroni and cheese.** We understand your sentimental feelings. This calorie- and fat-packed dish probably accounted for 60 percent of the solid food you ate in college, the other 40 percent being beer nuts and Buffalo wings. You survived, but why push your luck? If you're suffering a mac attack, consider a cup—*1* cup—of mac and cheese to be your entrée, and add two generous servings of vegetables.
- **Creamed spinach.** Your mother was right: Spinach is an important vegetable. But its importance comes to an end when it's swimming in a pool of cream. "Chances are, they're not putting effort into making it low-fat," says Susan Kayman, R.D., Dr.P.H., of the Kaiser Permanente Health Group in Oakland, California. Put some frozen spinach in the microwave instead. Or pick up a bag of fresh spinach and mix it with a bag of precut salad. Rinse before serving.

Before You Check Out

The serving size of many store meals leaves the typical guy wanting more, but that doesn't give you license to swallow three dinners at one sitting or to polish off a bag of cheese puffs later in the evening. If you suspect that your dinner won't fully tame your hunger, grab a can of minestrone or vegetable soup and a whole wheat roll. Or slice up a pear or a melon and top it with some low-fat yogurt, suggests Dr. Kayman. "That makes the dinner more satisfying without adding too many extra calories or too much fat." Here are some other things to check on before checking out.

Inspect your meat. Red or white? Base your choice on recent history. "When you're trying to decide which is better, you should think of what else you've had to eat that day," says Reimers. If you had a burger for lunch, make it a chicken dinner. "I've found that people who vary their eating habits tend to have better diets than people who stick strictly to foods they consider healthy," she notes.

Choose your drinking buddy. Unlike the meals at the drive-thru joint, none of these selections comes with a beverage. May we suggest a glass of milk? "A lot of guys don't drink enough milk because calcium is often stressed as being important only for women," says Reimers. In addition to keeping your skeleton solid, milk may fight colon cancer. If milk is not your cup of tea, try calcium-fortified orange juice.

Walk the produce aisle. The quantity of vegetables is often the weak link in supermarket meals; they should take up one-third to half of your plate. Compensate by grabbing a box of frozen vegetables before you leave the store, says Dr. Kayman. Broccoli, brussels sprouts, cauliflower, and spinach are crammed with nutrients. While dinner is heating up, pop the vegetables (in a covered dish with a little water) into the microwave.

Greater Strength through Food

Boost your muscle power by paying attention to what you eat between workouts.

Great workouts can give you more strength, more muscle, more speed, and more endurance. But so can watching TV, sleeping, and washing the car. That's right—you can build muscle, burn fat, and increase endurance even in your downtime.

Simply eating the right stuff between weight-lifting sessions can make a 15 to 25 percent difference in how much strength you gain, how much muscle you put on, and how much fat you take off, says Marcus Elliott, M.D., a sports-conditioning specialist in Santa Barbara, California.

For men who do a lot of cardiovascular exercise, the time off between workouts can be even more crucial. Eating before a long run or ride can increase endurance by more than 50 percent. And giving your body enough R and R between sessions can keep you on the road and off the DL.

The following nutrition and recuperation tips blaze the trail from your last workout to your next one. They'll show you what to eat, when to eat it, how long to wait, and what you'll gain, all without moving an extra muscle. And you'll notice the results almost immediately.

Add Muscle Before and After You Go to the Gym

The miracle of muscle growth—getting bigger and stronger after a workout—actually begins several hours before you pick up your first barbell. A study in the *Journal of Applied Physiology* found that your body's production of growth hormone, an important tool for muscle making, increases significantly when you eat a combination of carbohydrates and protein 2 hours before a hard workout and immediately after it.

Eating too soon before a workout might be a problem, though. A study at the University of California, Los Angeles, found that working out with undigested food in your gut can inhibit your body's production of growth hormone by up to 54 percent. If you must eat within 2 hours of starting your workout, it's better to eat carbohydrates than fat. But even eating carbohydrates can cut your growth-hormone release by 24 percent. "If your primary goal is to build or rebuild muscle, stop eating a few hours before you work out," Dr. Elliott says.

Right after exercise, your body enters what researchers call the "rapid phase of recovery." You call it "so hungry I could eat roadkill." It's time to chug down a shake or a sports drink that contains carbohydrates and protein, preferably in a four-to-one ratio, says exercise physiologist Edmund Burke, Ph.D., author of *Optimal Muscle Recovery*. Here's how this combination builds muscle.

- The protein helps repair damaged muscles after the workout; it helps your body build the tiny filaments that actually make your muscles bigger.
- The fluid in the sports drink floats nutrients to your muscles and carries away the garbage that makes your muscles sore—the lactic acid and carbon dioxide.
- The carbohydrates help your muscles refuel for the next workout.
- Together, the carbohydrates and protein create a surge in the hormone insulin, which injects your muscles with nutrients.

Eat a full meal 30 minutes to 2 hours after your workout. Go ahead and have the hunk of meat you crave, but add a baked potato, three slices of French bread, and a bowl of light ice cream for dessert. This will create a second wave of insulin to carry more nutrients to your muscles.

The object of weight training is to shock your muscles so much that they're scared to lift the same weights again. They'll grow bigger and stronger, so the next time you work out, it will be easier. But muscles need time to pull off this trick. Here's how much.

- If you're doing total-body workouts, rest 48 hours between sessions.
- If you're over 40, give yourself 3 days of rest between full-body sessions.
- If you're doing split routines (working different muscle groups on different days), give each muscle group at least 2 days' rest between workouts. Many men see results by waiting even longer—up to 5 days.

Drink Up and the Fat Goes Away

Caffeine loosens up your body's fat, which you can use for energy during a workout. But the fat won't burn without some carbohydrates for lighter fluid. So knock down two cups of coffee an hour before exercise, along with half a bagel, and you'll incinerate your flab, according to Jacqueline Berning, R.D., Ph.D., a nutritionist at the University of Colorado at Boulder.

After your workout, eating the wrong kind of carbohydrates can block your progress. Fast-acting energy foods, which your body burns almost immediately, create an insulin surge. This temporarily prevents your body from using fat for energy. So if you're trying to lose fat, eat slow-acting, low-octane carbohydrates at your postworkout meal: Your body will take a while to burn them. Examples include milk, yogurt, apples, oranges, pasta, and beans.

Another fat-burning trick: Eat some fat between workouts. "A low-fat diet, below 20 percent, lowers testosterone levels," Dr. Elliott says. Most active men need 25 percent fat. Lower testosterone means you build less muscle during your workouts, and that equals a missed opportunity to burn additional calories throughout the day, since adding muscle mass cranks up your metabolic rate.

To really burn fat, you'll need to do some type of exercise almost every day. Just don't do the same type of workout 2 days in a row. That way, your body will recover from weight lifting while you run, and recover from running while you lift.

Make Breakfast a Must

How much you benefit depends on how long you exercise, so eat the right foods before you hit the road. A study in *Medicine and Science in Sports and Exercise* found that trained cyclists who ate a meal of slow-acting carbohydrates (Kellogg's All-Bran cereal, an apple, and unsweetened yogurt) 30 minutes before exercise were able to pedal 59 percent longer than those who ate a meal of fast-acting carbohydrates (cornflakes, a banana, and low-fat milk).

As a general rule, if performance is your goal, you don't want much protein or fat in your stomach before running, cycling, or swimming. "Carbohydrates have the nutrients that you're going to digest most rapidly," says nutritionist Susan M. Kleiner, R.D., Ph.D., coauthor of *Power Eating*.

After exercise, you want to load your muscles with carbohydrates to refuel them for the next big push. Eat or drink a mix of fast-acting carbohydrates and protein to create an insulin surge, which will quickly replenish supplies of energy and nutrients.

Go for a run before breakfast, and by dinner your heart and lungs will already be in better shape. But you may need longer than that to refuel, and your muscles and joints may need extra time to repair themselves. Dr. Elliott suggests that if you've run, cycled, or swum one-quarter to one-half of your maximum distance, you can do it again 24 hours later. If you go more than 50 percent of your maximum, you need 48 hours to refuel fully. Your back, knees, ankles, and feet will repay you for the extra rest.

Many endurance athletes work out the day after a hard session, but if you do, make sure it's something different: a shorter run, a different type of cardiovascular activity, or weight lifting.

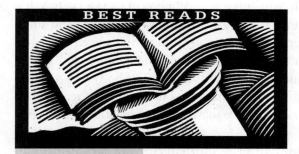

A Tooth-Protection Plan

The majority of advice about teeth centers around what you're not supposed to eat. Yet, according to Selene Yeager and the editors of Prevention Health Books in New Foods for Healing: Capture the Powerful Cures of More Than 100 Common Foods *(Rodale Press, 1998), eating nutritious foods is just as important in proper dental care. So make sure you get plenty of what they suggest and keep your teeth strong for life.*

Even though teeth are hard and bonelike, they're very much alive. Like your skin, muscles, or any other part of your body, they must be well-nourished to stay healthy. "In fact, selecting nutritious foods is probably as important as staying away from cavity-causing foods," says Dominick DePaola, D.D.S., Ph.D., president of Baylor College of Dentistry in Dallas.

While there's no substitute for regular brushing and flossing, choosing the right foods, particularly those that provide large amounts of calcium and vitamins A and C, will help keep your teeth and gums strong. At the same time, it's important not to bombard your teeth frequently with sugary, sticky snacks, which make it easy for cavity-causing bacteria to flourish, says Donna Oberg, R.D., a nutritionist with the dental health program of the Seattle-King County Department of Public Health in Kent, Washington.

Eating for Strong Teeth

Just as bones need calcium to stay strong, your teeth also depend on this essential mineral, especially during the early years. "Calcium-rich foods are extremely important," says William Kuttler, D.D.S., a dentist in private practice in Dubuque, Iowa. "Without calcium, teeth won't form." And in adults, calcium fortifies the bone that supports the teeth so they don't loosen over time.

Getting more dairy foods in your diet is about the best protection teeth can have. A glass of low-fat milk or a serving of yogurt, for example, contains about 300 milligrams of calcium each, which is about 30 percent of the Daily Value (DV). You can get somewhat smaller amounts from low-fat cheeses and some leafy green vegetables, like turnip greens, bok choy, and curly endive.

You need more than just calcium for good dental health, however. You also need a variety of vitamins, including vitamins C and A. The body uses vitamin C to make collagen, a tough protein fiber that keeps the gums strong. Vitamin A is used to form dentin, a layer of bonelike material just beneath the surface of the teeth.

It's easy to get enough of both of these nutrients in your diet. A half-cup serving of cooked broccoli, for example, has 58 milligrams of vitamin C, almost 97 percent of the DV. A half-cup serving of cantaloupe has 34 milligrams (57 percent of the DV), and a medium-size navel orange has 80 milligrams (133 percent of the DV).

The best way to get vitamin A is by eating foods that are high in beta-carotene, which is converted to vitamin A in the body. Sweet potatoes are a great source, with a half-cup providing over 21,000 international units of vitamin A, more than four times the DV. Incidentally, beta-carotene itself provides additional benefits. Studies suggest that people who have five or more servings a day of fruits and vegetables rich in beta-carotene have a lower risk for a variety of cancers, including oral cancer. Carrots are a great source of beta-carotene, with a half-cup of cooked carrots containing 12 milligrams, about 76 percent of the recommended daily amount. Other good sources of beta-carotene include kale and most of the yellow-orange winter squashes. (Despite its hue, acorn squash is a beta-carotene lightweight, with only 2 milligrams in a half-cup.)

Sticky Problems

While some foods help keep the insides of the teeth healthy, others aren't so good for the outsides. Sugary foods, for example, make it possible for large amounts of bacteria to flourish in the mouth. Over time, the bacteria and the acids they produce act almost like little dental drills, wearing away the surface of the teeth and allowing cavities to form, says Dr. Kuttler. And it's not just cookies, cakes, and candy bars that cause problems. A small Swedish study, for example, found that people who frequently ate high-carbohydrate foods like white bread and boiled potatoes, which contain natural sugars, were just as likely to have tooth decay as those who ate sweets.

Even fruit juices, which many people drink as a healthful alternative to sodas, can be a problem. "Juice is a very concentrated source of sugar," Dr. Kuttler explains. In fact, researchers in Switzerland found that grapefruit and apple juices did slightly more damage to teeth than cola did.

While sweet foods can be a problem, sticky foods are even worse, Dr. Kuttler says. The reason for this is that because such foods stick to the teeth, they make it easy for bacteria to remain in the mouth for long periods of time.

Obviously, you don't want to give up healthful high-carbohydrate foods, or even the occasional sweet. It's important, however, to take precautions. Just take a minute to brush your teeth after eating snacks, enjoying rice or a piece of bread, or having a sweet drink. Even if you can't brush, simply rinsing out your mouth with water will help remove sugars before the bacteria have time to do damage.

It's not only what you eat but how you eat that plays a role in keeping teeth strong. Your mouth naturally produces saliva every time you chew, so the more you chew—during a meal, for example, or while chewing gum—the more saliva there is to wash away sugars from the teeth, says Dr. Kuttler. As a bonus, saliva also contains calcium and phosphorus, which help neutralize tooth-damaging acids that form in the mouth after eating.

While you're at the dinner table, you may want to consider having a little cheese. Researchers aren't sure why, but eating cheese appears to play a role in preventing tooth decay. It may be that cheese contains compounds that neutralize acids in the mouth before they do damage, Dr. Kuttler says.

The SAD Diet

The most amazing fact from this excerpt from The Complete Idiot's Guide to Living Longer and Healthier *(Alpha Books, 1999) appears in the first sentence. With so many misguided eaters out there, the vast majority of people need to improve their diets. That's easier said than done, though. Fortunately, author Allan Magaziner, D.O., points out the major pitfalls in most Americans' diets and provides sensible solutions to get you within the experts' recommended dietary guidelines.*

Would you believe that even though 90 percent of our population thinks that they're eating a healthy diet, only 1 percent actually meets the dietary guidelines outlined in the food guide pyramid? Consider these dietary faux pas performed by the typical American on any given day.

- The average person eats only 1½ servings of vegetables and less than 1 serving of fruit.
- Forty-five percent have no fruit at all, and 22 percent eat no vegetables at all.
- Only 27 percent eat 3 or more servings of vegetables, and only 29 percent consume 2 or more servings of fruit.
- Overall, only 9 percent meet the U.S. Department of Agriculture's minimum recommendations of eating at least 5 servings of fruit and vegetables.

So even with all the bureaucratic rhetoric regarding what we should eat, we still haven't cut the mustard. Our Standard American Diet is just that, SAD. Not only are we not getting enough fruit, vegetables, and wholesome grains, but we're eating far too much refined and processed white food like white bread, enriched pasta, french-fried potatoes, and instant rice.

What else is wrong with our diet? For starters, we eat too many calories. And then we eat too many saturated fats and too much total fat, contributing to excess cholesterol in our diet. We also consume large amounts of quick and easy food. This is packaged, processed, and often fried food filled with food additives, preservatives, and artificial colorings and flavorings. Finally, we eat too much sugar, too much salt, too little fiber, and not enough variety of foods.

The bottom line is that we simply don't eat a balanced or wholesome diet. Even though the National Research Council recommends that our diets consist of 20 percent of calories from protein, 30 percent from fat, and 50 percent from carbohydrates, we simply aren't doing that. And on top of that, all of us have different needs. For example, a clerk in a department store has different dietary requirements from a professional athlete. One size doesn't fit all when it comes to our diets.

Even if you try to comply with the food pyramid diet, who really has the time, energy, or interest to tally up and consciously pay close attention to their daily food intake? And even if you meet the dietary recommendations, it's doubtful that anyone knows how much of the macronutrients (such as carbohydrates, fats, and proteins) or micronutrients (such as vitamins and minerals) he is really getting on any given day.

So what do you need to ensure that your diet isn't so SAD? You need to improve the quality of the foods you're eating. You need to eat a variety of foods that are fresh, not processed or refined. You should snack more on fruits and vegetables instead of ice cream, pies, cakes, and doughnuts. You need to introduce new, unfamiliar foods that you may not be used to eating. Eat more kiwifruit, mangoes, yellow or red peppers, spinach, melon, or perhaps grains (such as millet, barley, oats, couscous, and quinoa) and beans (such as navy, azuki, garbanzo, lima, or soy). Be creative, take chances, go to a vegetarian or even macrobiotic cooking class. You might even like it. Turn that SAD diet into a healthy, nutrient-dense, fiber-packed, wholesome, delicious, health-enhancing diet.

Avoiding Anti-Nutrients

Not only do we need to optimize our intake of foods rich in vitamins, minerals, amino acids, essential fatty acids, antioxidants, and phytonutrients but we really need to reduce our intake of foods that stress our bodies. These are the anti-nutrients.

Limit your intake of fried foods. The frying process generally heats oils at high temperatures, which promotes the formation of dangerous free radicals. It's much better if you can bake or broil your food, because these methods require less oil and there's little chance of any oils becoming rancid from continual reheating. Also try to avoid trans fatty acids, which are commonly found in margarine, shortening, cakes, pies, cookies, crackers, and other baked products and any hydrogenated vegetable oils; these are unhealthy. Trans fatty acids found in hydrogenated vegetable oils act like saturated fats and can raise your cholesterol level, increase your blood pressure, and perhaps make you more susceptible to cancer.

Trans fats account for up to 60 percent of the fat in many processed foods. The average American's intake is between 10 and 20 grams of trans fat per day. Try to keep your intake as close to zero as possible, since there is no safe dose and no known benefits to eating trans fatty acids. It has been estimated that these fats may contribute to 30,000 deaths each year as a result of heart disease.

So, is margarine, which is loaded with trans fats, your best bet? Absolutely not—unless you're an undertaker. According to the Nurses Health Study conducted at the Harvard School of Public Health, women who had the highest intake of margarine were at twice the risk for heart disease, compared to women who ate very few hydrogenated fats. Women who ate 4 teaspoons per day were 66 percent more likely to suffer from heart disease compared to those who ate less than 1 teaspoon each month. The message is clear: Avoid hydrogenated oils and trans fatty acids. The following list reveals some insightful information about those not-so-transparent trans fatty acids.

Food	TransFatty Acids (g)
French fries, large order	4.0–7.9
Packaged doughnut	5.0–6.0
Chocolate cake roll	2.0
Vegetable shortening (1 Tbsp)	3.0
Hard stick margarine (1 Tbsp)	2.0–4.6
Cracker	2.4
Cheese danish	2.2–5.2
Sugar cookies (2)	1.33
Pound cake (1 oz)	1.0–2.1
Dinner roll	.85
Mayonnaise (1 Tbsp)	.55
Butter (1 Tbsp)	.40

Limit your intake of caffeine. It has a diuretic effect and may wash out key nutrients. Caffeine is found not only in coffee but also in tea, soft drinks, and chocolate. One to two cups of coffee per day might be okay, but drinking more than three cups per day is not advisable.

Go easy on alcohol. Excessive alcohol intake can stress your liver and increase your risk of certain cancers, including esophageal, pancreatic, colon, and liver cancer. Alcohol also depletes B vitamins, vitamin C, and numerous trace minerals, not to mention the fact that it gives you extra unnecessary calories.

Taste your food before deciding whether you need salt. Most of the time, food has enough naturally occurring salt to make it palatable. Try adding spices, seasonings, and herbs to your food in place of table salt. If you're concerned about your blood pressure, you might want to try potassium salt as opposed to the more common sodium salt.

Don't be a chimney and continue smoking. Smoking accelerates aging and increases your risks for heart disease, stroke, high blood pressure, diabetes, and cancer. Plus, if you successfully quit, you'll have extra money to buy organic food and enjoy a night out at the movies.

Sugar and Spice and Everything Nice

Approximately 20 percent of our calories comes from sugar alone. White sugar, in particular—the type that you generally add to your cup of coffee in the

morning or that you use when baking a pie—is virtually devoid of any key vitamins and minerals. Sugar contains 16 calories per teaspoon and has no B vitamins, chromium, magnesium, zinc, or other trace elements that are necessary
to metabolize it. As a result, the sugar in your sugar jar essentially robs your body
of beneficial nutrients from healthy foods that you might be eating. To fully metabolize sugar, your body has to take B vitamins and other trace minerals from
healthy grains, beans, fruits, and vegetables instead of using them for more efficient and important purposes such as fighting infections, warding off allergies,
and preventing cancer or heart disease.

Be sure to read labels. Sugar is everywhere: in sodas, cake, pie, ice cream,
doughnuts, candy, chocolate, breakfast cereals, breads, ketchup, and even salad
dressings. And it may be disguised with an alias such as corn syrup, cornstarch,
or high fructose corn syrup.

Faux Finishes: Additives and Preservatives

While food additives and preservatives have their benefits, I recommend that
you do your best to limit your intake of them. These chemicals are generally used
in an effort to preserve food and prevent spoilage and retard mold growth. Some
people experience symptoms such as headaches, asthma, wheezing, dizziness, fatigue, or hives from some of these added ingredients. How to avoid them? It's
quite simple. Buy fresh food that's not packaged or prepared, and read food labels. A little bit of these chemicals won't hurt you, but the less you eat, the better
off you'll be.

This caution applies not only to food but also to your prescription medication. Drug manufacturers add food coloring and dye to their medications. Why?
Do you really care whether your antibiotic is white or pink? Some pharmacies
compound prescription medications so that they are completely free of artificial
colorings, flavorings, dyes, and preservatives. If you're concerned, ask your pharmacist to compound your medication without these unnecessary chemicals.

To Spray or Not to Spray

If you have ever tasted the difference between organically grown produce and
conventionally grown produce, you know why organically grown fruits and vegetables are gaining in popularity. Organic foods have not been sprayed with
chemical insecticides or pesticides. More natural forms of insect repellents and
fertilizers are used to keep these products nutrient-rich and delicious.

Although some people are skeptical of the merits of organic food, I am in favor of a toxin-free diet. Besides tasting better, organically grown fruits and vegetables also contain greater amounts of trace minerals. A recent study indicated that the amounts of calcium, magnesium, potassium, sodium, manganese, iron, and copper in five different vegetables were higher in those that were organically grown—in fact, they were as much as 50 percent to 390 percent greater!

A debate also rages about the potential health risks associated with pesticides, herbicides, and fungicides. These chemicals are stored in your fatty tissue and stay there for many years. They can accumulate in your brain, liver, and in virtually all the cells in your body. Do we really need them? Of course not. If possible, try to find a local grocer or farmer who is promoting fruits and vegetables as well as grains and beans that are not sprayed with chemical pesticides. The produce generally costs a bit more (sometimes 10 to 30 percent more, depending on the food), but you'll taste the difference.

Of particular concern is the fact that pesticide exposure may contribute to weakening your immune system and making you prone to colds or infections. Pesticides have also been linked to headaches, fatigue, skin rashes, muscle aches, and pain, and possibly even some cancers.

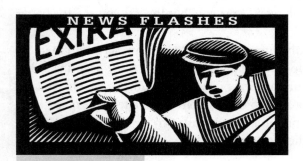

Too Much Iron Can Be Fatal

NEW YORK CITY—Unfortunately for guys, food manufacturers still fortify many staples (such as cereals and breads) with iron. Although this can be helpful to women, who sometimes lack the mineral because of heavy menstrual periods, an iron-rich diet can be toxic to men. Men under 50 are five times more likely than women to show symptoms of hemochromatosis, a deadly genetic disease that causes the organs to store too much iron. It's one of the most common hereditary diseases in the United States—about 1.5 million people have it—and it can cause impotence, diabetes, sterility, and liver damage.

"Men with hemochromatosis often have high iron levels in their twenties and thirties, and can die in their forties," says Victor Herbert, M.D., of Mount Sinai School of Medicine of the City University of New York. "If it's discovered early, though, you can lower your iron levels before too much damage is done." To test for hemochromatosis, ask your doctor to check your blood's ferritin and transferrin saturation levels, he advises. If both are high, you may donate blood weekly until your iron levels drop, and then monthly for the rest of your (much longer) life. Meanwhile, ditch those iron-fortified foods, and never take iron supplements.

Stop Cell Damage with Honey

URBANA-CHAMPAIGN, Ill.—A University of Illinois study found that dark, thick honey is high in antioxidants. Researchers measured 14 types of honey and found higher levels of antioxidants in dark, thick varieties. Antioxidants, which include vitamins C and E and beta-carotene, are believed to help prevent cell damage that can lead to certain cancers and heart disease. "By using honey exclusively instead of sugar, you can significantly increase your daily intake of antioxidants," says May Berenbaum, Ph.D. The top types of honey: buckwheat, sunflower, and Christmasberry. Look for them at health food stores.

Heavy Soda Consumption Can Lead to Bone Loss

BELTSVILLE, Md.—Never mind what it does to your teeth; drinking soda may weaken your bones. Researchers at the USDA had 11 men drink five cans of cola every day for 3 months. At the end of the study, the men had lost about 10 percent more phosphorus through their urine than normal, and they had absorbed less calcium. "Drinking large amounts of fructose changes how your body metabolizes the minerals responsible for healthy bones," says Forrest Nielsen, Ph.D., the study leader. "I wouldn't drink more than two cans of soda per day." Too much soda could lead to bone deterioration and an increase in injuries and breaks, he notes.

Wheat Bran May Top Others in Beating Colon Cancer

ATHENS, Ga.—Researchers at the University of Georgia report that wheat bran may be a better colon cancer fighter than oat or corn bran. Ideally, the fiber in bran should stay in your colon long enough to attach to and move out any cancer-causing compounds, but not so long that it causes gas and bloating. Lab tests performed with corn, oat, and wheat brans showed that wheat bran struck the best balance between colon cleansing and gut comfort, says one of the researchers, Scott Martin, Ph.D. Kellogg's All-Bran and Post Raisin Bran cereals are good sources of wheat bran.

Increasing Dairy Exposure Can Alleviate Lactose Intolerance

CHICAGO—Most people who think they are lactose intolerant really aren't, and they don't need to cut dairy products out of their diets, according to a research review in the *Journal of the American Dietetic Association*. People who have trouble digesting dairy foods often have a very low level of the enzyme lactase in their bodies. "Without enough lactase, your body is unable to digest lactose—the sugar in milk—and you end up feeling bloated and sick," says the review author, Lois D. McBean. Fortunately, many people with low lactase can improve their ability to tolerate lactose by gradually increasing their exposure to dairy products. Try drinking a cup of milk with meals or eating aged cheeses. Or eat yogurt with active cultures—it contains bacteria that can help you digest lactose.

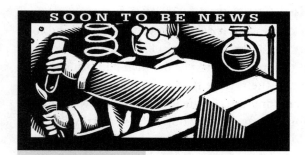

Healthier Eating through Super Tomatoes?

Genetically altered tomatoes can provide 10 to 25 times as much beta-carotene as regular tomatoes. "We crossed a beta-carotene-rich wild tomato with existing tomato breeds to make the new lines," says John Stommel, Ph.D., a USDA plant geneticist. The result was a tomato toting about 8,000 micrograms of beta-carotene—an antioxidant that may strengthen the immune system and keep your eyes healthy. That's about 77 percent of the amount of beta-carotene found in a medium-size carrot.

Specially labeled tomatoes, sauces, and juices should be in stores in a year.

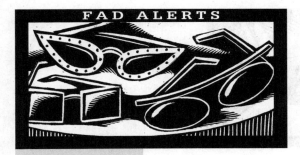

Taurine Drink

 The latest octane booster to push shaky nutritional claims is called, appropriately, Red Bull. Its maker says it will "revitalize the body and mind" with a 1,000-milligram shot of taurine, an amino acid that helps your body metabolize fuel. But drinking taurine won't pep you up, says Beth Bussey, R.D., a nutritionist at the University of Alabama in Tuscaloosa. Your body already produces plenty of it, and you simply pass the excess in your urine.

The lightly carbonated drink also packs a titanic payload of B vitamins—B_{12}, B_6, and niacin. This can turn your urine bright yellow, but "megadoses of niacin and B_6 are not known to enhance mood or create an energy boost," says Marla Reicks, Ph.D., a nutritionist at the University of Minnesota in Minneapolis–St. Paul. Any energy perk comes from its 80 milligrams of caffeine (more than a half-cup of coffee has). Stick to java, especially because Red Bull costs about $2 a can and tastes like a liquid cold lozenge.

Cherry Burgers

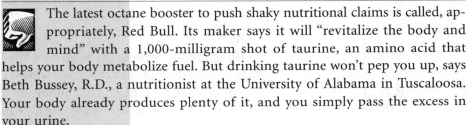 A study at Michigan State University in East Lansing found that hamburgers that contain tart-cherry particles have significantly fewer carcinogens than beef-only burgers. J. Ian Gray, Ph.D., a coauthor of the study, compared regular all-beef patties with burgers made of beef and 11.5 percent tart-cherry particles. Dr. Gray found that adding cherries to beef slowed the deterioration of fat compounds and reduced the formation of suspected cancer-causing substances, called heterocyclic aromatic amines, by roughly 75 percent. Premade cherry burgers are available in some grocery stores and on the Web at www.plevas.com. One brand, Plevalean, actually tastes pretty close to the real thing. You can make your own burgers by adding ¼ cup diced fresh cherries to ¼ pound beef.

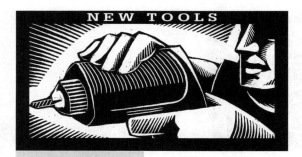

Zestier Grilling

Tasty Burrito

If you give your grill a workout starting in early spring, you've probably had your fill of the usual red-meat suspects by midsummer. You could just drown a few drumsticks in barbecue sauce, but why not give the bird a bit of Southwestern finesse? Karen Woods, a chef and caterer in Santa Fe, New Mexico, tells how to build a simple, low-fat chicken burrito topped with a spicy salsa that makes the most of summer vegetables.

Salsa

½	cup avocado cubes
½	cup diced fresh plum tomatoes
1	tablespoon finely diced red onion
1	jalapeño pepper, seeded and chopped (wear plastic gloves when handling)
3	tablespoons chopped fresh cilantro
½	teaspoon ground cumin
1	garlic clove, minced
	Juice of 1 lime
	Salt and freshly ground black pepper (to taste)

Burritos

4	boneless, skinless chicken breasts
	Juice of 1 lime
	Freshly ground black pepper (to taste)
4	flour tortillas (8" diameter)

To make the salsa: Combine the avocado, tomatoes, onion, jalapeño, cilantro, cumin, garlic, lime juice, salt, and ground black pepper in a medium serving bowl. Toss gently, cover, and refrigerate until the burritos are ready.

To make the burritos: Coat each chicken breast with lime juice and season with pepper. Grill the breasts on both sides until the meat is no longer pink or a thermometer inserted in the thickest portion registers 160°F. Thinly slice each chicken breast and arrange the slices in the center of a tortilla. Roll up the tortilla and top it with salsa. Makes 4 servings.

Per serving: 278 calories, 8 g fat (25% of calories), 30 g protein, 23 g carbohydrates

Better Barbecuing

Grill Tools

Any fool can barbecue with an egg spatula and a salad fork. Where's the fun in that? If you can't gild a simple pursuit with frivolous equipment, it's hardly worth pulling out the briquettes on a sunny Sunday afternoon. Tote this briefcase-size 18-piece Brookstone grill set to your next barbecue, and the gape-mouthed guests will clear your path to the coals. These heavy stainless-steel utensils are prison-quality mess tools; most have long wooden handles to keep you away from the dangerously high fire you've built. The 30-inch meat machete shows you're serious, but the four pairs of wooden corncob handles nestled in their own custom divots are pure overkill—that's why we like them so much. $100. Call Brookstone at (800) 351-7222.

Safer Meat

Instant-Read Thermometers

Only a thermometer can guarantee that your meat won't bite you back. But that oversize thumbtack your mother stuck into the rump roast can take up to 2 minutes to register—enough time for a burger to petrify. Here are two of the new instant-read thermometers.

Atkins Mini-Digital Thermometer. Insert this probe halfway into your meat, and 10 seconds later, you'll see the temp on an easy-to-read digital display. Unlike conventional meat thermometers that must be inserted sideways into burgers, the Atkins can be stuck into the top of any burger—just make sure it reaches the center of the patty. $20. Available at restaurant supply outlets, or call (800) 284-2842.

T-Stick Hamburger Cooking Thermometer. Only a $150 digital thermometer can beat the 5-second readout time of the T-Stick. Your burger is a safe 160°F when the dot on this disposable white plastic stick turns black. $3 for 12, or $12 for 60. Call Environmentally Sound Products at (800) 886-5432.

Spicier Eating

Asian Seasonings

The selection of Chinese seasonings at your local grocery store probably stops pretty far from Beijing. To find the real ingredients that oriental chefs use, call the Spice Merchant, a small mail-order service in Jackson Hole, Wyoming. The $50 Shelf Stocker kit has all the basics needed to make a Chinese meal, including specialty items like hot Szechuan bean sauce and dried shiitake mushrooms. Call (800) 551-5999 to request a catalog.

Healthier Drinking

Smoothies

Not only is there no free lunch, there's no free breakfast or dinner, either. Everything you eat has a price—in cash, calories, or useless fat—starting with your first meal of the day.

Want to come out ahead when you're barely out of bed? Take a blender, 90 seconds, and a few ingredients, and you can drink more good food at breakfast than most guys eat all day.

Here are five healthy smoothies, one for each workday. Each one targets a different problem. They'll help protect you from cancer, fight heart disease, keep you energized, increase your brainpower, and even help you recover from a binge. And they're a breeze to make: Just dump in the ingredients, blend for a minute or two, decant (optional), and drink.

Prostate Protector. This soy milk–based concoction provides a hefty dose of genistein, a compound that can prevent prostate cancer and an enlarged prostate. Ruby-red grapefruit contains lycopene, the nutrient that reduces prostate cancer risk by as much as 35 percent. And according to a recent Swiss study, the combination of lycopene and vitamin E (that's what the wheat germ is for) inhibits prostate cancer cell growth by nearly 90 percent.

> 1 cup vanilla soy milk
> ½ cup ruby-red grapefruit juice
> 1 cup ripe honeydew chunks
> 2 tablespoons wheat germ
>   Honey (to taste)

236 calories, 3.6 g fat (13.7% of calories), 4 g fiber, 8.6 g protein, 46 g carbohydrates

Artery Aid. The ground flaxseed in this mix attacks bad, low-density lipoprotein (LDL) cholesterol with fiber (6 grams per ¼ cup) and lots of omega-3 fatty acids. Every gram or two of soluble fiber you eat each day lowers your LDL by about 1 percent, and omega-3's lower heart attack risk by more than 50 percent. (Ground flaxseed is sold in health food stores and some supermarkets.) This shake will also supply nearly half your Recommended Dietary Allowance of potassium, which helps prevent high blood pressure.

> 8   ounces low-fat vanilla yogurt
> 2   tablespoons ground flaxseed
> 1   cup sliced fresh or frozen peaches
>   Honey (to taste)

407 calories, 10.8 g fat (23.9% of calories), 6.8 g fiber, 16.6 g protein, 65 g carbohydrates

Endurance Shake. When the finish line is 10 kilometers away, you need to draw on more carbohydrates than your morning bowl of Froot Loops provided. You also need protein and fat. In a recent study, cyclists who drank a prerace beverage consisting of four parts carbohydrates and one part protein cycled 66 percent farther than when they quaffed an all-carbohydrate sports drink. And when researchers added a little extra fat to runners' diets, they lasted 23 percent longer on endurance runs than they did on low-fat diets.

> 1   banana, sliced
> ½   cup orange juice
> 8   ounces low-fat vanilla yogurt
> 4   ounces crushed pineapple
> 2   tablespoons peanut butter

644 calories, 21.3 g fat (29.7% of calories), 6 g fiber, 22.4 g protein, 98.9 g carbohydrates

Brain Builder. You could down a cup of coffee to jump-start your brain. But caffeine depletes your stores of B vitamins, the very nutrients you need to keep your mind sharp. Instead, feed your head with this recipe. Not only does it provide those badly needed B's, it also delivers a shot of protein to help produce the wake-up chemicals dopamine and norepinephrine. The milk in the mix contains choline to help fire up your memory. Along with the vitamin C in the fruit and orange juice, choline can also help prevent the mental deterioration associated with Alzheimer's and Parkinson's diseases.

1 cup fat-free milk
2 tablespoons frozen orange-juice concentrate
1 cup strawberries
1 kiwifruit

222 calories, 1.4 g fat (5.7% of calories), 6.7 g fiber, 10.7 g protein, 44.5 g carbohydrates

Hangover Helper. Use this liquid meal to fight alcohol-induced dehydration. It's loaded with vitamin C to help combat binge-related cell damage, and the fructose in the fruit juices helps speed the metabolism of liquor. Upset stomach? The ginger in ginger ale will help quell the motion sickness caused by your spinning bedroom. And some experts say the acidophilus bacteria in the yogurt may get your gut back in chemical balance.

1   cup tangerine/orange blended juice
1   tablespoon lime juice
½   cup low-fat vanilla yogurt
½   cup Canada Dry ginger ale (or any other ginger ale that contains real ginger)
    Sprig of mint

246 calories, 2.3 g fat (8.4% of calories), 0 g fiber, 4.6 g protein, 53.7 g carbohydrates

A New Way to Lower Cholesterol

Benecol

A new margarine can help lower your cholesterol levels. In a study at the Mayo Clinic in Rochester, Minnesota, 79 subjects with mildly elevated cholesterol ate margarine containing stanol ester—a plant substance that inhibits cholesterol absorption—three times a day. Their daily intake: 4½ tablespoons. After 8 weeks, their low-density lipoprotein ("bad") cholesterol levels had dropped by 14 percent. Six weeks after they stopped eating the margarine, the subjects' cholesterol had climbed back to the old levels, according to Lowell Dale, M.D., one of the study's researchers.

Marketed as Benecol, the margarine can also be used for cooking. Look for it at your local supermarket.

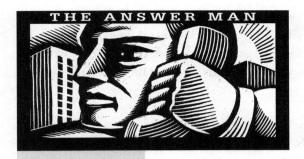

Fishy Question

When I order grilled salmon at a restaurant, it's sometimes served with the skin. Does the skin contain some of those helpful fish oils I'm always reading about, or is it just loaded with fat?
—J. F., Lake Charles, La.

"It doesn't matter if you eat the skin," says Martha Daviglus, M.D., assistant professor of preventive medicine at Northwestern University in Chicago. "But there is no nutritional benefit at all in the skin, only in the flesh." That flesh contains a very high concentration of omega-3 fatty acids, which, studies have shown, can help prevent heart disease. More recent studies have shown that omega-3's may help fight depression, too.

Vegetarian Daughter

My teenage daughter has declared herself a strict vegetarian: no eggs, dairy products, or anything else that comes from an animal. Can this possibly be healthy?
—C. B., Colts Neck, N.J.

She may be healthier than you are. "Vegetarian diets are often low in fat and high in fiber; they can lower your risk of heart disease, high blood pressure, diabetes, and some forms of cancer," says Tina Ruggiero, R.D., a registered dietitian in New York City.

By boycotting eggs and meat, however, your daughter is missing out on complete proteins—foods that deliver the nine essential amino acids the body needs. This is easy to fix if she mixes and matches a variety of beans, grains, vegetables, and fruits at each meal. One combination that provides the necessary amino acids is legumes and grains; you can get this duo in such meals as rice and beans, bean tacos, a peanut-butter-and-jelly sandwich, and meatless chili. Another protein-rich combination is grains with nuts or seeds, such as basmati rice with nuts or falafel.

Your daughter's diet might also leave her deficient in calcium (because she won't eat dairy products) and vitamin B_{12} (found in meat). She can take in calcium by eating lots of broccoli, fortified orange juice, and fortified soy milk. Since there aren't any strict vegetarian, or vegan, foods that contain B_{12}, a daily multivitamin is also a good idea.

Faster Healing

I recently broke my right hand. What foods can I eat to help the bone heal as quickly as possible? Will supplements help?
—F. Y., Moscow, Idaho

Bones can take longer to heal if you're deficient in calcium and vitamin D, says Robert Heaney, M.D., professor of medicine at Creighton University in Omaha, Nebraska. Unless you drink milk several times a day, you're probably not getting enough of either one. A cup of skim milk provides 30 percent of the calcium you need each day and 25 percent of the vitamin D, so 4 cups a day will provide enough of both. Other good sources of calcium are cheese, yogurt, broccoli, and green leafy vegetables. Because a normal, healthy diet supplies these nutrients, Dr. Heaney doesn't recommend taking supplements.

Not-So-Real Cheese

What exactly is pasteurized processed cheese food? Is real cheese better for me?
—T. M., Syracuse, N.Y.

Along with Tang, Spam, and Fruit Roll-Ups, processed cheese food is one of the great technological marvels of our age. Cheese food begins its life as some kind of natural cheese (often Cheddar) that is combined with emulsifying salts and sometimes dyes and flavoring agents, says Larry Steenson, Ph.D., director of science and technology at the International Dairy Foods Association. Then it's heat-processed to create a smooth, gel-like substance that's perfectly uniform in color and texture—which is why that chunk of Velveeta melts over your nachos without separating.

Nutritionally speaking, both cheese food and natural cheeses are high in fat and calories: An ounce of either processed American or natural Cheddar has about 110 calories and 9 grams of fat. But natural cheeses are slightly more nutritious. An ounce of Cheddar has 7 grams of protein and 204 milligrams of calcium, compared with American's 6 grams of protein and 174 milligrams of calcium. Natural cheeses also tend to be lower in sodium. In addition, if you have problems digesting dairy products, naturally aged cheeses are a better choice since enzymes used in the aging process have already broken down some of the lactose.

Pills Aren't the Answer

My doctor put me on cholesterol-lowering drugs 4 months ago, and my total cholesterol has dropped to 180. Since that's below the recommended level, can't I now eat whatever I want? If not, why not?

—J. R., Paducah, Ky.

You may think you've found a way to protect your heart while maintaining a diet of BLTs, fried mozzarella, and snack foods that end with the letters *ito*. You haven't.

"Don't kid yourself," says Sidney C. Smith Jr., M.D., past president of the American Heart Association and professor and chief of cardiology at the University of North Carolina at Chapel Hill. "Although you may be able to keep your cholesterol numbers down this way, you'll need a much higher dosage of the drugs than if you were following a low-fat diet. And the higher the dosage, the greater your risk of developing side effects, such as chronic muscle pain and liver damage. A high-fat diet also leads to a high-fat body, and that's bad for your heart no matter how low your cholesterol is."

The whole point of lowering your cholesterol is to reduce your overall risk of developing heart disease. If you want to do that, you need to eat right, exercise regularly, avoid smoking, and control your blood pressure, says Dr. Smith. Unless you do all those things, there is no pill in the world that can keep your heart healthy.

Fiberless Fruit

I don't want to eat pesticides, so I always peel my fruit. Am I losing any nutritional benefits by cutting off the skin?

—S. L., Harrisburg, Penna.

The majority of nutrients found in fruit exist in the flesh itself or just under the skin, according to Nancy Clark, R.D., a registered dietitian at SportsMedicine Brookline in Massachusetts. What you're really losing with the peel is fiber, so you need to add beans or high-fiber cereals to your diet. By the way, peeling does eliminate most of the pesticides, but so does a good rinsing with plain water.

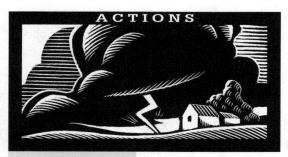

Diet contributes to 4 of the top 10 causes of death in the United States. Experts estimate that Americans could save more than $23 billion a year on hospitalization costs alone if we took on a more healthy diet.

But food doesn't just play a part in your death; it greatly impacts your quality of life. Other chronic diseases related to diet—cataracts, memory loss, diabetes, obesity, and high blood pressure—might not kill you directly, but they sure won't make life more enjoyable.

View food as more than fuel. View food as a potent healing agent and disease fighter. If you do, you may be pleasantly surprised at how quickly your meal choices can lead to a better, stronger, healthier you—not just in the long term but also day-to-day.

Here are some ways to hit the road to healthier and more enjoyable eating.

1. **Eat just one.** If you include a fruit or a vegetable each time you eat, you'll steadily improve your health, says Ken Goldberg, M.D., founder and director of the Male Health Institute in Dallas and author of *How Men Can Live as Long as Women.*

The 30-year Framingham Heart Study by Harvard researchers found that the risk of stroke among 832 men ages 45 to 65 became lower with each additional serving of fruits and vegetables they ate.

And lowered stroke risk is only one benefit. Eating more fruits and vegetables also lowers your risk for colon cancer and heart disease, says Dr. Goldberg.

2. **Get the red out.** Given the option, choose fish, turkey, or chicken instead of red meat. A landmark study of almost 48,000 male health professionals found that the men who ate the most red meat had a significantly higher risk of advanced prostate cancer than those who ate the least.

3. **Stop, drop, and live.** A side benefit of eating more fruits and vegetables and less fatty red meat is that you'll probably shed a few pounds. Even the least bit of waist whittling can add to your life. In another landmark study—this one of nearly 20,000 men over 22 years—researchers found that being just 2 to 6 percent over your ideal weight increases your risk of cardiovascular disease. Being as much as 20 percent over increases your risk to more than 2½ times that of ideal-weight men.

4. **Bring on the red stuff.** Tomato sauce, especially when cooked with even the tiniest bit of olive oil, seems to guard against both colon and prostate cancers. Some evidence suggests that it may protect against cancers of the stomach and esophagus as well. Plus, this special sauce may even contribute to agility as we age.

5. **Don't blow off broccoli.** Broccoli is fabulously full of immune system–building vitamin C. And it has a fistful of the phytochemicals thought to fight cancer. Plus, there's a variety of healthy ways to stomach it: steamed, stir-fried, blanched, baked, and raw—even with yogurt dip.

6. **Keep kidney beans handy.** Kidney beans boast the highest, healthiest fiber mix of any member of the legume family—almost 6 grams per ½-cup serving. They're especially high in heart-protecting folate, too.

Of the fiber, 2.8 grams is cholesterol-lowering, blood glucose–controlling soluble fiber. Kidney beans are associated with a lower risk of heart disease and stroke, and with protection from colon cancer, says James W. Anderson, M.D., professor of medicine and clinical nutrition at the University of Kentucky College of Medicine in Lexington.

7. **Reach for ginger relief.** Ginger, the cooking spice and the flavor in real ginger ale, is a great stomach soother and a pleasant motion-sickness preventive, says Varro E. Tyler, Ph.D., distinguished professor emeritus of pharmacognosy at Purdue University in West Lafayette, Indiana. This root can stop nausea quickly. You can make a tea with ½ to 1 teaspoon of grated fresh ginger, or with 1 teaspoon of ground ginger.

8. **Strip away the silk.** To grill corn, pull the husks halfway down and remove the silk. Pull the husks back up over the cob and tie the ends shut with twine or with long, thin pieces of husk. Soak the ears in cold water for 30 minutes. Grill the corn in the husks for about 20 minutes, turning often.

9. **Become a microwave magician.** Anything that can blister a frozen hot dog in 38 seconds deserves unquestioned respect. Here are some tips for using that reactor in your kitchen.

- Keep paper towels and brown bags out. They sometimes contain metal fibers, which can start fires.
- Move thick foods to the edge of the dish. The heat is more intense there.
- Debone meat. Microwaves can't penetrate bone, so the meat nearby will remain cold. Heat thick meat slowly, at half-power.
- Salt after cooking. Salt granules attract microwaves, burning the food and causing freckles. If you want to brown chicken or pork evenly, brush it lightly with soy sauce.
- Don't undercook your chicken. When you pierce the bird and the juice runs clear, not pink, it's done.
- Microwave vegetables briefly. Heat them for 15 seconds at a time, checking to make sure they don't get too soft. Overcooking destroys nutrients.

10. **Chew away heartburn before it hits.** After you finish that fried burrito-enchilada combo, try popping a stick of gum in your mouth—and not just to stifle your spicy breath. Chewing gum for half an hour after meals can prevent or reduce heartburn, according to a study from the University of Alabama at Birmingham. "Chewing increases saliva flow, and the saliva neutralizes stomach acid and washes it away from your esophagus," says study leader and gastroenterologist Robert Marks, M.D.

11. **Eat your fat early.** If you want to lose the belly, you need to eat less fat. But if you suddenly try to cut all the lard out of your breakfast and lunch—even if you fill up on a huge salad—you might end up with a worse blubber craving than Captain Ahab. In a study at Ohio State University in Columbus, 25 men drank a shake made with either whole milk or skim milk for lunch, every day for a week. The guys who drank the leaner (but just as large) shakes consistently ate more fat during the rest of the day.

"They didn't know the fat content of their lunches, yet they unconsciously chose foods that would balance out their fat intakes," says John Allred, Ph.D., the study author, who adds that further research might reveal exactly how your body monitors your fat consumption. Meanwhile, to lose weight, cut back on fat gradually and eat a little fat (say, olive oil or cheese) in early meals so you don't shift into fat-scavenger mode later.

12. **Reach for the supplement.** USDA researchers have found that a fish-oil supplement may provide the same health benefits as a diet high in fish. Ten men were given 6 grams daily of an oil rich in the omega-3 fatty acid docosahexaenoic acid (DHA). That's equivalent to 11 pounds of salmon a day. After 3 months, the men's high-density lipoprotein ("good") cholesterol levels were 26 percent higher, and their triglyceride levels were 15 percent lower. "Since DHA appears to be more potent in its pure form, it may be even more effective as a supplemental pill than in fish," says Gary J. Nelson, Ph.D., the study author. Look for supplements that are labeled "DHA," not just "omega-3 fatty acids."

13. **Serve up shish kebabs.** At your next cookout, resist the urge to serve up your signature charred hot dogs. Instead, make shish kebabs. Here's how.

- Use twin steel skewers. Two prongs keep the chunks more secure when you turn them on the grill. You can buy skewers in any kitchen store. If you'd rather use wooden skewers, soak them in water for 30 minutes before grilling.
- Pick cubed tenderloin. It's the juiciest cut of beef, and 3 ounces contains only 11 grams of fat. Chicken breast is even leaner.
- Make a fiery marinade. Mix spoonfuls of garlic powder, onion powder, ground cumin, ground red pepper, and Worcestershire sauce in a resealable plastic bag until it forms a paste. Toss in the meat and shake until it's well-coated.
- Be inventive. Between chunks of meat, use garlic cloves, portobello mushrooms, shallots, or large pitted olives. Dried apricots or figs work well with beef.
- Sear fresh fruit first. Mangoes, kiwifruit, and bananas work best with chicken, but grill them separately for 2 minutes so they don't fall apart.
- Set it ablaze. The meat is done when a meat thermometer says its core has reached 170°F. With chicken, the juices must run clear. Put the shish kebabs in a serving dish, douse them with warm cognac or brandy, and touch a lit match to them. They'll burn for a few minutes, leaving juicy meat under a crusty coating. Serve stout or porter with beef, and pilsner or lager with chicken or fish.

14. **Find the frozen veggies.** The frozen-food aisle in the supermarket holds more than waffles and ice cream: It's a mecca of vegetables. Frozen vegetables have just as much nutrition—if not more—than fresh, says Melanie R. Polk of the American Institute for Cancer Research in Washington, D.C. Search for medleys that offer five or six different kinds of vegetables. Make them as a side dish, or toss them into pasta dishes, soups, and stir-fry meals.

15. **Pile it on.** Even a basic sandwich has room for more servings of vegetables. Use a piece or two of lean meat and low-fat cheese, but stuff the bread with dark green lettuce, tomatoes, and onions, says Laurie Meyer, R.D., a nutritionist in Milwaukee.

16. **Buy seasonal and long-lived fruits.** Buy a variety of fresh fruits often so you can benefit from the multitude of nutrients and phytochemicals. Especially stock up on apples and oranges, Polk says. Left in the refrigerator, these fruits keep for weeks. Buy a bunch of both so that you're always sure to have fruit on hand.

17. **Seek out alternatives.** Love tacos? Try them with chicken or beans. Have a craving for chili? Throw in some turkey instead of beef. "You don't have to get rid of meat, but try to use more fish and skinless poultry," says Meyer. Chicken, beans, turkey, and fish give you the meaty feel without the fat. If you really want to try something new, search for ostrich or buffalo meat. "It tastes like beef but has the fat content of chicken," notes Meyer.

18. **Split it.** If you're eating at a deli or a restaurant that thinks a portion size should feed a small country, order one meal and split it with a friend.

19. **Load on the spice.** By adding a little bit of flavoring to meats and vegetables, you can enhance the taste without adding fat, Meyer says. Season vegetables and meats with herbs and spices. Cook with flavored vinegars and with sauces such as soy and teriyaki. Use low-fat salad dressings as meat marinades.

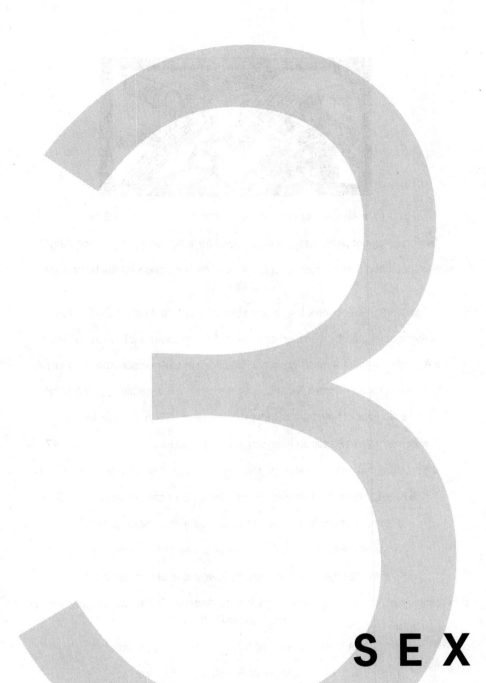

3

SEX

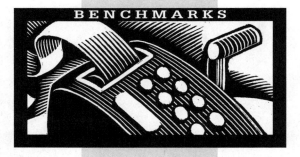

■ Average age of first sex in the United States: 15.8

■ Percentage of penile tissue a man loses between the ages of 21 and 73: 24

■ How the United States ranks among industrial democracies with the highest rates of sexual infidelity: 1

■ Average erect penis length of a stallion (horse, that is): 2 feet 6 inches

■ Average length of a man's erect penis, according to American men: 10 inches

■ Average length of a man's erect penis, according to American women: 4 inches

■ Percentage of women satisfied with the size of their partners' penises: 58

■ Number of times per month most men ages 25 to 34 have sex: 3

■ Percentage of American men who say they like sex better than money: 47

■ Percentage of American women who say they enjoy sex more than money: 26

■ Average number of thrusts required for a 10-minute sex session: 500

■ Number of condoms used every second in the United States: 14

■ Percentage of men who believe in love at first sight: 66

■ Percentage of women who believe in love at first sight: 57

■ Percentage of American men who name Pamela Anderson as the woman they would most like to have sex with: 36

■ Average duration of American sex: 25.3 minutes

■ Average duration of French sex: 18.8 minutes

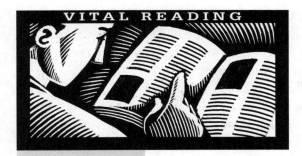

VITAL READING

Seven Habits You Should Acquire

These pointers keep sex from becoming routine.

Hey, habits, even bad ones, take time to perfect. You don't just pick them up overnight. So the fact that you've had more than your fair share of sex in this life, while undoubtedly a great source of pride to you, probably means that over the years you've developed a few bad habits—maybe learned to cut a few corners here and there in the bedroom. Happens to the best. Show us a gorgeous woman, and we'll show you a man who's making love to her on autopilot at least once in a while.

The problem here is that women, under the misguided impression that we men have delicate egos, are not always inclined to point out ways we can improve our lovemaking. So the bad habits endure.

Replacing your bad sexual habits with some of the better ones here will result in a much happier and more satisfied partner, which, being the selfless sort that you are, is the only thing that really interests you. It could also, by the way, result in bedpost-rattling, plaster-loosening, forget-your-own-name, animalistic fun for you, too. In case you're interested.

Habit #1: Be handy, man.

When it comes to using your hands to get her worked up, you can't afford to be all thumbs, at least according to the book *The Guide to Getting It On!* So the next time your fingers are doing their love thing, make sure you follow these tips.

Get them in the right position. When a woman masturbates, she often rests her wrist on her lower abdomen just above the pubic bone. If this is what your partner does, try to do the same, since it will affect the way your fingers feel on her vulva. Try lying parallel to your partner and reaching your arm over her body until your fingers contact her crotch. This allows your fingers to approach from the same angle that hers do.

Wait for it to come to you. Great lovers know to start with light, gentle caresses that barely touch the inner thighs and pubic hair. Don't go any farther until she spreads her legs or until her pelvis begins to arch upward. Then tease and caress until the lips of her vulva invite your fingers inside.

Flick your wrist. Men typically use only one finger when they get down around the action zone. It's best to get your entire wrist into the motion, even if only one finger is actually touching her vulva. This is a subtle and important detail that the great ones all know.

Habit #2: Stay in training.

"A man can learn a lot about being a better lover through masturbation, even if he has a regular partner," says Peter Sandor Gardos, Ph.D., a clinical sexologist in San Francisco. "One of men's biggest concerns during sex is that they'll come too soon. Regular masturbation is the perfect way to learn to recognize the signs that you're getting close to orgasm." Here's how to get the most out of Solo Orgasm 101.

Slow down. "The fear of being found out motivates boys to learn to masturbate to orgasm as quickly as possible," says Patricia Love, Ed.D., a marriage and family therapist in Houston and author of *Hot Monogamy*. The trouble is, these quickies condition your sexual responses in such a way that you end up climaxing much faster than you'd like to with a partner. An occasional lightning orgasm is okay, but try to set aside some time when you can relax and masturbate for 20 minutes or so.

Lighten up. Another danger of high-speed wanking is that a jackhammer stroke creates sensations that can't be reproduced when you're not the only one in the room. "Some men get so used to the hard, fast strokes that they have trouble climaxing with a partner," says Barbara Keesling, Ph.D., a sex therapist in Orange, California, and author of *Super Sexual Orgasm*.

To master a new stroke, try switching hands, which will make you very conscious of every move you make and defeat any "automatic" movements.

Habit #3: Broaden your horizons.

An effective lover knows there's more to sex than intercourse. "He doesn't simply grab a woman's breasts and then dive for her crotch," says Robert Birch, Ph.D., a marital and sex therapist in Columbus, Ohio. Instead, he "sees intercourse as one of many options."

Sex therapists recommend many possibilities, from using sex toys to rubbing your penis on different parts of your partner's body to watching her masturbate. "The essential attitude—especially in a long-term relationship—is that nothing in particular has to happen during any sex act," says Constance Avery-Clark, Ph.D., a clinical psychologist in Coral Springs, Florida.

Habit #4: Float like a butterfly.

They may not want to admit it, but women like receiving oral sex as much as we do. If you've already figured out how to make your partner hear colors, we salute you. But if you could use a bit more time in the lab, try this technique: It's the fabled Venus butterfly, described here by Ava Cadell, Ph.D., a clinical sexologist in Los Angeles.

Spend some time kissing and touching until your partner starts to become aroused, then gently pull back the hood of her clitoris. Stimulate the clitoris with short, then long, strokes with either your tongue or your moistened fingers. Ask your partner to tell you when she's reached at least 8 on an excitement scale of 1 to 10.

Then, with small, circular motions, stimulate the entire outside area of the vagina with your tongue and your fingers until she's back down to 5.

Then, go back to the clitoris. When she reaches 8 again, place the palm of your hand against her genitals and slide one finger into her vagina. With your fingertip, tap a spot about 2 inches inside her vagina, on the upper wall (home of the elusive G-spot—some women have it and some don't, but either way, this will feel good).

Just keep stroking or licking her clitoris while tapping her G-spot. She'll let you know when it's time to stop.

Habit #5: Keep her waiting.

Teasing doesn't come naturally to most men, but it can be very appealing to women. Why rush the greatest thing in life? Instead, enjoy it more. . . .

Take 10 times longer. The stereotypical guy watches his mate undress and then pounces on her like a linebacker on a loose ball. He grabs hold of her breasts and works them like pizza dough, and soon she's bored out of her mind. So, if you want to make a big impression, surprise her with your slowness. The key: Build steadily and specifically to a nipple crescendo for her, says Linda DeVillers, Ph.D., a sex therapist and author of *Love Skills*. Start at the outermost rim of the nipple and slowly spin inward. As your finger travels, you should notice the rim around her nipple (the areola) darken and the nipple itself stiffen. Place a finger on each side of the nipple and push down lightly, pulling your fingers apart as you go. Making the nipple taut (and ready!) in this way will heighten the sensation for her when you start to lick and tickle it a few moments later.

Start early in the day. "Call your lover at work and tell her what you'd like to do to her tonight when she gets home," suggests Dr. Gardos. You'll both be thinking about sex for hours.

Habit #6: Catch her off guard.

You may have magic hands, but if you make love the same way, time after time, sooner or later she's going to find it as exciting as a rerun of *This Old House*. "When a woman anticipates every move a man is going to make," says John Gray, Ph.D., author of *Men Are from Mars, Women Are from Venus*, "she may no longer become excited by sex—and this is very common." Here's how to make a few bedroom improvements.

Try new positions. "My number one advice for men is: Change your sexual positions frequently," says Dr. Cadell. "Her orgasm will feel different in every position, and she'll be grateful for your creativity."

Get away from it all. "Changing the environment is very important for a woman," says Dr. Gray. "If you can't afford a hotel, camp out. It's not the location so much as the feeling that she doesn't have to worry about the details, that you're doing the thinking. That gets her out of her mind and into her body."

Habit #7: Play at the pump.

While you're trying all those new and varied positions (woohoo!), don't forget about the most basic technique of intercourse: the thrusting of your penis. "Monotonous pumping can have a numbing effect on the woman, especially if she's not aroused enough to respond to intense sensation," says Felice Dunas, Ph.D., author of *Passion Play*. Variations in the depth, speed, rhythm, and timing of your pelvic thrusts can dramatically enhance the experience for both of you. Dr. Dunas suggests starting with mostly shallow, slow thrusts; as your partner becomes more aroused, mix in a higher percentage of deeper thrusts. To really keep her on her toes, try some brief pauses between thrusts.

Handle with Care

Skip these eight mistakes to avoid trouble down there.

On one level, men are always thinking about their penises, but on another level—maintenance and proper care—they completely ignore them. Hell, the way some of us act, you'd think a penis was as indestructible as your nephew's Tonka truck.

Well, it isn't, and men learn that lesson the hard way every day. Some of them wind up in the emergency room, where doctors snap Polaroids and start typing contributions to the *Journal of Urology* even before the bleeding stops. Other guys treat themselves at home and wear baggy pants for a week. Either way, many suffer lasting damage. In one study, men who took a shot between the legs were more than three times as likely to become impotent or to develop Peyronie's disease—an embarrassing and sometimes painful curve of the penis—as men who didn't.

Want to make sure you don't become one of the casualties? Then avoid these eight common moves that could cripple your unit.

Mistake #1: Forcing down what's gone up. You wake up with a rock-hard erection and have to pee. So you go into the bathroom and push the big guy downward, right? "That's a bad idea," says Paul Gleich, M.D., chairman of the department of urology at Regions Hospital in St. Paul, Minnesota. Putting downward pressure on an erect penis, whether you're standing in front of the john or trying to force it into a tight pair of Levi's, strains the suspensory ligaments, the two long tendons that attach your penis to your pubic bone and provide leverage for it to become erect. If these tendons are stretched too far, they'll lose their ability to hoist your member, resulting in erections that point out or down instead of up. The best way to deal with an unwanted erection is to wait until it subsides.

Mistake #2: Coercing it into sex before it's ready. Like your old high-school sweetheart, your penis does not respond well to premature attempts at intercourse. "Any time you're trying to penetrate or thrust with a penis that's not fully erect, you're susceptible to bending and buckling injuries," says Gerald Jordan, M.D., professor of urology at Eastern Virginia Medical School and director of the Devine Center for Genitourinary Reconstruction surgery, both in Norfolk. You can actually damage the structures inside your penis that fill with blood when you get an erection. The result? A penis that permanently bends, sometimes painfully, in one direction or the other.

If penetration is difficult, then it's also dangerous. Try giving your partner something she probably wants more of anyway: foreplay.

Mistake #3: Unzipping too quickly. You understand the danger of operating sharp metal teeth in close proximity to your penis, and you're careful to tuck everything neatly away before you zip. But how careful are you when you unzip? Most zipper injuries actually occur on the downstroke, when you're probably not paying attention.

If this happens to you, try to work yourself loose by pulling the zipper in the direction it came from, in one swift motion. Don't fiddle; you'll end up making matters worse. Then assess the damage and, if necessary, apply antiseptic cream and a bandage to stop the bleeding. "Zipper injuries are rarely anything more than skin injuries. They don't cause lasting harm, but they cause great pain," says Dr. Gleich. If you can't unhook yourself, you'll have to go to an emergency room, where they'll give you an anesthetic and take the zipper apart with metal clippers.

Mistake #4: Lathering up with a stand-in lubricant. You've always prided yourself on innovation. So when you and your mate are ready to get down to business and you discover that your tube of K-Y Jelly is flat, you head for the medicine cabinet and come back with Dippity-Do. No problem, right? Think again. "This is simply not an area of the body that's made for chemical application," says Charles V. Pollack Jr., M.D., chairman of the department of emergency medicine at Maricopa Medical Center in Phoenix. "A few years ago, I treated a very unlucky man who had masturbated with hair gel. He had a severe allergic reaction and ended up with second-degree chemical burns on his penis. He spent 14 days in our burn center."

And that's just one case. Other doctors have treated sexual do-it-yourselfers who have experimented with a wide range of household supplies. Deodorant, Windex—the possibilities are endless.

Mistake #5: Playing Trigger to her Annie Oakley. You and your mate are happily going at it when suddenly there's a slip, then an audible cracking noise and the worst pain you've ever experienced.

Penile fracture—just saying the name hurts. "It's probably the most common severe penile injury we see," says Dr. Gleich, "and it's almost always caused by an accident during intercourse, when the penis is jammed against an immovable object, such as her pelvic bone." These accidents are most common during "rodeo sex," when your partner is bouncing around on top of you. To protect yourself, make sure that if she's on top, she doesn't lift more than an inch or two off of you on the upstroke. And tell her never to lean back against the direction of your erection while you're inserted. Also, be careful when changing positions; it's usually better to withdraw before you pick her up or flip her over.

If you do fracture yourself, you'll know. Your penis will turn purple and swell up like an eggplant. Don't dawdle: Go quickly to an emergency room. "Some men delay seeking treatment for days because they hope the problem will go away on its own," says Dr. Gleich.

Mistake #6: Taking it back to nature. The great outdoors is full of peril even when your pants are on. Take them off, and you're really asking for trouble. Here are three irritants to avoid.

1. The sun. "The penis is rarely exposed to the sun, so it's pretty easy to overdo it the first time you strip off your swimsuit," says Michael Carius, M.D., chairman of the department of emergency medicine at Norwalk Hospital in Norwalk, Connecticut. Worse, exposing your penis to ultraviolet rays (from the sun or tanning beds) can make its skin tougher, leading to rough, scaly patches and decreased sensitivity.

2. Poison ivy. If you're determined to make love in the great outdoors, check the ground carefully for three-leaved foliage. Nothing will ruin your week like a rash that you can't scratch in public.

3. Animal teeth. "Animals may go for the crotch when they attack because they know it's a vulnerable area," says Dr. Gleich.

Dr. Pollack tells the tale of "a guy who, while he was naked, was playing with his pet rattlesnake. He managed to anger the snake, and his penis was swollen and painful by the time I saw him. He ended up losing about half of it because of the venom."

Mistake #7: Having it surgically enlarged. These days, about $6,000 is all it takes to buy your way to a bigger penis. At least, that's the cost in cash. Believe us, you'll pay a sexual price as well for the extra inch (and this is the max, by the way) that the doctor can give you. "The penis-lengthening procedures involve snipping the suspensory ligaments in the abdomen. Unfortunately, snipping these ligaments also means you'll have a wobblier erection, and therefore a greater chance of buckling and fracture injuries," says Irwin Goldstein, M.D., professor of urology at Boston University Medical Center.

If you also opt for a girth-enhancing procedure, you can expect a lumpy erection—the result of fat injections that clump in spots. And that's on a good day. Some cosmetic surgeons have butchered so many erections that they've created a whole new subspecialty: urologists who try to undo the damage done by their clumsy peers.

"Unless you have a penis that's so short you have trouble urinating or inseminating a partner, you shouldn't even consider this surgery," says Dr. Goldstein. We're talking about penises that are less than 3 inches long when erect.

Mistake #8: Sticking it where it doesn't belong. You know all about the dangers of sexually transmitted diseases, so we'll spare you the lecture about sleeping with a strange partner. But there are two other places to watch out for.

1. The mouth of any woman you wouldn't trust with your ATM code. "Remember, you're putting yourself in an extremely vulnerable situation when you let another human being put her teeth in such close proximity to your penis," says Dr. Pollack. If you have any reason to believe she's susceptible to seizures or vengeful outbursts, confine your attentions to those areas of her body that are free of incisors. And don't ever have oral sex in a moving vehicle, especially if you're driving.

2. Any nonhuman orifice. This topic barely merits discussion, except to say that guys who look to other species and appliances for sexual satisfaction deserve what's coming to them. Dr. Pollack once had a patient who rubbed himself with raw hamburger in order to entice his dog to a little oral action. "Sure enough, one day the dog got a little carried away and chewed him up pretty well," he says. Another man suffered a similar fate after seeking satisfaction from the hose of a canister-type vacuum cleaner that contained a hidden fan blade.

The Naked Truth

What women won't tell you about sex.

In general, you may not have too many complaints about your wife or girlfriend hiding her thoughts and feelings. In fact, you may think she has altogether too much to say about her family, your family, the size of her butt, and the state of the neighbors' marriage. But there's one subject that doesn't get enough airtime, at least not in down-and-dirty detail. The subject, of course, is sex.

No matter how well you know a woman, you can bet she has certain opinions about your sex life that simply don't come up in conversation. Chalk it up to her delicate nature, her puritanical upbringing, or her reluctance to damage your fragile ego, but when it comes to the stuff you really need to know, she's not talking. Here are a few things women would like you to know—as long as they don't have to tell you themselves.

1. The missionary position sucks. True, this position (you on top, her down below) is a classic. But so are the Stooges, whoopee cushions, and *Star Trek* reruns, and you know how most women feel about those.

"Most men think that if they stick it in you, you'll be screaming with orgasm if they keep at it long enough," says Ruth, 30. It's just not so. No matter how much you pump, nothing is going to happen unless her clitoris is involved. And that's physically impossible if you're lying on top.

Sure, forward-and-back motion brings a man to orgasm, something you probably figured out in junior high. But a woman needs some attention to the periphery. Even the most tireless humping and pumping isn't going to make it happen.

What should you do? Get creative. Don't be afraid to suggest a few different positions. (Trust me, if her orgasm is on the line, she'll be willing.) Think doggie style. Or her on top. Or side by side. Or her legs on your shoulders. Push your flexibility, and hers, to the limit. Use your hands, your penis, or anything else that's handy to stimulate the clitoris, no matter what position you're in. She'll show and tell you how she wants to be touched down there. If she doesn't, ask.

2. She doesn't know any more about the G-spot than you do. "It's a myth!" shouted an exasperated George on one of the last episodes of *Seinfeld*. Clearly the words of a man who has tried and failed to find the G-spot. And no wonder: Ask three women whether they have a G-spot, and you'll hear three different answers. Some women know they have one, some are sure they don't, and some are as lost as George. "I can't find my own," says Vicky, 32. "I know it's supposed to be a place in the vaginal canal, but I haven't been able to find it yet. And it's not for lack of trying."

   "It's not a magic button," says Lonnie Barbach, Ph.D., a sex therapist in Mill Valley, California.

3. Oral sex does not equal orgasm. You want the truth, so here goes: Your partner may love it when you stimulate her orally, but if you think it's a sure way to bring her to orgasm, think again. As Julie, 31, says, some men seem to think of oral sex as a time-saver, as in, "I know she's not really turned on yet, but if I give her oral sex for exactly 30 seconds, we can cut right to the good stuff." That's not the way it is. Oral sex feels great, but it doesn't change a woman's basic sexual wiring, which usually dictates that sexual satisfaction takes time.

   Here's another bulletin from the oral-sex front: Though some women really do have breathtaking orgasms during oral sex, there are plenty of others who find the whole process a bit intimidating, especially with a new partner. This can put a woman under pressure, says Julie. "If I get the sense that a guy finds it gross or tedious, I feel like I should hurry up and come, which pretty much guarantees that I won't."

   So what's a man to do? Make sure your partner knows that going down on her is a huge turn-on for you. Do whatever you have to do to make that point: Wax poetic, make happy noises, break into song. And if you really don't enjoy this particular activity? Don't do it. A woman can tell when you're just doing her a favor, and there's no quicker way to put a damper on her sexual excitement. There are a million other ways you can make her happy.

4. She fantasizes, too, but not the way you do. Women aren't above the occasional erotic daydream, but contrary to what you might expect, most don't get hot and bothered about the ripped 19-year-olds who make a living modeling boxer briefs. "Those boys are beautiful, but they just don't do it for me sexually," says Tricia, 29. Men may get off on the beauty of a centerfold model, but when a woman fantasizes, she concentrates less on the appearance of her dream man and more on the raw passion he brings to the bedroom.

"My fantasies are all about intensity," says Tricia. "I might be visualizing someone from work or the guy who teaches my night-school class, neither of whom is that great-looking. But in every case, my dream man is absolutely crazed with lust."

Women's opinions on the subject are virtually unanimous: The men in their beds may play it cool, but the men they fantasize about do just the opposite. "The guy in my fantasies looks like my boyfriend, but he acts totally different," says Kathleen, 34. "Mark is reserved in bed, but in my fantasies he's a complete wild man."

5. She wants to hear that she's great in bed. If you feel uncomfortable telling a woman she's great in the sack, you're not alone. "It's our whole culture," says Marty Klein, Ph.D., a family counselor and sex therapist in Palo Alto, California. "Is it a compliment to tell a woman she's good in bed? Or is it a sexist, insensitive statement for which she'll toss you out of the house? Many men have learned to keep quiet about this."

For the record, when you tell her she's good at sex, she takes it as a compliment. She has an ego, too. "Not all loving sex has to be pristine," says Carolyn, 32. "Women like more than roses and candlelight. We're game for anything, as long as we know you respect us." Just make sure your delivery is sincere, and use your best judgment when using vernacular. "You're the hottest chick I ever banged" might work for the odd woman (the very odd woman), but it won't work for most.

6. She thinks you're fat. Sometimes the truth hurts. The irony here is that many men (usually the same idiots who tease their wives about gaining weight) are under the illusion that they can let themselves go and the women in their lives won't care. Dream on, butterball. She'll still love you, but she won't want to see you naked.

"If he isn't careful about his weight or if he doesn't present himself in a way that's attractive to her, he's sending a message that he doesn't care about her," says Dr. Barbach. So why should she want to sleep with him? Show her that you're willing to put some effort into it and that you're willing to work as hard as she does at making yourself look more attractive.

It's not just a matter of appearance; it's also a health issue. There's nothing erotic about hearing a man pant if he sounds like he's about to have a coronary. So take a long, hard look in the mirror, and if you don't like what you see, do something about it. You'll feel better, and the sex will be better.

7. You've never really pleased her sexually. If you do hear this, you'll hear it only once—over her shoulder as she heads out the door. This is one time when you should ignore what she has to say. A woman who attacks your sexual prowess does so for one reason: It's the single most hurtful thing she can think of to say, and at this moment, hurting you is what she wants to do.

Is she telling the truth? Don't even think about it. When someone hurls a grenade, you don't examine it to make sure it's really a grenade. You duck. Besides, once a woman throws this one at you, the truth of it no longer matters, because she has no intention of ever sleeping with you again. What it takes to satisfy her is no longer your problem. Remember, even if it's true that you never rang her bell, the next woman who sleeps in your bed may be shrieking like a car alarm.

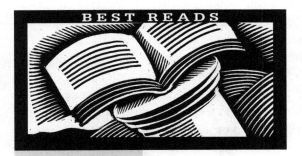

BEST READS

Discovering Viagra

The impotence-treatment drug Viagra burst onto the scene in the summer of 1998, and it has proven to be a miracle pill for millions of men. How did researchers make this amazing discovery? In this excerpt from The Virility Solution: Everything

You Need to Know about the FDA-Approved Potency Pill That Can Restore and Enhance Male Sexuality *(Simon and Schuster, 1998), authors Steven Lamm, M.D., and Gerald Secor Couzens sketch out the events that led to Viagra's commercial debut.*

Testing a potential mass-market drug is no small matter. It takes time, plenty of money, and patience. When a pharmaceutical company believes it has a marketable drug, it must be submitted to rigorous scientific trials. They consist of actual tests on human subjects and can take a decade or more to complete, with time spent to assemble, correlate, and disseminate the data. Pharmaceutical companies estimate that taking a new medication from the research phase through each of the three, sometimes four, individual experimental trials, to the final submission of the data to the Food and Drug Administration costs $500 million on average. For all the time and money spent, the pharmaceutical company is afforded some protection from competitors. Once a drug gets FDA approval, the company then has 2 decades in which to exclusively produce and sell that drug.

The procedure for drug trials is always the same. Each promising drug starts out with a relatively small Phase I trial in which the new medication is offered to a select group of patients who have not been helped by conventional therapy. This is not without risk: Although the drugs have been tested on animals, toxicity to humans is, at this point, unknown. Phase I trials are usually limited to just a dozen or so patients and generally last up to a year.

If the drug appears to be effective and has acceptable side effects, Phase II begins. Now, dozens of people will receive the drug, while dozens more will take placebos (inert substances). At this time, the researchers are looking at the safety and side-effect profile, but they especially want to know if the experimental drug is more effective than both the placebo and any current therapy used to treat the same ailment. If the drug still seems to be working, then Phase III trials start in which hundreds of subjects, some of whom receive the drug, some of whom get a placebo, are used. Neither group, nor the administering physicians, know who is taking the drug and who is taking the placebo. Researchers examine the side effects and effectiveness very closely and also seek to determine optimal dosages of the drug. By Phase IV, the drug has been proven to be effective and researchers are fine-tuning the treatment on test subjects, not checking for efficacy, but rather seeking to determine whether or not any disturbing side effects appear.

Time-consuming as they are, these medical trials are very important. They strive to prove whether the drug works the way researchers claim it will. They also check to make sure that, when dosage recommendations are followed carefully, the patient will be helped. In the end, the overall safety of a drug is a more crucial consideration than its efficacy.

The Viagra Tests

The tests on Viagra (sildenafil) were no different than those of any other drug. In the first human trial of the drug, a dozen men in England who were experiencing erectile dysfunction (ED) took it three times a day for a week. The results were extremely encouraging, but researchers had to pose some realistic questions: Does anyone really want to take a pill three times daily? And who could afford such a costly treatment?

Another short trial was begun. This time, the dozen men took a single dose every day. Remarkably, 10 of them showed positive results, and the researchers concluded that the drug was "a well-tolerated and efficacious oral therapy and represents a new class of peripherally acting drugs for the treatment of this condition."

Phase II drug trials spread beyond the west of England to other parts of the United Kingdom as well as France and Sweden. In one study, 42 men between the ages of 34 and 70, all of whom had experienced ED for at least 3 years, were divided into two groups. Half took Viagra in daily doses of 25, 50, or 75 milligrams while the others received a placebo. Later, the two groups switched pills. After 28 days, more than 90 percent of the men reported significantly improved sexual performance. This was confirmed by the answers they provided on detailed sexual-activity questionnaires. Not only were they filled out by the men taking part in the study, they were answered by their partners as well. It turned out that the men who experienced profound improvement had been taking Viagra.

Then a much more extensive study was begun. This time, 351 patients between the ages of 24 and 70 participated. The men were randomly assigned to take the pill at one of three doses (10, 25, or 50 milligrams) or a placebo. After 28 days, almost 90 percent of the men taking the 50-milligram pill reported a threefold improvement in the quality of their sex lives. They cited satisfaction with the frequency, hardness, and duration of their erections.

"The drug has given me back my life," one man said. "It has changed the way I think about myself. I'm a new man."

Viagra had a powerful effect on the men who tried it, and when the Phase II trial ended and the supply of the drug was stopped, there were a lot of complaints and protests from the test subjects. In fact, one test subject, who had developed ED years earlier, pleaded to be allowed to continue using the drug. Viagra, he said, had altered his life. In his case, the researchers relented and gave it to him. He was, after all, almost 90.

For Phase III, the trials were moved to the United States under the direction of Dr. Tom Lue, a noted San Francisco urologist. Now, unlike the highly successful European trials that had specifically excluded any man whose ED had a physiological basis, the American tests focused solely on men with physical problems. Subjects with atherosclerosis, or a nerve-related problem such as diabetes mellitus, were chosen. The results reinforced the power of Viagra. The European trials proved that it could help men whose ED was contributed to by anxiety or emotional problems. Now the American trials showed that ED related to physiological problems could also be overcome.

In the American study, 416 men with ED problems were randomly chosen to receive either a placebo or a 5-, 25-, 50-, or 100-milligram daily dose of Viagra over an 8-week period. Once again, when the study was ended, a questionnaire was used to assess sexual satisfaction. More than 70 percent of the men answered that 50 milligrams of Viagra improved their erections. More than 75 percent said that double that dosage imparted the desired effect.

According to Dr. Harin Padma-Nathan, associate professor in the department of urology at the University of Southern California in Los Angeles, who was also a key researcher in the Viagra trials, the drug had far-reaching effects. It was able to specifically target and greatly enhance a man's ability to have and maintain an erection, improve orgasm, and enhance the overall quality of sexual intercourse.

The American study also addressed the possible side effects of the drug. Every medication has the potential to cause discomfort, which is sometimes mild, and other times severe. That's why it's always important to ask your doctor about any medication you are about to take. Once in a while, the possible reactions are so off-putting and difficult to live with that a patient will decide to forgo treatment. In the case of the cure for ED, that is unlikely to happen.

The potential side effects for men who take Viagra include:

Headaches. They occur in less than 10 percent of subjects.

Flushing, or reddening of the face. This occurs in less than 10 percent of men taking it.

Dyspepsia, or gastrointestinal disorder. This problem occurs in less than 10 percent of test subjects.

Myalgia, or muscle pain. This is experienced by less than 10 percent of men.

Slight alteration in color vision. This has not been reported in men taking up to 100 milligrams, in either the American or European trials. It has occurred, however, in test doses over 100 milligrams, which far exceeds the recommended prescription of 50 milligrams. When it did happen in test subjects, it lasted from several minutes to a few hours. It is not true color blindness, but rather a slight problem in discriminating among blue-green hues.

Interaction with other drugs. Because of adverse side effects, men taking a nitrate-based drug such as sublingual nitroglycerin or isosorbide dinitrate (Isordil) cannot use the drug.

Viagra had much to recommend it, with few, if any, drawbacks, and Dr. Lue presented the results of his study to a packed audience at the annual meeting of the American Urological Society in New Orleans in 1997. "Sildenafil," he told his fellow physicians, "is an effective, well-tolerated oral treatment for patients with ED associated with a broad range of etiologies."

One of the most significant comments about Viagra was made by a leading ED expert whose specialization included psychiatry. "The evidence that Viagra is an effective treatment is overwhelming and ushers in a whole new era," stated Raymond C. Rosen, professor of psychiatry and medicine and codirector of the Center of Sexual and Marital Health at the University of Medicine and Dentistry of New Jersey-Robert Wood Johnson Medical School in Newark. "It will finally move ED treatment into the realm of primary-care medicine. Millions of men will be helped."

At last, a pill for ED had been developed. Quick-acting, virtually free of side effects, and easy to take, it was the miracle cure men had been hoping for since ED was first known.

Sex and the Middle-Age Male

Middle age brings more than crises about what has been accomplished in life to date. It also brings about physical changes as one's body ages. Regrettably, some of the changes affect your sexual equipment. And while these changes are inevitable, that doesn't mean an end to your sexual life. Far from it, points out Art Hister, M.D., in this excerpt from his book Midlife Man: A Not-So-Threatening Guide to Health and Sex for Man at His Peak *(Greystone Books, 1998).*

Leonard Cohen, a man who has clearly been there and certainly done that (when I come back, I hope it's as a sour, lined, black-garbed poet), has complained in song that he aches in places where he used to play. Although most of us have not been fortunate enough to play nearly as often as Leonard has and certainly not on the same squad that Leonard managed to be drafted for, the reality is that even if we never quite made it onto the first-string team, most middle-age guys are "aching" in places that once used to be ache-free.

Now before you leap to a fallacious conclusion, let me quickly interpose that I'm absolutely certain that Leonard is using "ache" in a metaphorical sense. It's not so much that middle-age guys experience physical pain in the old playground; it's more that our seesaws don't go as high as they used to when we were younger. Some guys are even finding that they cannot get their seesaws off the ground any longer, the countervailing weight, either emotional or physical, having become too heavy to be lifted without appropriate assistance. And that is why, of course, Viagra has become this era's hula hoop and pet rock.

Sexual Changes in Midlife: Good to the Last Droop

What does happen to sexual functioning in middle age in men? Not much, but too much. For a start, a man's testicles shrink slightly as he ages (and no, I don't know anyone who has actually had theirs measured, nor do I know of any health plan that would pay for this procedure should you choose to have it done), they don't ride as high as they used to, the aging male's scrotum tends not to shrink as much when he becomes aroused, and the number of testosterone-producing cells begins to drop. There is also a smaller volume of pre-ejaculatory secretions, sperm production and semen volume fall, and there is a small drop-off in the percentage of mature sperm that are most capable of fertilizing an anxious yet hopeful ovum. Overall, however, most middle-age men still produce enough sperm to be able to impregnate a partner, if not quite on demand, then at least with effort, in time. ("With effort, in time," by the way, is the Hister family motto, at least for the male side of the family.)

In addition, erections begin to change in midlife. Now I realize that many of you, especially the younger men, might have trouble understanding that last bit. For most younger guys, after all, an erection is much like an elevator in a three-story tenement building: It goes up and it goes down; the view while it's in use is generally nonvarying; and aside from the speed at which your elevator delivers you from the depths of the basement to the exhilaration of the penthouse, there really isn't much else to appreciate or criticize about it. And usually, that's the way it goes in the early years. Up and down, up and down, on command, when in demand, zipping rapidly between floors, delivering its soon-to-be-ecstatic cargo to the luxurious upstairs suites whenever called on to carry the weight, and requiring minimal maintenance, not even any regular lubrication for that matter.

Even the most pampered and well-maintained elevator, however, can sometimes get stuck between floors. It might even malfunction on occasion by lingering on the lower-level floors. Worst of all, like HAL, the computer in *2001: A Space Odyssey*, the elevator might even develop a mind of its own and prefer to stay grounded most of the time, despite its handler's best attempts to get it moving upward into service. That's how it is with erections, too, so during middle age, not only do many men begin to suffer from occasional bouts of impotence but even a midlife man who is always able (with effort, in time) to get hard enough to do his duty tends to suffer a bit of loss of upward mobility of his penis because of changes in the blood vessels that are responsible for creating and maintaining an erection. These changes also lead to a slight alteration in the angle of the erection.

Middle age also brings changes to the "quality" of an erection. Not only does it take most middle-age guys longer to achieve even a garden-variety, run-of-the-mill erection, but in contrast to when they were young, when a rock-hard erection immediately sprang up after even the vaguest erotic thought, in midlife some men may require direct physical stimulation to get an erection, or they may not hit full hardness until they are in place. This is because erections tend to become less firm (much like other body parts of the middle-age owner of those erections), the kind of erections that men often describe as softer or weaker. How do we know that, you ask. Because the people who study these things actually have a way of measuring the strength of erections. (Those of you reading this chapter to your kids as a bedtime story might want to skip the next part.) In *Clock of Ages*, Dr. John Medina claims that "ejaculatory distance" drops off from "2 feet in young men to only minimal dribbling distance in the elderly," and I'll bet you that until you read that, you had absolutely no idea that they even held that kind of competition. Well, they clearly do, and I'll bet that it's a sellout every time.

For some middle-age men, even with physical stimulation—to paraphrase Gertrude Stein's comment about Oakland—there is often no there, there. In other words, middle age is when increasing numbers of men begin to be visited by that unwelcome guest known as impotence, who is inevitably greeted like a death figure in a Woody Allen film, come to call on the wrong guy at the wrong time. For men who begin to be troubled by intermittent but increasingly frequent visits from this frightening apparition, a diamond-hard erection becomes elusive, and for a small but growing number of men, it becomes rarer to experience a trouble-free sexual episode than to discover a television talk show host with at least a double-digit IQ.

Midlife man also finds that his orgasm is often shorter. "But how much shorter can it get?" asked my smirking wife, proving how little attention she actually pays to what I tell her. It's orgasm that they're talking about, not foreplay. With increasing age, a man's erection also detumesces faster; that is, his rocket plummets to Earth more quickly than it did in the old days, and he can't relaunch nearly as rapidly for a second flight.

These generally gradual changes are universal with advancing years, and no man is immune, but clearly they don't affect all men equally. Furthermore, no matter how mild or severe the changes may be, men respond to them in very different ways. After all, the brain, which usually includes the mind, is still the biggest and certainly the most important sexual organ for men. As a result, some guys are devastated by even the slightest change in their sexual apparatus or functioning, while others seem to absorb significant changes with only minimal complaints. Now that Viagra is available, however, even these guys are appearing in doctors' offices in amazing numbers to get help stiffening their resolve.

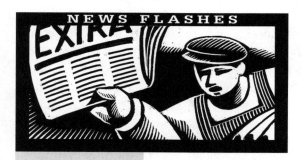

Antibiotics May Solve Some Cases of Infertility

HOUSTON—Bacterial infections may be a more common cause of infertility than previously thought. In a study presented at the annual meeting of the American Society for Reproductive Medicine, researchers isolated two types of bacteria from infertile men's semen and introduced them into healthy sperm samples. Within 3 hours, 40 percent of the sperm were unable to swim. "If these findings are confirmed, infertile men could benefit from specific testing to rule out this type of infection," says Larry Lipshultz, M.D., professor of urology at Baylor College of Medicine. "In that case, antibiotics may help restore sperm function."

Taller Men Are Conceived in the Summer

VIENNA, Austria—Researchers at the University of Vienna analyzed data from more than 500,000 Austrian army recruits and found something bizarre: On average, men born in the spring were taller than men born in the fall. To be specific, men with April birthdays were about ¼ inch taller than men born in October. Gerhard Weber, Ph.D., the lead study author, believes that the height difference is related to sunlight. "The amount of melatonin released into the body is related to the amount and intensity of sunlight the body encounters. And melatonin may have an effect on the body's growth hormones," he says.

Faster HIV Test Results Now Available

WASHINGTON, D.C.—Every year, about 25 million people are tested in clinics for HIV. But since conventional tests require two blood samples and take 2 weeks to process, a full one-quarter of people tested don't return for their results. Now, there's no need for a lengthy wait: A clinic test can determine if you're

HIV negative in about 10 minutes. The Public Health Service is letting clinics share the results of the initial "rapid" blood test with patients; they reserve the second round of testing for people who test positive.

Polyurethane Condoms Are Riskier Than Latex

SACRAMENTO—Researchers at the California Family Health Council recently reported that polyurethane condoms are more likely than latex condoms to break and slip off. Researchers gave 805 couples either polyurethane or latex condoms to test for 6 months. The polyurethane condoms failed 5.2 percent of the time, compared with 0.6 percent for the latex. "If you're allergic to latex, polyurethane condoms are still your best protection against pregnancy and sexually transmitted diseases," says James Trussell, Ph.D., director of population research at Princeton University. But Dr. Trussell recommends applying a water-based lubricant to minimize the chance of friction tears and using a diaphragm or spermicide as a backup to prevent pregnancy.

Researchers Discover New Cause of Infertility

BUFFALO—A newly identified sperm defect may cause infertility. The culprit? Premature release of acrosome enzymes, which soften the covering of the egg to allow sperm to penetrate and fertilize it. Researchers at the State University of New York at Buffalo studied 250 infertile couples and found that 40 percent of the men had prematurely released acrosome enzymes. "Now we can better judge the proper functioning of sperm," says Lani Burkman, Ph.D., the lead researcher. "And if the sperm are defective, we can recommend in vitro fertilization, donor sperm, or sperm injection."

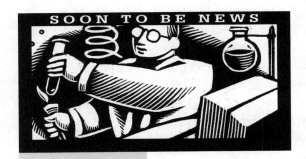

Gel Replacing the Patch?

For men struggling with itchy testosterone patches, relief is on the horizon. A Chicago company called Unimed announced its latest round of trials on Androgel, a clear testosterone gel that's rubbed on the chest and upper arms. Unimed believes that its product may be as effective as current methods of supplementation and that it causes less discomfort.

Unimed plans to file for FDA approval in the next few months.

Speedier Viagra?

For those who want it all and want it now, researchers at Pfizer are teaming up with a company called Scherer Corporation to develop a new form of Viagra that would dissolve in your mouth, speeding the active ingredients to your bloodstream in just minutes instead of the full hour the pill now needs to take effect.

Pfizer says any new form of Viagra is still years away from the market.

Go to the Brain to End Impotence?

According to a study at the University of Arizona in Tucson, a new impotence treatment may do the trick when other options fail. Researchers injected 10 impotent men with Melanotan-II and a placebo. In eight of the subjects, Melanotan-II produced an erection for an average of 38 minutes; placebo erections lasted an average of 3 minutes. Unlike Viagra, which works by increasing bloodflow to the penis, Melanotan-II treats psychological and other forms of impotence by stimulating the brain to cause an erection, says Hunter Wessells, M.D., one of the researchers. "It may even produce multiple erections," he says.

Clinical trials on an oral form of Melanotan-II are expected to begin this year.

Rub-On Relief?

In about a year, impotent men who can't use Viagra may be able to enjoy sex with the help of a new rub-on drug. Researchers at Boston University have developed a gel, called Topiglan, that spurs erections. It contains alprostadil, an impotence drug that has long been used in injectables, such as Caverject. A patented hydrocarbon in Topiglan helps the alprostadil slip through skin cells to reach the corpus cavernosum (the tissue that traps blood to form an erection), says Irwin Goldstein, M.D., professor of urology at Boston University Medical Center. In a preliminary study performed by Dr. Goldstein, 114 impotent men applied Topiglan or a placebo gel to the heads of their penises, then watched adult films. Within 45 minutes, 69 percent of the Topiglan group had erections, compared with only 20 percent of the group that used the placebo gel. "Topiglan could help men who either can't use Viagra or are only partially helped by it," says Dr. Goldstein.

So far, Topiglan's only reported side effect is a warm sensation on the penis. Trials for FDA approval should begin soon.

Sperm to Deliver Vaccines?

Researchers at the University of Southern California in Los Angeles think they've found the perfect vehicle to transport vaccines for chlamydia, genital warts, and HIV into women: sperm. According to Virginia Scofield, Ph.D., an immunologist, women may eventually be able to insert vaccines for sexually transmitted diseases into their vaginas via a foam, and then—as a necessary second step—have sex. "The vaccine would lock onto sperm, and the sperm could ferry the vaccine deep into the cervix to produce a potent, local immunization," says Dr. Scofield. Several "intercourse-delivered" vaccines are under development, she says. The method might also work for birth-control drugs.

If tests remain on track, products could be on the market within 5 years.

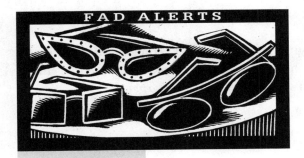

Yohimbe

Pausinystalia yohimbe is widely sold as a natural alternative for treating impotence. It's thought that yohimbe can dilate blood vessels, increasing bloodflow to the penis. A review in the *Journal of Urology* of seven clinical trials including 419 impotent men found that a prescription version of the herb was more effective in producing erections than a placebo was. But yohimbe preparations may carry some serious side effects, says Donald D. Hensrud, M.D., assistant professor of preventive medicine and nutrition at the Mayo Clinic in Rochester, Minnesota.

First of all, yohimbe may react dangerously with a substance found in wine and cheese, causing high blood pressure, nausea, and vomiting. Second, "it can cause anxiety and sleeplessness, and even psychotic reactions in people who are predisposed to mental disorders," says Dr. Hensrud.

But chances are, you won't have to worry about any of that, because "there's almost a 100 percent chance that the yohimbe product you purchase over the counter will be worthless," says Varro E. Tyler, Ph.D., distinguished professor emeritus of pharmacognosy at Purdue University in West Lafayette, Indiana. An analysis of 26 commercial yohimbe products found that 17 contained insignificant amounts of the herb, or none at all.

Finally, it's not smart to use yohimbe to self-treat sexual dysfunction. Even if it does work, its apparent ability to induce erections may be largely due to the placebo effect, which is notoriously strong where herbal remedies are concerned. And impotence can be a symptom of psychological problems or a serious undiagnosed disorder, such as diabetes or heart disease. See a doctor.

Muira-Puama

 It's hard to go wrong with a remedy that has been nicknamed potency wood. Studies suggest that it's safe and effective as both an aphrodisiac and an erection booster. When 262 men took 1 to 2.5 grams of muira-puama extract a day for 2 weeks, 51 percent reported better erections and 62 percent said it helped their libidos. There were no reports of side effects.

"I haven't reviewed the original study myself, but I confess that if I had erection problems, I might try this herb," says James A. Duke, Ph.D., retired ethnobotanist and herbal expert, and author of *The Green Pharmacy*.

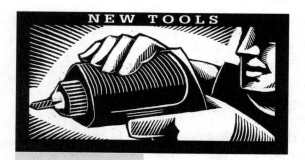

NEW TOOLS

Better Sex for Him and Her

Shared Sensation Condom

Trojan banged a loud drum for its Shared Sensation condom ($8 per box of 12) when it came out. It's the first latex condom that combines a flared head (to give you more wiggle room) and a slightly ribbed, nubby shaft (to give her more zing with every thrust). So it's part prophylactic, part sex toy.

The baggy head is a nice feature; the friction between penis and plastic feels better than with other condoms. But *Men's Health* magazine's women testers didn't notice any greater pleasure. "It wasn't until afterward, when I read the package, that I even knew the ribs were there," said one female volunteer. Trojan says the ribs should lightly brush her clitoris, but the condom's bumps (which start about 3 inches from the tip) are way too subtle. "When sex-toy manufacturers put bumps and ridges on novelty condoms, they're at least five times more prominent than the ones on the Shared Sensation condom," says Luanne Cole Weston, Ph.D., a sex therapist in California.

If you'd like to try the Shared Sensation, call (800) 487-6526 for a free condom.

Less-Risky Riding

Bicycle Saddle

Since several published articles have suggested that bicycle saddles can cause impotence by crushing arteries that deliver blood to the penis, the cycling industry has been working to produce a safer seat. There are many designs, but none as sleek and apparently effective as the Specialized Body Geometry Comp. The Specialized company and Roger Minkow, M.D., a physician and ergonomic designer in Petaluma, California, developed this saddle to help shift weight to the pelvic bones and reduce arterial and nerve compression.

Robert Kessler, M.D., a urologist at Stanford University, has recommended the seat to 18 cyclists with numbness, pain, and erectile problems. "Almost all of them have had significant improvement," he says.

Unlike other ergonomic models, the saddle doesn't scream, "I have trouble getting it up!" You'll find both in most bike shops. Buy one for your mate, too, even if she rides a stationary bike. In a study from Boston University, 96 of 282 female cyclists (many of whom rode less than 5 hours a week) complained of clitoral numbness; a control group of 51 female runners reported no such problem.

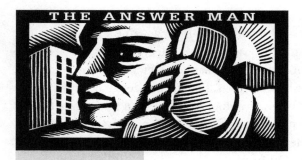

Caught in the Act

Our kids caught us having sex. It was pretty upsetting to them. What should we say or do in this situation?
—C. W., McLean, Va.

For starters, how about "Barney's downstairs and he wants a damn hug!" Actually, it's more important to know what not to say or do, advises Mark F. Schwartz, Sc.D., and Lori D. Galperin, clinical co-directors of the Masters and Johnson sexual therapy clinic in St. Louis. If your kids were upset, we imagine that you two jumped around like lunatics trying to gather up your privates and spent sexual aids. Big goof. That affirmed that something hugely bad was going on, and though they probably won't barge into your room again soon, they're no doubt wondering just what kind of evil has invaded your souls. Take them aside and give them the "Daddy wasn't hurting Mommy" spiel, along with a few sneak previews of the pubescent sex talk. Once they're nodding with insight, let them go. Cinemax will make it all click soon enough.

To prevent this reaction in your kids, act like teenagers in front of them every day. Hug, kiss, hold hands, play "I can pin you on the rug." It'll prepare the youngsters for the day they may accidentally find you grappling in a sweaty, convulsive fit of animalistic copulation. "If kids see parents showing physical affection, physical contact won't be such a shock," says Dr. Schwartz. They'll just assume that your usual horseplay has graduated to an intensity that requires a mattress.

No Place to Go

I had a vasectomy 6 years ago. What has happened to the billions of sperm my body has produced since?
—D. C., Corvallis, Ore.

If a man has had a vasectomy, his sperm swim around aimlessly in the epididymis, a long, narrow tube that's coiled up between the testicles and the vas deferens (the sperm-carrying tube that's clipped in a vasectomy), says Marc Goldstein, M.D., professor of urology and director of the Center for Male Reproductive Medicine and Microsurgery at New York Hospital–Cornell Medical Center in New York City. After a few days, the sperm die and their tiny corpses are shuttled off by the body's waste-removal system.

The only possible complication occurs if you decide to have the vasectomy reversed. In most men who have had vasectomies, a few sperm leak out into the bloodstream. When this happens, your body may perceive the sperm as intruders—like viruses or bacteria—and start producing antisperm antibodies to combat them. (Studies show that about half of all men who have had vasectomies eventually develop these antibodies.) The antibodies won't hurt you, but if you do decide to have your vasectomy reversed, the antibodies may alter your sperm and keep you infertile.

Late Comer

It usually takes me about 25 minutes of thrusting to have satisfying sex. But after 10 minutes, my wife starts complaining of pain and asks me to stop. What can I do to help her go longer?
—N. T., El Paso, Tex.

Your wife's vaginal secretions are water-based, so they evaporate during sex. If she doesn't stay highly aroused, she won't replenish those secretions fast enough to stay well-lubricated. And, frankly, dry sex hurts. Use a lubricant, available in drugstores.

By the way, the mere thought of 25 minutes of steady pounding is probably turning her off, so try to reach orgasm in less time. One trick is to contract and release your butt muscles as you thrust; it can trigger a faster ejaculation.

Low Desire

Ever since I had a vasectomy, my sexual desire has waned. Are these two things related?
—D. V., Cincinnati

Maybe, but it's probably temporary. Your testicles are still functioning and producing male sex hormones, but your decreased libido might be psychological; some men feel anxious about losing their fertility. Talk to your partner about this, or confide in a male friend who has undergone the snip. Odds are, you'll rebound.

If your vasectomy was more than a year ago, however, something else could be the culprit. See your doctor or a urologist. Some men experience testicular pain after sex up to 6 months after a vasectomy, and that can certainly dampen desire. If you have pain, tell your doctor.

Tasty Spermicide

My new girlfriend says she will perform oral sex on me only if I wear a condom and if she knows that the spermicide on the outside of the condom isn't harmful to her. I'm ready to do my part. Can you help me out on the spermicide deal?

—K. S., Santa Rosa, Calif.

"If your girlfriend is willing to endure the ghastly taste of spermicide, then fine," says William Kassler, M.D., a medical epidemiologist with the Centers for Disease Control's division of sexually transmitted disease prevention. "Spermicide can, at worst, burn a little on the mouth, but it's not dangerous in terms of allergic reactions. She won't get sick if she swallows it. This is a matter of—dare I say—taste.

"The question is why your girlfriend would want you to use a condom with spermicide during oral sex. Psychologically, it may make her feel better, and the spermicide does provide a very small amount of protection against disease transfer if the condom breaks, but that normally doesn't happen during oral sex."

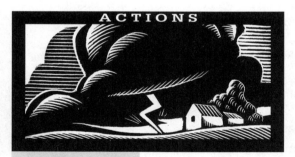

ACTIONS

If something is worth doing, then it's worth doing well. And sex is something that's always worth doing. Problem is, not everybody does it well.

Sure, some guys might argue that there's no such thing as bad sex. And, yes, even awkward, poorly timed groping sessions are more fun than watching TV. But there's no mistaking a really good night of passion, when everything goes off without a hitch and you can actually hear the fireworks when it's over. With that in mind, here are some tips to help you experience that every time you muss up the sheets.

1. **Seek out a new place.** "Having sex in new locations can create new fantasies that may lead to more powerful orgasms," says Michael Seiler, Ph.D., a

Chicago sex therapist. Start simply—say, by having sex in your car while it's parked in the garage—and work your way up.

Some hints for making it work: If you're hurried, be sure you and your partner dress for speed by forgoing undies and any garments with complicated buttons or zippers. If you're standing, rear-entry sex will usually work best, especially if you can get your partner to lean forward, bracing herself on a wall, desk, or tree.

2. **Look elsewhere for stimulation.** Most men don't realize how sensitive the male breast can be. The fact is, her breasts and yours are remarkably similar. "The only real difference in breast construction between the sexes is the amount of glandular and fat tissue," says Sondra Lynne Carter, M.D., a gynecologist in New York City.

3. **Get stand-up erections.** "We routinely ask our impotent patients to stand when we administer erection-causing drugs, simply because gravity improves bloodflow to the penis and helps harden erections in some men," says Wayne Hellstrom, M.D., associate professor of urology at Tulane University in New Orleans. It may also intensify orgasms by increasing muscle tension in the pelvis.

4. **Plan sex all day.** Virtually all of us, including many who say they aren't often turned on, experience surges of sexual energy during the day. The key to firing up your libido is to hang on to these surges for a few seconds each time they hit, says Bernie Zilbergeld, Ph.D., a San Francisco sex therapist and author of *The New Male Sexuality*. The next time something you see, hear, smell, or remember causes a twinge of desire, let your imagination roam. Imagine the feel of your partner's lips, hands, breasts, or vagina. Mentally recreate the texture, the temperature, the way your bodies connect. An hour or two later, close your eyes and recall that image for a few seconds. Continue in this way every hour or two during the day, whenever you have seconds to "simmer."

5. **Keep your eye on the balls.** It's a real mistake to neglect your testicles. "The skin that covers the scrotum is made from the same embryonic tissue that, in women, forms the outer vaginal lips. There are a lot of nerve endings there," says Barbara Keesling, Ph.D., a sex therapist in Orange, California, and author of *Super Sexual Orgasm*. Some experts even speculate that gently massaging the testicles may help increase testosterone production.

6. **Use common scents.** Just the smell of certain foods and flowers can increase bloodflow to your genitalia, says Alan R. Hirsch, M.D., neurological director of the Smell and Taste Treatment and Research Foundation in Chicago and author of *Scentsational Sex*. His study found that for men, the magic scents are pumpkin pie, black licorice, and oranges, each of which increases bloodflow to the penis by 20 to 40 percent. For her, try cucumber and Good & Plenty licorice candy.

"Eating these foods is by far the most efficient way to introduce them to the nose, and the effects occur within about a minute," says Dr. Hirsch. Since more blood to your genitals could mean improved sensation, make a well-planned pre-sex snack part of your ritual.

7. **Have a tall one.** When you were younger, you downed a beer or two to help you prepare for sex. Now you know better. Alcohol can act as a depressant and may make it more difficult for you to get an erection. Instead, drink a tall glass of water about 30 minutes before calling it a night. "It sounds almost too good to be true, but this simple step could make all the difference in getting and maintaining an erection," says Earl Mindell, R.Ph., Ph.D., professor of nutrition at Pacific Western University in Los Angeles.

8. **Get a leg up.** Research has shown that one of the most favored sexual positions is a version of the missionary position that has you placing your legs outside your partner's legs instead of between them. On a scale of 1 to 10, men rate this a 9.5 for pleasure (because her vagina is tight) and women rate it an 8.5 (since muscle tension is increased when her legs are flat and together).

One word of advice: A dab of lubricant will help prevent her pubic hair from irritating the shaft of your penis.

9. **Find your rhythm.** The key to a good sexual rhythm is finding a thrusting pattern that alternates several shallow thrusts with every deep one. It's a matter of pneumatics, says Douglas Abrams Arava, a San Francisco–based expert in ancient sexuality and coauthor of *The Multi-Orgasmic Man*. "Every deep thrust pushes air out of the vagina, creating a vacuum that the shallow thrusts intensify," he explains. Start with one deep thrust for every five to seven shallow strokes, and as your arousal levels build, add more and more deep thrusts to the mix. Be sure to keep an inch or so of your penis inside her at all times to avoid breaking the seal of the vacuum.

10. **Exercise together.** There's no better aphrodisiac than an invigorating workout. Aerobic activity, such as running, bicycling, or swimming, increases brain activity in the left hemisphere and produces feel-good chemicals called endorphins. Catch that biochemical wave, and you'll increase your desire, arousal, and orgasm intensity, according to Linda DeVillers, Ph.D., a sex therapist and author of *Love Skills*.

1 1. **Put time on your side.** The secret to good "handy" foreplay, say Robert and Leah Schwartz, authors of *The One Hour Orgasm*, is to pretend that her clitoris is a clock. Your finger is the hour hand. After using a gentle up-and-down motion to get her relaxed and excited, place your finger at the 10 o'clock position. Stroke gently, working toward 1 o'clock (that's most women's most sensitive spot). If she's very aroused, the head of her clitoris may be too sensitive to stimulate directly. In that case, play your clock game with the clitoral hood down.

1 2. **Enjoy an occasional quickie.** Remember, not every sexual encounter has to be long and drawn out. Even if your lives are hectic, you could be overlooking opportunities if you tune out sexual thoughts unless the time and place are "right." Be open to spontaneous overtures, and don't worry if she doesn't have an orgasm. Many women don't mind having sex every now and then without climax.

1 3. **Sweeten your semen.** If your mate objects to the taste of your seminal fluid, you might try skipping the spices and bringing on the fruit. Although sour semen can be caused by a prostate infection, it's usually the result of favoring highly acidic foods (tomatoes, tomato sauce) or spicy fare (onions, garlic, oregano, thyme, basil) or of drinking lots of caffeinated beverages or alcohol.

On the other hand, men with diets high in natural sugars, especially fruits, are reportedly blessed with sweeter seminal fluids, says Judith Seifer, Ph.D., past president of the American Association of Sex Educators, Counselors, and Therapists. Since the effect of what you eat takes roughly 12 to 24 hours to show up in your semen, make eating fruit a habit.

1 4. **Care for your glans.** If you're without a foreskin, exposure to the elements might be taking its toll on the head of your penis, reducing its sensitivity. The foreskin's first duty is to keep the glans soft and supple. You can't grow a new foreskin, but you can replicate its effects with simple moisturizing hand lotion. Look for a brand free of potentially irritating perfumes or additives. Also wear comfortable, absorbent cotton underwear, and to prevent chafing, use plenty of lubricant during sex.

1 5. **Please your prostate.** There's a simple, fail-safe sexual technique that can result in longer, stronger, harder erections and explosively pleasurable orgasms. The catch: It's a little hard to reach.

The nerves surrounding your prostate are hot-wired to your penis: When you massage the gland, you may actually feel the pleasure in your penis, says John D. Perry, Ph.D., coauthor of *The G-Spot*. You or your partner can massage your prostate indirectly by pressing firmly on the stretch of skin between the base of your scrotum and your anus.

16. **Ride high.** The coital alignment technique (CAT) may not have a sexy name, but don't let that throw you. When couples make love in this position, 90 percent report more intense orgasms, and 60 percent say it boosts their libidos.

Starting from the missionary position, slowly slide forward so you're "riding high" with your pelvis slightly above hers. This puts the shaft of your penis in touch with her clitoris and puts pressure on the base of your penis, indirectly stimulating your sensitive prostate. Relax your upper body, lowering it onto her torso and releasing the tension in your shoulders and neck. Rather than thrust, the two of you simply rock back and forth: She tips her pelvis up, and you push with just enough force to tip it back down. She should focus on directing her swing so she feels pressure on her clitoris.

17. **Use condom sense.** Every guy who's ever fumbled with a condom can vouch for the fact that they're real mood dampeners, or worse, erection dampeners. So before you even unbutton her blouse, carefully rip open the foil wrapper and lay the rolled condom on top. If it's cold, warm the condom by lightly breathing on it, or ask your partner to snuggle it between her thighs until it's room temperature. Then, when you're fully erect and ready for penetration, place a dab or two of water-based (never oil-based, since it weakens the condom) lubricant in the centermost inside part of the rolled-up condom. This extra lubricant will encourage the latex near the head to slide around in a pleasurable way.

18. **Play with toys.** One of the best ways to electrify your sex life? Use batteries. No longer the mark of lonely, raincoat-clad men, sex toys are most often used by married, monogamous couples who already enjoy pretty good sex, according to surveys.

19. **Tell her what you want.** Too often, compatible partners end up having mediocre sex because they assume sex is supposed to happen "naturally," without any need for words. That's not how it works. Remember, she will never know exactly what it's like to have a penis, just as you'll never really understand the clitoris. The next time she's missing the mark, employ one of these subtle tactics to get her back on track.

- Share your dreams. She can't blame you for what you dream. If you've been aching to try something new but think it's too kinky to ask for straight up, start with, "I had the craziest dream last night. . . ." Gauge her reaction, and if she's game, bring the dream to life.

• Talk dirty. Don't be afraid to speak during sex. As long as you're not acting like a drill sergeant in bed, she'll probably appreciate a few pointers on technique. And don't forget that well-placed moans, sighs, and screams can work even better than words. "Most men dramatically underdo sounds of pleasure," says Dr. DeVillers.

20. **Just let it happen.** A simple technique to make orgasms more intense: Let them be. As you feel yourself approaching climax, keep focused and maintain your rhythm, but resist the urge to clench down or speed up. "Let it come to you rather than chasing it," advises Edward W. Eichel, the psychotherapist who invented the coital alignment technique. Those who have experimented with the technique say that a "letting it just happen" approach to orgasm yields powerful results for both partners.

4

WEIGHT LOSS

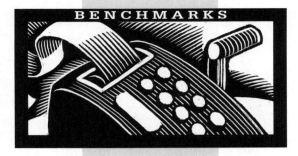

BENCHMARKS

■ Chance that an American adult is obese: 1 in 4

■ Percentage of men between the ages of 20 and 34 who are overweight: 22.8

■ Between ages 35 and 44: 35.7

■ Quarts of ice cream eaten by the average Southerner each year: 12

■ By the average New Englander: 23

■ Number of men who suffocated as a result of obesity in a 1-year period: 705

■ Number of calories burned in an average kiss: 9

■ Average number of calories an executive burns in an hour working in his office: 105

■ Number of calories in 1 pound of fat: 3,500

■ The average American man's percentage of body fat: 18

■ Muscle burns 17 to 25 times as many calories as fat

■ Number of pounds typically gained each year after age 40: 1 to 2

■ Average number of pounds gained by Americans between Thanksgiving and New Year's: 6

■ Number of pounds a 170-pound man can lose in 1 year by taking his dog for a 20-minute walk every day: 7

■ By pedaling a stationary bike at a moderate pace for an hour every day: 19

■ Number of calories the American College of Sports Medicine recommends burning per week for weight loss: 1,000 to 2,000

■ Typical number of pounds lost in 1 day by college football players during two-a-day workouts: 7

■ Estimated percentage of American fifth graders who are overweight: 33

■ Percentage of men who lie about their weight: 11

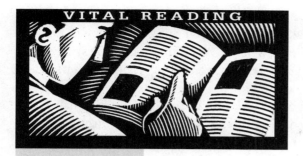

Lose It for Good

Seven roadblocks to shedding weight, and how to get past them.

Day after day, you do everything you can to exhaust, expunge, excommunicate, and exile the fat around your midsection. And morning after morning, you wake up to find it's still there.

But are you really doing all you can to lose it? Some experts point out the following seven ways in which men routinely give themselves the middle linger. Start now, and you can count your losses this week and beyond.

Beware the Too-Restrictive Diet Plan

If your eating plan doesn't fit you and your food preferences, your diet is done for. "People sabotage their weight-control efforts when they deprive themselves too much," says Anne Fletcher, R.D., a registered dietitian and author of *Thin for Life* and *Eating Thin for Life*. "They deny themselves and obsess about it. It's better to give in occasionally and indulge within reason. In fact, you should plan for it."

Fletcher studied 208 weight-loss "masters" who had lost at least 20 pounds each and kept it off for 3 or more years. She found that most of these people were particularly good at one thing: dealing with cravings. Here's how the best weight losers deliver themselves not into temptation.

Use stopgap measures. Create a system for limiting the amount of fun foods you eat at a time—buying 1 to 2 ounces of candy instead of a bag, for example, or buying the smallest container of ice cream as opposed to an industrial drum.

Make trade-offs. If you decide to eat a slice or two of deep-dish pepperoni pizza, give up something else high in fat you were going to eat that day.

Don't even start. Although it makes sense to allow yourself treats occasionally, more than half of the best weight losers just avoid the foods that they know will trigger an orgy of overeating.

Don't Work Out Just So You Can Pig Out

If you're like many physically active men, you think that going to the gym regularly will keep you from gaining weight. "We call it the 'gym-fix syndrome,' " says James Kenney, R.D., Ph.D., nutrition-research specialist at the Pritikin Longevity Center in Santa Monica, California.

Let's say you go to the gym after work. You warm up by walking half a mile on the treadmill. You've burned 50 calories. (We're assuming throughout this example that you weigh 190 pounds. You'll burn more if you weigh more, less if you weigh less.) Then you run 2 miles at a 7-minute-mile pace. That's 275 calories. You follow that with 20 minutes of weight training, burning 200 calories more. You've completed a great workout and burned 525 calories. Good for you.

Then you stop on the way home for a burger, fries, and a shake. In 5 to 10 minutes, you throw down 1,200 calories—more than twice what you burned in an hour at the gym. Some men can get away with this because of youth, genetics, or massive amounts of calorie-consuming muscle. The average guy can't.

"Fast food is such a concentrated source of energy, it's like rocket fuel," says Dr. Kenney. "The problem with most Americans is that they eat rocket fuel and then they sit on the launchpad."

Here are three suggestions on how to buy satisfying post-workout food from a drive-thru window. (You'll probably need two servings to feel full, but keep in mind that the nutrition information that follows is based on only one.)

McDonald's. Eat the Grilled Chicken Deluxe (300 calories, 5 grams of fat if you request it without mayonnaise, 27 grams of protein). Avoid the Quarter Pounder with Cheese (530 calories, 30 grams of fat, 28 grams of protein).

Arby's. Eat the Roast Turkey Deluxe Light sandwich (260 calories, 7 grams of fat, 20 grams of protein). Avoid the Bac'n Cheddar Deluxe sandwich (539 calories, 34 grams of fat, 22 grams of protein).

Taco Bell. Eat the Grilled Chicken Burrito (410 calories, 15 grams of fat, 17 grams of protein). Avoid the Mexican Pizza (570 calories, 35 grams of fat, 16 grams of protein).

Don't Replace Calories You Didn't Burn

Sports drinks and sports bars are fixtures in health clubs today. But unless you skip a meal somewhere, the drinks and bars will add hundreds of calories to your daily intake. "If you're doing extreme endurance sports in hot weather, you may need them," says Ross E. Andersen, Ph.D., a weight-loss researcher at Johns Hopkins University in Baltimore. "But if you're eating a well-balanced diet, with fruits and vegetables and lots of fluids, there shouldn't be a need for these types of replacements."

Remember, water quenches thirst, and there's nothing an energy bar can give you that you can't take in from real food.

Acknowledge That You Might Not Exercise Enough

The majority of the men in the National Weight-Control Registry—a study of people who have lost 30 pounds or more and kept it off for at least a year—burn 2,000 or more calories a week through exercise. For a 190-pound man, that means running or walking a little more than 13 miles.

The sort-of-bad news is that some men do become fit enough to run those miles, but they still don't lose all the weight they would like to lose. Indeed, exercise has a point of diminishing returns for weight loss. "The first 500 calories you burn daily will have a major impact on your body weight," says Dr. Kenney. "The second will have less. The third probably won't have any. You're just increasing your risk of an exercise-related injury."

If you get to the point in your exercise program where you're burning more than 1,000 calories in a single workout and you still haven't lost as much weight as you'd hoped, don't sweat it. "As long as you maintain your fitness, being a little bit overweight doesn't affect your mortality very much," says Larry Gibbons, M.D., president and medical director of the Cooper Clinic in Dallas. "If you lose weight through exercise, that's great. But if you don't, don't lose sleep over it."

On the other hand, if you don't burn anything close to 2,000 calories a week during exercise, you should probably start sweating it. Now.

Are You the Accidental Fat Guy?

Sometimes you take in almost as many calories by accident as you do on purpose. Do any of these describe you?

- You work in an office in which every employee's birthday is celebrated with cake, and it wouldn't be friendly to skip the festivities. One large slice of cake: 300 to 400 unexpected calories.
- Your planning meeting runs through the lunch hour. The boss sends out for pizza. Even though you normally have a turkey sandwich for lunch, you don't think it would be good for your career to eat something other than what the boss is having. Half a pizza might be 800 to 1,000 calories—that's twice as many as your sandwich has.

- One of your co-workers keeps a bowl of candy outside her cubicle. You can't stop by to say hello without grabbing a handful. Four bite-size pieces of chocolate: 200 or more calories.
- Your kids never finish their Chicken McNuggets and french fries. Rather than throwing the food into the trash, you gobble it. Three congealed nuggets and half a small order of fries: 250 calories.
- You're hanging out with some friends on a Sunday afternoon, watching the Packers demolish the hometown 11. Somehow the chip bowl ends up in front of you. "You down about 750 calories without blinking an eye," says Georgia Kostas, R.D., a registered dietitian and nutrition director at the Cooper Clinic. She calculates an average of 50 chips per sitting, at 15 calories a chip.

In each of these situations, there's some pressure to eat what everyone else is eating. So what's a weight-conscious guy to do? "Make some adjustments later on," says Penny Kris-Etherton, Ph.D., R.D., nutrition professor at Pennsylvania State University in University Park. "If you eat cake at work, skip dessert that night." If you eat more than you expected to at lunch, eat less than you normally would at dinnertime.

Handle Holiday Bingeing

There is a way to control your eating during the holidays: Keep a food diary. In one study, participants were encouraged to keep one through Thanksgiving, Christmas, and New Year's Day, and also for 7 nonholiday weeks. Overall, the participants gained 500 percent more weight during holiday weeks than during nonholiday weeks, but the best monitors—those who recorded most of what they ate—actually managed to lose weight through the holidays.

If you decide to keep a food diary, here's what to record in it.
- What you eat
- When you eat it
- How much of it you eat
- How many calories and fat grams the food contains (If you don't have time to look these figures up, estimate.)

You Might Be Cutting Fat, but Not Calories

The 155 men in the National Weight-Control Registry keep the fat in their diets below the recommended maximum of 30 percent of total calories. Still, if you're cutting fat but not losing weight, maybe you've fallen into the old trap:

Some men simply replace high-fat foods with greater volumes of low-fat stuff, rewarding themselves with a box of low-fat cookies because they passed on a doughnut. "Calories are the bottom line," says Barbara Rolls, Ph.D., professor of nutrition at Pennsylvania State University. "If you're going to lose weight, you have to eat fewer calories."

Here are three ways to cut fat and calories.

1. Eat soup or a salad, which take up stomach space and make you feel full.
2. Eat the food you want in its least-processed state—a whole baked potato instead of french fries, or fresh or frozen corn instead of corn chips, for example. You'll be able to eat more while taking in fewer calories.
3. Eat fruits and vegetables at every meal. They fill you up and are loaded with vitamins and other nutrients.

Take Your Choice

There are really only three ways to lose weight.

For all the hoo-ha over stomach stapling and cabbage-soup diets and good old-fashioned drugs, there are only three safe, effective, and realistic ways to lose weight: eat less, exercise more, or eat less and exercise more. Studies have found that all three methods work, at least temporarily, so the important questions are: Which one will work best for you? And which one will give you the best shot at permanent weight loss?

Here's a look at the big three and what each requires to help you lose weight and keep it off.

Exercise Only

Ever had a super-buff friend who worked out 2 hours a day so he could eat anything he wanted and never gain weight? No matter how much you resent him, your fit friend is onto something. Exercise burns calories. Burn more calories than you consume, and you lose weight. If you work off 3,500 more calories than your body absorbs, you've lost a pound. Since most men burn between 100 and 130 calories per mile when walking or running (doesn't matter which you do; running simply gets you through the mile faster), all you need to do to lose a pound is walk or run 27 to 35 miles. Easy, huh?

Let's do the math: If you walk for an hour a day and cover 3 miles during that hour, you burn . . . well, you don't burn much—between 300 and 400 calories. Even if you do that every day, you're going to lose less than a pound a week.

So chances are, your eating-with-impunity friend does some combination of strength training and aerobic exercise. That changes the equation. Weight lifting burns some calories, but the real benefits occur after you've finished your workout. Here's how.

The muscles you build in the weight room use more calories on a minute-to-minute basis than fat does. A pound of fat might need only a calorie or two to maintain itself during an average day, but a pound of lean muscle needs 35 to 50 calories. Let's say that, over the course of a year, you put on 10 pounds of muscle. That muscle could burn 350 to 500 calories a day just by being on your body. That's more than a pound of fat every month.

Be forewarned: Since muscle is denser than fat, you may actually put on some pounds as you begin building your body. But don't worry; the newly added muscle takes up less space than fat, so you will actually look firmer.

Here's how the exercise-only plan stacks up.

Difficulty: high. The biggest weight-loss benefits come from training longer, harder, or both. "Think of how hard it is to burn 1,000 calories versus how easy it is to eat 1,000 calories," points out Dixie Stanforth, a lecturer in the department of kinesiology at the University of Texas at Austin.

Speed of weight loss: slow to very slow. To lose a pound a week with aerobic exercise, the average guy will need to devote more than an hour a day, 7 days a week. Losing weight by lifting weights is even slower, since the real benefits don't kick in until you've built a considerable amount of muscle. If you combine the two, the time frame for weight loss will be somewhere in the middle.

Sustainability of weight loss: very high if you continue your exercise program, very low if you abandon it. About 50 percent of those who start an exercise program abandon it within 6 months, according to Stanforth.

Diet Only

The previous section may have stopped you cold with the time it requires. Sure, you could work out for an hour a day—but when the heck would you do your job, speak to your wife, play with your kids, and download pictures of Alyssa Milano? If your life is truly that overbooked, you may be tempted to try to lose 10 pounds by merely altering your diet.

You can do this quickly, or you can do it slowly. "A typical man can lose 10 pounds in a 4-day fast," says Michael Hewitt, Ph.D., director of exercise physiology at the Canyon Ranch spa in Tucson.

Sound good? Here's why it's not: Of those 10 pounds, only 2 are fat. The rest of the weight is water, which your body will quickly regain. Another problem is that all diets, including fasting, make you feel deprived, and that's a difficult way to live long-term. Also, a calorie-depriving diet tends to make your body think it's starving. One of the ways your body reacts is to feed off your muscles.

It gets worse. In the previous section, you saw how building muscle increases your metabolism—the speed with which your body uses energy on a minute-to-minute basis. Losing muscle has the opposite effect: Your body's metabolic rate downshifts, and any food you eat after you go off the strict diet is actually more likely to be stored as fat than it was before. How's that for a deal? You starve yourself, and you end up fatter.

Still, the diet-alone method does have its proponents, as long as the dietary changes aren't too radical. "I wouldn't cut more than 500 calories out of the daily diet," says Wayne C. Miller, Ph.D., professor of exercise science and nutrition at George Washington University Medical Center in Washington, D.C. Since it's roughly the equivalent of a large bag of french fries, 500 calories a day doesn't seem so unreasonable, especially if your current eating habits aren't particularly ascetic.

You say you don't eat fast food and you still can't lose weight? There are other dietary modifications almost any guy can make. Drinking diet soda instead of regular Coke or Pepsi might save several hundred calories a day (each serving has about 156 calories). Putting mustard on your sandwich instead of mayonnaise could save close to 100 calories. Drinking light beer instead of Swamp Turkey Dark Deeds Amber could save you about 50 calories per round.

Difficulty: moderate. Almost anyone can psych himself up enough to eat less for a short period of time.

Speed of weight loss: fast to very fast, especially at first. Many gimmick diets—for example, those that encourage a very high protein intake—will cause you to lose a lot of water weight initially, which looks great on the scale.

Sustainability of weight loss: very low. Eventually, you'll eat a piece of chocolate cake at a birthday party, or drink a few beers and then go to White Castle and order some cheese fries. You'll get sick of going to restaurants with friends and being the only one to ask for dressing on the side. Small wonder that short-term diets fail more than 95 percent of the time.

Diet Plus Exercise

The obvious conclusion is that if you take something from column A and something from column B—say, you burn 250 calories a day exercising and eat 250 fewer calories a day—you can lose a pound a week without living at the gym or suffering the indignity of life without pizza. On top of that, you look better because exercise has given you some muscle to replace the lost fat.

Unfortunately, exercise plus diet isn't the miracle weight-loss method you might think. When Dr. Miller analyzed 25 years of weight-loss research, he found that dieters lost about 23.5 pounds in 15 weeks while dieters who exercised lost 24.2 pounds in 13½ weeks. Better, but not overwhelmingly better. In one 8-week study, dieters lost the same amount of weight—about 10 pounds—whether or not they exercised.

So why does almost everyone recommend the deluxe combo for weight loss? Because if you want to stay slim, nothing else comes close to working as well.

Mary Lou Klem, Ph.D., heads up research for the National Weight-Control Registry, the largest continuing study of weight losers. In her study, she says, "nearly 90 percent of successful losers used both diet and exercise to get the weight off and keep it off."

"In the long run, most forms of exercise tend to reduce appetite," notes Stanforth, although she suspects the biggest motivation to keep weight off is the memory of what came before. "You feel better, you look better, and you know what it's like not to feel that way."

Here's the final tally on diet plus exercise.

Difficulty: moderate. You don't have to become a bodybuilder or marathoner to make this work. You don't have to starve yourself or deprive yourself of your favorite foods. But you do have to exercise discipline and moderation: Order a mushroom pizza instead of double-cheese and pepperoni or take a trip to the gym instead of having lunch out with your co-workers. You don't have to exercise an hour or more a day, but you do have to fit in about 30 to 45 minutes' worth, four or five times a week.

Speed of weight loss: moderately fast. If you spend a lot of your exercise time in the weight room, you'll still have to deal with the fact that the added muscle will slow down overall weight loss. And if you don't spend time in the weight room, you may be disappointed that the weight you lose comes from everywhere—including your chest and shoulders—making you thinner but perhaps not as athletic-looking as you'd like.

Sustainability of weight loss: very high. That is, if you stick with the program.

The Best for Less

To make the diet-plus-exercise plan work, aim to lose about 12 to 16 ounces per week—in other words, a pound a week at most. "It takes time to change your lifestyle, and weight loss will follow that," says G. Ken Goodrick, Ph.D., assistant professor of medicine at Baylor College of Medicine in Houston and coauthor of *Living without Dieting.* This combo plan will empower you to shake those pounds and keep them off for good.

"Guys shouldn't worry about counting calories," says Dr. Goodrick. "They should really try to eat foods that are low in sugar and fat. I wouldn't ask any guy to count calories—unless he's an accountant."

These are the guidelines Dr. Goodrick recommends.

- Increase your fiber intake. High-fiber cereals and whole grains make you feel fuller longer.
- Eat more fruits and vegetables.
- Make complex carbohydrates (whole-grain breads, pasta, rice, and spuds) the centerpiece of every meal.
- Eliminate foods that are high in saturated fat and refined sugar.
- Eat moderate-size portions, not servings that would stuff Henry VIII.

We asked Dr. Hewitt to put together a sample program. This workout schedule is ideal for men who are used to exercising and playing sports.

Monday
Cardio: 40 minutes
Strength: none
Flexibility: 51 minutes

Tuesday
Cardio: 20 minutes
Strength: 20 minutes
Flexibility: 51 minutes

Wednesday
Rest

Thursday
Cardio: 20 minutes
Strength: 20 minutes
Flexibility: 51 minutes

Friday
Cardio: 40 minutes
Strength: none
Flexibility: 51 minutes

Saturday
Cardio: 90 minutes
Strength: 20 minutes
Flexibility: 51 minutes

Sunday
Rest

To ensure that you get the maximum benefit from exercise, here are some guidelines to follow.

Cardiovascular exercise: During the 20-minute sessions, do something strenuous—running, cycling, rowing—so that you burn about 300 calories. For example, a 175-pound man running 9-minute miles burns 18.4 calories per minute. In 20 minutes, that's 368 calories burned.

For the 40-minute workouts, you can do something that's pure cardio or something more playful, such as pickup basketball, tennis, or inline skating. Aim to burn 400 to 700 calories.

For the 90-minute Saturday session, do something fun, like taking a long hike or bike ride, sea kayaking, or playing golf (walk the course and carry your clubs).

Strength: Concentrate on the major muscle groups (legs, back, chest), since you're trying to increase muscle mass. You can work the smaller, vanity muscles (biceps, triceps, calves) after you've lost the weight.

Do six or seven exercises using either free weights or machines. Do 2 or 3 sets of each exercise with a weight that's heavy enough to fatigue your muscles within 8 to 12 repetitions.

Flexibility: Identify the four or five stretches that are most challenging for you. (Hint: Most men have incredibly tight hamstrings.) Perform these stretches at the end of every workout, holding each one for 30 seconds.

A limited number of stretches done consistently is far more effective than 20 stretches done once in a while, Dr. Hewitt says.

Workouts for Your Stomach

Fill up and watch the pounds disappear.

Your stomach is a good employee, but it's a lousy boss. When you're giving it orders about when to work and what to do, it serves your nutritional needs well. But when your gut is growling demands for increased overtime and cheaper raw materials, it only fattens your bottom line. And in this case, that's a bad thing. What you need are strategies to make sure your stomach is working for you, not vice versa.

Though plenty of physical and psychological factors are involved in hunger—for instance, the speed with which the body uses food, the efficiency of glucose use, and external cues—there's probably no single reason for your emptiness between meals. You're eating enough to keep yourself alive. Heck, you're probably eating enough to keep your entire family alive. You simply don't feel full between one meal and the next.

The eight eating strategies listed below can help in that department, filling you up without popping the top button on your Dockers. Try all eight as a day-long meal plan, or learn why each suggested food fills you up, so you can achieve the same effect with other foods.

You may find yourself missing the social scene around the pastry cart and the candy machine. But trust us—the attention drawn by your lean and not-so-hungry body will make up for it.

Strategy #1: Boost Your Fiber

Increasing your fiber consumption is the best way to stifle belly growl. Fiber, ounce for ounce, is probably the single most filling food item you can consume. For one thing, foods rich in fiber generally have to be chewed more and take longer to consume, so your brain has time to realize that you're eating and turns off the hunger switch sooner. Then, once it's in your stomach, fiber takes up a lot of space, making you feel full. This feeling stays with you longer because fiber takes more time to travel through the long and winding road of your digestive tract than most foods do.

"As fiber works to move things through the gut, it actually attracts water from other points in the body, and that requires some time," says Leslie Bonci, R.D., a registered dietitian at Allegheny General Hospital in Pittsburgh and a spokeswoman for the American Dietetic Association. This "water drain" means that you have to drink more when you eat high-fiber foods. Those extra fluids you take in, meanwhile, will also help your body hold on to that filled-up feeling.

Ask an expert which food makes you feel the fullest, and chances are, the answer will be oatmeal. Oatmeal is a soluble fiber, which means that it attracts fluid and stays in the stomach longer than insoluble fiber. It's generally served hot, which slows down the digestive process further, and it takes up a lot of room. In addition, a recent study at Pennsylvania State University in University Park has shown that oatmeal sustains your blood sugar levels longer than many other foods, which means it won't leave you jittery and ravenous just about the time the snack cart rolls around.

Practical advice:
- Eat old-fashioned oatmeal instead of the chopped-up, ready-in-a-minute variety. Less refinement means that your body will have to work a little harder to process the food. (If you have a microwave, even the slow kind of oatmeal cooks in 3 minutes or less.)
- Cook a half-cup of oats according to the package directions, then top it with 4 ounces of skim milk and a tablespoon of brown sugar.

Alternatives: Other foods with different flavors and textures from oatmeal have many of its benefits. Cold oat cereals are good substitutes, as are cereals made from barley. The less processed the cereal, the better; stay away from puffed or sugary cereals.

Strategy #2: Pick Fruit

If you eat a grapefruit with your oatmeal, you'll be adding the benefits of an entirely different fiber, called pectin, which has an almost magical ability to make you feel less hungry throughout the day. In a recent study reported in the *Journal of the American College of Nutrition*, subjects drank plain orange juice or orange juice spiked with pectin for breakfast. The people who got the loaded juice felt fuller after drinking it than those who got the juice without pectin, and the difference between the two groups persisted for more than 4 hours. It didn't take much, either: People who consumed as little as 5 grams of pectin felt just as full as people who glugged down 20. (A grapefruit has slightly more than 3 grams.)

Practical advice:

- Pawn your serrated grapefruit spoon. Much of grapefruit's fiber is in its white pith, so peel the fruit and eat it as you would an orange. For the same reason, grapefruit juice isn't as filling as the fruit itself.

Alternatives: When you get sick of grapefruit, substitute another fruit, such as an orange, an apple, a peach, or strawberries, all of which contain pectin.

Strategy #3: Make Sure You're Satisfied

If you start your day with a bowl of oatmeal and a grapefruit, you're getting lots of carbohydrates but not much of the protein that is far more satiating. "Your metabolism adjusts very rapidly to changes in protein intake," says Richard Mattes, R.D., Ph.D., professor of foods and nutrition at Purdue University in West Lafayette, Indiana.

Practical advice:

- Spread 2 tablespoons of peanut butter on a slice of whole-wheat toast for breakfast, or smear it on celery for a snack if your energy level heads south around midmorning. (Psychological benefit: You'll work so hard chewing the celery and peanut butter that you may be able to convince yourself you're burning more calories than you're taking in.)
- If you prefer to go for genuine peanut butter rather than the reduced-fat version, it won't be a dietary disaster. The overall calories are almost the same; the low-fat spread contains fewer calories from fat, but makes up for that with more sugar than the regular stuff.

Alternatives: A slice of light cheese, such as Swiss or provolone, is a good substitute topping for your bread.

Strategy #4: Eat the Right Kind of Fat

Okay, maybe it's a little weird to be recommending fat in a nutrition article. But some studies are now suggesting that fat signals your body to take a longer break between meals, according to Barbara Rolls, Ph.D., professor of nutrition at Pennsylvania State University in University Park. And hey, it doesn't bother us.

The key is a substance called cholecystokinin, also known as CCK. This acronym may look like it belongs on the jersey of an East European hockey player, but CCK is actually a hormone in your small intestine that creates satiety, the feeling that your needs have been fulfilled. (Your dietary needs, anyway; other needs have their own hormones.) Carbohydrates, protein, and fat all trigger the release of CCK, but fat is the most effective trigger.

Cheese quesadillas make a good example for our purposes; they're easy and quick to prepare, and they're a "combo food"—they contain plenty of carbohydrates, protein, and fat.

Practical advice:
- To make cheese quesadillas, melt ½ cup of shredded cheese between two 6-inch corn tortillas. Top it off with ¼ cup of salsa. Skip the sour cream. You don't need to release that much CCK.
- Don't make cheese quesadillas at home to reheat later for lunch; you'll end up with something about as appealing as an oily rag. Instead, pack the tortillas and cheese separately (buying grated cheese will save time and make cleanup easier), and stash a bottle of salsa in the office refrigerator. The lunchroom microwave will have them ready in seconds.
- In a hurry? Drive to Taco Bell and have their quesadillas, even though they're made with flour tortillas instead of the slightly bulkier corn variety.

Alternatives: Stuff 3 ounces of water-packed tuna into a 6-inch piece of pita bread for a lunch alternative that's easier to make, with many of the same benefits. If the tuna cries out to you for moisture, soothe it with 1 tablespoon of light mayo.

Strategy #5: Soup Up Your Meals

Many people see soup as an unsatisfying and spectacularly unexciting food—the nutritional analogue of a PG-13 sex scene. But a hearty soup such as beef minestrone can do a fine job of filling you up. Like oatmeal, a vegetable-bean soup has plenty of fiber, so it stays with you for a while. The beans and beef stock provide protein. And heck, there's just a lot of it. "It conveys some satiety immediately because it takes up a lot of room in the gut," says Bonci, "and it continues to convey it for a longer period of time because of the fiber and protein it contains."

Practical advice:
- No need to make homemade soup; Campbell's or Progresso is just fine, according to Bonci. With a can opener, a bowl, and a microwave, you can have it ready in a couple of minutes.

Alternatives: Other filling soups include beef barley, potato, black bean, lentil, and split pea. You get the idea.

Strategy #6: Have a Good Stiff Drink

Like soup, a fruit smoothie is a liquid-food hybrid that takes up a lot of internal real estate but doesn't add too many calories to your daily tally. You're probably not going to scarf down a smoothie in one or two gulps, as you would a bag of M&M's or some other sugary snack, so your body has time to realize that it's being fed. And the fiber in the fruit makes it hang around a while in your belly.

Practical advice:

- To make a strawberry-banana smoothie, blend together 8 ounces of nonfat vanilla yogurt, ½ cup of frozen or fresh unsweetened strawberries, a small banana, and 4 ounces of orange juice. When you're finished, this will blend down to about a 12-ounce drink.
- You can make your smoothie at home and drink it in the office, but store it in a Thermos or some other insulated container so it stays cool (courtesy of the frozen strawberries) until you're ready for it.
- Commercially made smoothies work just as well, but be sure to choose ones that include low-fat or nonfat yogurt or milk, not regular yogurt or ice cream.
- Size counts. An 8- to 12-ounce smoothie is a good snack. Beyond that, your calorie count really starts climbing.

Alternatives: If you want a dessertlike snack, frozen yogurt or a Creamsicle won't kill you in the calorie department. Those who don't mind sticking to the fruit route can snack on cottage cheese and fruit. (Low-fat cottage cheese is best.)

Strategy #7: Take Your Time

Too many of the foods you can order for dinner are just too easy to eat. A juicy burger on a soft white bun, the whole production dripping with secret sauce, can be inhaled in a minute or less. But unless you're a sword swallower, you'll have to take your time with cubes of chicken breast barbecued on skewers.

"You rarely see someone overindulge in a high-protein, high-carbohydrate food like white-meat chicken," notes Dr. Mattes. Add some grilled vegetables, and you have a satisfying high-protein, high-fiber dinner. If you marinate the kebabs in vinegar and olive oil before you grill them, you'll win the nutritional trifecta of protein, carbohydrate, and fat.

Practical advice:
- Marinate 6 ounces of cubed boneless, skinless chicken breast plus vegetables (zucchini, red pepper, mushrooms, onions, cherry tomatoes, and broccoli are all popular choices) in ¼ cup of light vinaigrette. The chicken may take longer to cook, so put the meat and vegetables on separate skewers. Grill on your barbecue.
- If you're short on time, buy precut vegetables, or stick to ones that don't need to be sliced, such as mushrooms, cherry tomatoes, and baby squash.

Alternatives: You can do a lot of things with the same basic ingredients. How about a nice stir-fry of chicken and vegetables, served over rice or pasta? Or chicken fajitas? Or chicken and vegetables in pita bread?

Strategy #8: Go for the Spuds

A baked potato makes a nice complement to kebabs, for several reasons. First, it has two kinds of fiber: soluble in the "meat" of the spud, and insoluble in the skin. Soluble fiber, like that in oatmeal, is the whistle-stop campaigner of the nutritional world. It moves slowly through your digestive system, making lots of new friends and taking them along. Insoluble fiber is a plant-based conquistador. It just wants to carve a path from here to there and is willing to bludgeon into submission anything that gets in its way. Insoluble fiber doesn't stick around as long, but that's not a bad thing: It keeps things moving in the digestive system, preventing constipation.

A baked potato with a low-fat or fat-free topping has a low energy density (few calories for its weight). Researchers are realizing that energy density plays an important role in satiety. "This energy-density idea is new, and there are a lot of studies in progress right now trying to tease it out," says Dr. Rolls. One study that she recently conducted suggests that consuming foods with low energy density—ones with lots of volume but few calories—will control your hunger just as well as the same volume of food with more calories.

Practical advice:
- To microwave a potato, wash but don't dry it. Poke a few holes in the skin with a fork. Wrap the spud in microwaveable plastic wrap, then nuke it on high power for 8 to 9 minutes. Some microwave ovens even idiot-proof the process with a setting for baked potatoes.

Alternatives: Bake an occasional sweet potato or a creamy Yukon gold potato for some variety. Try different toppings, too: a butter-flavored spray, Parmesan cheese, reduced-fat ranch dressing, or salsa, for instance. Or go for one of the many common and exotic grains available in supermarkets, such as barley, bulgur, or couscous.

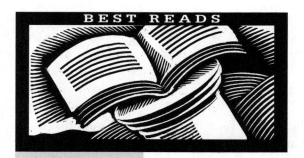

The Secret to Permanent Weight Control

Wouldn't it be nice if this book excerpt was about a newly discovered pill that could melt the pounds off forever? Some year it might be, but not this one. What Joseph Mason does clear up in this excerpt from his book Let My Heart Attack Save Your Life: A Simple, Sound, Workable Weight Management Plan *(John Wiley & Sons, 1998) are the misconceptions about how calories are burned. By concentrating on the activities that burn the majority of calories, one can achieve steady and permanent weight loss.*

Did you ever say, "How can Jane or Dick eat so much and stay so thin?" We have all known people who ate a lot and stayed thin. We may have heard that their metabolisms were high, but what exactly does that mean? We need to understand how our metabolisms work.

In earlier chapters, I discussed where calories come from and how they function as our energy source. How are these calories used? Exercise? Most people are surprised to learn that very few calories are used during exercise.

Calories are used in three ways: digesting food, physical activity, and basal metabolic rate (BMR).

The percentage of your total calories each of these uses remains fairly constant: digestion uses 10 percent, physical activity uses 25 percent, and basal metabolic rate uses 65 percent. While you can't change the percentage of each of these uses, you can change your calorie demand, and thus, alter the total calories required by your body. A person who consumes 1,000 calories a day uses 10 percent, or 100 calories, to digest that food, and a person who consumes 3,000 calories uses 10 percent, or 300 calories, to digest that food. While digestion stays at 10 percent, the number of calories used to burn the food you eat increases from 100 to 300 calories by eating more. You need to find a way to burn more calories without eating more.

The second use of calories is physical activity—all physical activity. Getting up out of your chair and going to the refrigerator is physical activity; so is going for a walk. The number of calories you use depends on your body weight and time. A person who weighs 200 pounds and walks for 10 minutes uses more calories than a person who weighs 150 pounds and walks for 10 minutes. All of your physical activities in a day use only about 25 percent of the total calories you consume. This means the physical activity from driving to the store, washing dishes, changing the channel on the television—everything—only accounts for 25 percent of your total calories, and this even includes that 15 to 30 minutes of aerobic exercise three to five times a week.

So far, I've only accounted for 35 percent (10 percent for digestion and 25 percent for physical activity) of the calories you consume. What is the big user of calories?

Pay attention, because here is one of the secrets to permanent weight loss and control.

Approximately 65 percent of the calories consumed in a day are used to supply the energy for the basic work of the body's cells to maintain life. This is energy used to keep the heart beating, the lungs breathing, all cells conducting activities, and the nerves generating their continuous streams of electrical impulses. Basically, it's all the functions that support life 24 hours a day, even while you sleep. This is called the basal metabolic rate.

Basal Metabolic Rate

Your BMR can be measured in a laboratory while you are lying down and not digesting any food. By eliminating digestion and physical activity, electronic instruments can measure your calorie expenditure that is needed to support life. How can two people who are the same age, sex, height, and weight burn different amounts of calories while they are just lying down? How can Jane or Dick eat so much and stay thin?

If you are accustomed to highlighting certain passages in a book with a yellow marker the way students do, then get ready to do that. How does a person obtain a high BMR? What's the secret? It's no secret to a nutritionist or dietitian. The key is the amount of lean body tissue or fat-free mass you have. Even when we sleep, lean tissue is more active metabolically than fat tissue. A person with lean tissue instead of fat tissue burns more calories and, therefore, gets to eat more calories. So Jane and Dick have more lean body tissue.

If you exercise and burn 200 calories every other day, the important point to remember is that you are keeping your muscles lean. Consequently, these muscles are using more calories the rest of the day, even at night.

It's the calorie demand of their BMRs that keeps the fat people fat and the thin people thin. Overweight people with lots of fat tissue will have a low calorie demand for their BMRs. On the other hand, people with more lean tissue will have a high calorie demand for their BMRs. And as you now know, your BMR accounts for 65 percent of your total calories.

The good news is that you can change your BMR. An overweight person can get thin, but it takes knowledge, commitment, and time. The longer you have been overweight, the longer it takes to become thin. But it is easy, once you have the know-how.

You should not try to lose too much weight too fast. Fasting and dieting lower your basal metabolic rate, which is the opposite of what you want to do. Your body thinks there is a food shortage, and it slows down your BMR so you can survive on fewer calories. Although you may lose a lot of weight, much of it will be muscle and not fat. If you decide to lose a lot of weight in a hurry, don't throw away your old clothes, because the fat will be back. Ask Oprah Winfrey.

I mention Oprah Winfrey as an example because she is nationally recognized and most people are familiar with her rapid weight loss. Many people have done exactly the same thing. When she lost a lot of weight in a short time, she lost muscle along with fat and her BMR slowed down. Chances are, at her lowest weight, she was existing on very few calories. Who could stay on such a low calorie count?

If you lose weight gradually (½ to 1 pound a week), you have two important advantages. First, your body doesn't think there's a food shortage, and your BMR doesn't slow down. Second, you lose fat and not muscle.

If you add moderate exercise, your muscles become leaner, thereby raising your BMR. A higher BMR means you get to eat more.

I couldn't possibly go on without making a public apology to Oprah Winfrey. She is a person to be admired, especially for her work on child abuse. I in no way meant to defame her. I mentioned her only because of the thousands of people who have done exactly the same thing. Estimates are that 90 percent of the people who lose a lot of weight in a short time fail and go right back to their old weights or higher. Some people even start to think they are supposed to be overweight; how absurd.

I wasn't supposed to be overweight. I couldn't lose weight because I didn't understand nutrition; it's as simple as that. I didn't have a psychological problem or a glandular problem, as many people imagine they do.

If you are overweight, I suggest you ask yourself two questions: Do fewer than 30 percent of my calories come from fat? Do I exercise the equivalent of a 30-minute walk three to five times a week?

The starting point for weight loss and control is a resounding "yes" to both of these questions.

Please don't fall victim to the celebrity who ballyhoos some weight-loss program or product. You're smart—give yourself credit. If it sounds dumb or too good to be true, then it is. I say to the celebrities who lend their names to diet programs, I feel you are doing a real disservice to your fans.

By now you realize that when you lose weight, you could be losing water, muscle, or fat. Only when you understand how to lose fat can you achieve permanent weight control.

Slow Weight Loss Burns Fat

Please remember this: Rapid weight loss gets rid of muscle. This lost muscle is no longer on your body to burn calories. If you don't stick to a low-calorie diet, you gain the weight back as fat. One pound of fat uses fewer calories than 1 pound of muscle. But the 1 pound of fat takes up more space on your body than 1 pound of muscle.

If you have trouble visualizing this, remember the old riddle: Which weighs more, a pound of feathers or a pound of steel? You're right, they both weigh a pound. Now, which one takes up more space? The pound of feathers would be about the size of a bed pillow. The pound of steel would be about the size of a golf ball. Muscle is like the golf ball and fat is like the pillow. When you lose muscle and replace it with fat, it's like tying all those pillows to various parts of your body. I know a man who is shaped like a pear because his lean mass was replaced by fat.

Do you have an unusual shape? Now you know why. Chances are, you have dieted before. I bet you lost 3, 4, or even 5 pounds in 1 week. Does this sound familiar? You didn't do your body any favors; you lost muscle! Are you eating fewer calories now than the first time you dieted? Of course you are; you have less muscle.

If you follow the guidelines in this book:

1. Your fat consumption will be less than 30 percent of total calories.
2. The weight (fat) will come off slowly—about 1 pound a week.
3. You will be eating more.
4. Muscle will be retained or increased.

Maintaining your ideal weight should be easy and fun. And you should take pride in the fact that you are knowledgeable about nutrition and your good health.

Dining on the Dash

One of the best ways to sabotage a lifestyle of good eating habits is to eat out. Yes, smart choices exist at everything from fast-food joints to the finest restaurants, but these foods aren't screaming out their healthiness. You have to be savvy and know what to avoid and what to eat when dining out. Shed Some Pounds the Lazy Way (Alpha Books, 1999) by Annette Cain and Becky Carlson is loaded with simple tips to help you make the right food choices. Here, the authors address the always troublesome venture of eating outside the home.

You are the last car in line, and you vacillate between staying there or parking and placing your order inside. You're not sure which will be faster, but you decide to stick to the drive-thru since you're already there anyway. After a few minutes of idling, you trade money for food and you're on your way. Sound familiar?

It seems the busier we get, the more we depend on drive-thrus, restaurants, vending machines, and prepared meals for our daily nourishment. Relying on these sources may save us time, yet it can also preserve our poundage (and then some). Now, we don't expect you to give up this convenient mode of consumption, but there are some rules to follow to steer you in the right direction.

Fast Food: You Don't Have to Fast

The good news is that fast-food restaurants are not off-limits. You can order a meal at any of these joints without blowing your fat budget. Of course, we're not talking about a double-decker burger with a giant order of french fries (that could be 2 days' worth of fat). We mean choosing a menu item that is low in fat.

Here are some pointers for selecting fast-food meals that can make you happy and healthy, too.

- Most fast-food restaurants use regular processed cheese, which is high in fat and calories. Get in the habit of omitting the cheese from any item that you order.
- Order your muffins, biscuits, or sandwiches without any butter, mayonnaise, or mayonnaise-based sauces.
- Choose a broiled chicken sandwich over a hamburger or a breaded, deep-fried chicken or fish sandwich.
- Avoid the deluxe or jumbo versions of any menu items. Always choose the smallest size offered (it's usually regular).

- If fried chicken is your only choice, choose the regular coating over the extra crispy type and make sure you peel the skin off.
- When selecting a pizza, opt for a thin crust and tell them to go easy on the cheese. If you add an extra topping, make sure it's veggies (but tell them to hold the olives).
- If a fast-food restaurant offers potatoes, order yours plain.
- Consult the fast-food nutrition guides to find out if your favorite menu items are healthy. Try to keep your fast-food meal around 500 to 600 calories and 12 to 18 grams of fat.

Out to Lunch (or Any Meal, for That Matter)

Dining out can be a daunting experience when you are trying to shed some pounds. You know how it is . . . you're tempted by the dessert tray practically the minute you walk into the place; you're never quite sure how much fat the chef uses behind closed doors; and virtually everything on the menu sounds enticing.

This wouldn't be such a problem if you dined out once or twice a month; you could have whatever your heart desires (they probably won't let you buy the whole dessert cart). But if you eat more than two or three meals a week in restaurants, you need to be more selective.

Here are some tips to help you dine out without a dash of concern.

- Try to restrict alcoholic drinks. Alcohol is not only loaded with empty calories but it can also increase your appetite and decrease your self-control. Choose a wine spritzer, lite or nonalcoholic beer, or a virgin Bloody Mary. Always ask for a glass of water as soon as you're seated.
- Limit yourself to one piece of bread or one handful of chips.
- Appetizers can be on both sides of the fat fence. Stay away from items that are deep-fried or full of cheese. Gravitate toward consommés, soups, vegetable platters, or shrimp cocktails.
- Ordering two appetizers instead of an entrée can help you keep your portion sizes small.
- When you're at the salad bar, fill your plate with lots of raw veggies, and pass on the prepared salads like potato, pasta, or oil-marinated veggies. Use seeds, croutons, bacon bits, and hard-boiled eggs sparingly.
- Always ask for your dressing and sauces on the side. Then you can dip your fork in them to get a little flavor with each bite.
- The healthiest ways for the chef to prepare your main dish (chicken, fish, or meat) are baked, broiled, grilled (no butter), or poached.

- Avoid menu items that contain words like *scalloped*, *deep-fried*, *au gratin*, *bearnaise*, or *hollandaise sauce*.
- If you must succumb to the dessert tray, choose items like fresh fruit, sorbets, or angel food cake. Share your dessert with your companion(s).
- When ordering your mocha or latte, be sure to ask for nonfat milk. You won't miss a thing with this request except for fat and calories.

Going Out but Not out of Control

Some of the hardest times to make healthy food choices are when you are invited out to parties, weddings, and other social functions—mostly because you have to look pretty hard to find some morsels that haven't been drowned in fat and calories (other than the boring crudités tray). But there is a way to indulge without losing control. You just need to plan your course of action.

These simple strategies will keep you on course.

- The best way to handle food in social situations is to take small (maybe even tiny) amounts of what's offered.
- At a party buffet, if they offer a choice of plate size, use the smaller one. Pass on any refills.
- Try to stay away from the hors d'oeuvres table. Focus your attention on the company and audience rather than just the food.
- Avoid alcohol and choose no-calorie beverages instead. Try a glass of seltzer with cranberry juice and a squeeze of lime or a nonalcoholic beer.
- When you know you're going to be eating rich foods that night, choose to eat healthy, low-fat meals during the day. Be sure that you aren't starving when you go out, though; this could make you overindulge. Have a light snack before you go out to take the edge off your appetite.
- You can always stick to the crudités tray if you want to be extra good.
- Whenever there's dancing, be sure to bring your boogie shoes to burn up the extra calories.

The Workday Grub

It usually happens between 2:30 and 3:00 in the afternoon . . . your stomach or your brain (you're not sure which one) decides you are hungry and leaves you in a state of rumbling and grumbling. You nod off, hoping this may quiet them down, only to dream that the candy bars in the vending machine are fighting over which one will be next to take the big plunge. Of course, they want you to pick the winner. . . .

This is just one of the scenarios you may toil with at work. Eating healthy on the job can be a labored process. It could be a matter of not having enough time or even having too much. Or it may be those tempting morsels hanging out amongst your memos.

Here are some ways to keep your workday grub healthy without making eating a chore.

- It's best to steer clear of vending machines. If you're hungry, chances are, you'll think that all of the candy bars should be winners. Most items in vending machines are losers when it comes to being low in fat, calories, sugar, and sodium.
- Stock your desk with low-fat snacks at the beginning of each week.
- Keep a bottle of water at your desk and drink from it throughout the day.
- If you know you are going to be spending your lunch hour at work, try to prepare a healthy meal the night before. This will keep you from skipping lunch or going out for more fattening fare.
- Skip the doughnuts, croissants, and muffins at those breakfast meetings— they're loaded with fat and calories. Choose some fruit, fruit juice, or a bagel, instead.

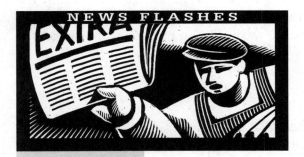

Lack of Zinc Linked to Obesity

NEW YORK CITY—Zinc deficiency may be a cause of obesity, according to a study published in the *Journal of the American College of Nutrition*. Nine men were placed on a high-zinc diet for 12 weeks and then on a zinc-restricted diet until their levels fell below normal. Researchers measured the leptin—a hormone thought to affect feelings of fullness—in the subjects' blood. Leptin levels increased by 1.5 nanograms per milliliter (ng/ml) when zinc levels were high, and decreased by 0.5 ng/ml when they were low. "Leptin decreases appetite and increases energy expenditure," says Christos S. Mantzoros, M.D., the lead researcher.

"But it fails to do so in obese people." Your daily diet should include at least 15 milligrams of zinc.

Small Weight Gains Are Still Hazardous to Your Heart

STOCKHOLM, Sweden—Even a slight weight gain can increase your odds of dying from heart disease. Researchers recorded the weights of 6,874 middle-age men, along with their reported weights at age 20, then tracked their health for the next 20 years. The men who weighed 4 percent to 10 percent more at middle age than they did at age 20 had a 60 percent greater risk of dying of heart disease than did the men whose weight held steady.

Walking Will Keep Off the Pounds for Years

HOUSTON—You don't need to start running 10-Ks to keep your gut inside your pants. Just walk. A study of 500 NASA employees (average age 40) found that people who walked every day, even if they didn't change their diets, gained no weight over a 10-year period. The typical 170- to 180-pound man in the study who walked just 2¼ miles per day (about a 30-minute stroll) or 16 miles per week had gained only a pound or two after 10 years. But the participants who managed only about an hour's worth of activity per week had piled on 14 to 20 pounds in the same period. Men who weigh less than 180 pounds will need to walk a little more to keep their weight the same; heavier guys will require less mileage. If hoofing it isn't your thing, 7 hours a week of any activity that burns about 350 calories per hour (such as waxing the car or cleaning the garage) will do the job.

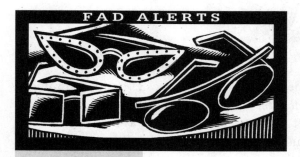

FAD ALERTS

Calorie Monitors

It's easier to keep trudging through a 3-mile run (or walk) when you know how many calories you're burning. That's why we gladly strapped on the Polar SmartEdge calorie monitor ($199). The chest band measures your pulse rate by sensing your heart's electrical impulses, and the monitor uses that statistic to estimate the calories you're burning. But is it accurate? Not really, says Daniel Kosich, Ph.D., an exercise physiologist in Denver who tested the SmartEdge for *Men's Health* magazine. Depending on factors such as your aerobic fitness level and the type of activity you're doing, you'll burn calories differently, he says.

"Though the calorie count isn't necessarily accurate, it's close enough to use for motivation," says Carol Garber, Ph.D., associate professor of medicine at Brown University in Providence, Rhode Island. (She tested the device against laboratory monitors on men who ran on treadmills.) The Polar company acknowledges that the SmartEdge has a 10 percent margin of error: If it reads 500 calories, you've probably fried at least 450.

Sugar Busters!

 According to the bestselling book *Sugar Busters!*, if you eliminate refined sugar and high-glycemic carbohydrates—foods that spike your blood sugar—you'll be able to "enjoy steak, eggs, cheese, even wine—as you get healthy and lose weight."

The book's theme centers around the theory "cut sugar to trim fat." Glucose, or blood sugar, is the body's main source of energy. It's also stored in the liver and muscles. But when you eat more sugar or high-glycemic foods than your body needs or can store, insulin converts the excess glucose to fat. It may even help block the conversion of fat back into glucose. Refined sugars and other glucose-boosting foods, such as pasta, potatoes, corn, and beer, are off-limits to *Sugar Busters!* buyers. You're also encouraged to exercise and to moderate your intake of fat and of lean meat.

The catch is that, by itself, simply eating less sugar will not make you lose weight. "Their theory is overly simplified," suggests JoAnn Manson, M.D., endocrinologist and researcher at Harvard Medical School. "You can consume a lot of calories without eating refined sugars and carbohydrates. You'll still gain weight."

The reason that some people will lose weight on this diet is that many foods that raise blood sugar also tend to be high in calories. Cut them out and don't increase total calories, and you'll drop pounds.

If you want to save the cost of the book, replace foods that tip the glucose scales with foods that are lower in calories and higher in fiber. For example, exchange white rice, white bread, and pasta for their whole-grain counterparts, and trade in your baked potatoes for sweet potatoes. Foods that pack more nutrients for their size and take longer to digest will make you feel fuller, too. Beer and ice cream are okay in moderation.

Calorad

Calorad claims that just 1 tablespoon at night "feeds the body with a collagen protein supplement, helping the body lose excess fat and toxins naturally."

A 1-month supply of the liquid supplement costs $55. Essentially Yours Industries, the 4-year-old company that markets Calorad, has more than 300,000 "independent business associates" who distribute and sell the dietary supplement.

The collagen formula found in Calorad supposedly enhances the body's "natural mechanism of rejuvenation and repair" while you sleep, which helps it build lean muscle mass and burn more calories. Take 1 tablespoon of Calorad with water just before bed, and don't eat or drink anything but water for 3 hours before you take it. There's no need to exercise or alter your regular diet in any way.

They have one thing right—lean muscle does burn calories. But gulping a glass of collagen won't build calorie-burning muscle.

"In reality, you need many different high-quality proteins (strings of amino acids), and you also have to exercise," says Peter D. Vash, M.D., associate clinical professor of medicine at the University of California, Los Angeles. "That's why taking Calorad right before you go to bed is of little value for building muscle and of less value for promoting fat loss."

Also, "collagen hydrolysat," the ingredient listed on the Calorad label, is the scientific name for gelatin (think unflavored Jell-O), according to David Pearson, Ph.D., an exercise physiologist and associate professor at the Ball State University human performance laboratory in Muncie, Indiana. Pearson and others who studied gelatin's effects on joint health found nothing in gelatin that can help build muscle or reduce weight.

If you want to save $55, eat high-quality proteins and move some dumbbells. "Tuna, chicken breast, tofu, and beans are good sources of muscle-building proteins," says Dr. Vash.

Meridia

The program claims you can "lose weight and keep it off." Meridia is a legitimate prescription drug that works by regulating the brain's appetite control center. Those who take the drug and make appropriate changes in their habits can expect to lose up to 10 percent of their weight.

More than $80 million has been spent on Meridia since it reached pharmacies 2 years ago, according to Knoll Pharmaceutical Company.

"It acts on neurotransmitters in the brain and makes you feel full sooner, so you eat less," says Louis Aronne, M.D., a Meridia clinical investigator and the director of New York Presbyterian Hospital's comprehensive weight-control program. The drug should be taken once a day in conjunction with a healthful diet and a daily exercise program.

Meridia works, but it's not for the person who has put on just a few extra pounds. It's a prescription appetite suppressant intended for those who are at least 25 percent overweight. Studies show that it slightly increases blood pressure in some people, so those with hypertension should use it with caution.

If you have a lot of weight to lose, see your doctor to determine whether Meridia or another weight-loss medication is right for you. Otherwise, have a complete physical exam, and then begin to exercise more and change your diet.

Fit America

 This program touts itself as "The All-Natural Answer for Weight Control." Pop the Fit America herbal supplements and follow the recommended food plan to lose between 10 and 18 pounds per month. In 1997, Fit America grossed more than $33 million in retail sales. A 35-day supply of supplements costs $139.

The combination of 10 herbs—astragalus, bitter orange, cascara sagrada, foti, ginkgo, English hawthorn, henna, licorice root, ma huang, and valerian root—is supposed to "help suppress the appetite, regulate the bowels and kidneys, and stimulate the metabolism so the body utilizes the foods consumed more efficiently." Fit America recommends that you start by taking one gray herbal capsule twice a day and one peach-colored herbal tablet once a day. You are encouraged to increase the dosage of the gray herbal capsules gradually, but not to take more than eight in one day. Followers of the Fit America plan are also advised to eat a high-protein, low-carbohydrate diet, with no limit on their intake of fruits and vegetables.

"Cascara sagrada and henna are both laxatives," says Steven Margolis, M.D., clinical instructor of alternative medicine at Wayne State University in Detroit and at William Beaumont Hospital in Troy, Michigan. "You'll end up spending a lot of time in the bathroom." That's where you're most likely to lose weight, too. Worse, two of the herbs in the Fit America supplements—licorice root and ma huang—may have dangerous side effects. "Although these herbs are reported to boost metabolism and suppress appetite, they can also increase blood pressure, making this supplement potentially harmful to those who have hypertension," Dr. Margolis says.

If you want to save $139, "drink a glass of vegetable juice, grapefruit juice, or anything else that has some bulk in it to suppress your appetite," says Kathleen Zelman, R.D., a nutritional consultant and a spokeswoman for the American Dietetic Association. Also, avoid a high-protein diet (it's tough on your kidneys), and eat more high-fiber vegetables and carbohydrates for a natural laxative effect. As for increasing your metabolism, there's only one effective method short of medication: exercise.

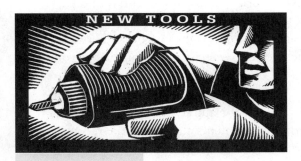

Quicker Ideal-Weight Calculation

Mayo Clinic Web Site

To help you more accurately pinpoint the weight that's healthiest for you, the Mayo Clinic network now offers a free service on the Web. After you answer questions about your height, weight, exercise habits, and health, the site calculates your ideal weight. To check it out, go to www.mayohealth.org and search for the term "weight assessment."

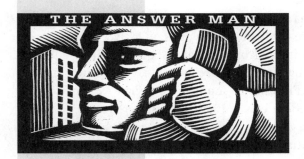

Run the Weight Off

I always hear how weight lifting supposedly speeds up the metabolism and aerobics doesn't. So why are most runners rail-thin and a lot of heavy lifters fat dudes?

—L. B., East Lansing, Mich.

Your question has more to do with energy than with metabolism, according to Len Kravitz, Ph.D., an exercise physiologist at the University of Mississippi in Oxford. "You'd have to consume 4,000 to 6,000 calories to offset the energy output required to run 5 to 10 miles a day. These guys can't feed themselves enough. Metabolism really isn't an issue at this level."

It is true that weight training can increase your metabolism by as much as 10 percent, says Dr. Kravitz. Muscles contain fat- and carbohydrate-burning "stoves." When you increase the size of your muscles, you're increasing the size of these stoves. That's how you increase metabolism. But weight lifters still don't expend as much energy as distance runners.

Faulty Binge Theory

My skin-and-bones buddy says he's able to stay thin because he satisfies his junk-food cravings with one binge day a week. He claims the body can't digest all that fat at once, and most of the bad stuff just moves through the digestive tract unabsorbed. Who's the bigger idiot—him for thinking it's true or me for almost believing him?
—T. M., Milwaukee

You're both candidates for donkey ears. The body is quite capable of absorbing all the calories you put into it, according to Mark Kantor, Ph.D., associate professor and extension specialist in nutrition and food science at the University of Maryland at College Park. "Body weight and body fat are determined by the amount of calories that go in—namely the food you eat—versus the amount of calories that you burn up," he explains. "Eating the foods all at once makes little difference." Your pal's theory, in fact, may be the opposite of what actually occurs. Research shows that three meals spread out over the day are easier for the body to burn. "If you're going to eat lots of fatty burgers or whatever," Dr. Kantor says, "there may be an advantage to spreading them out over several days."

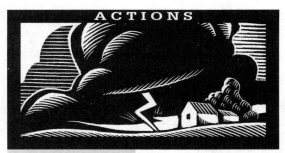

When you diet, you aren't just combating a few pounds of fat. You're squaring off against a large, sophisticated organism that doesn't take kindly to starvation. On-again, off-again dieting trains your enzymes to take a defensive posture: They start socking away fat whenever your body threatens to lose weight, says Michael Colgan, Ph.D., president of the Colgan Institute of nutritional science in Encinitas, California, and author of *Optimum Sports Nutrition*. Endlessly munching on carrot and celery sticks is no way to exist. To lose weight and to keep it off, you have to make small changes over time. That way, you can develop good eating and lifestyle habits to maintain a healthy weight for life. Here are some tips to get you on the right track.

1. **Wash dishes by hand.** Instead of always turning to the dishwasher, do it the old-fashioned way. You'll burn an average of 94 extra calories per day—the equivalent of about 9 pounds over the course of a year.

2. **Close your ears.** Place your finger on the harder part of your ear near your cheekbones. Hold that part of your ear between your thumb and forefinger and press. This is the hunger acupressure point on the ear, says David Nickel, a doctor of Oriental medicine, a certified acupuncturist in Santa Monica, California; and author of *Acupressure for Athletes*. Pressing this point should help control compulsive eating, which will help you lose weight, he adds. Hold the point for 5 seconds, then let go for 5. Continue these 5-second intervals for about a minute.

3. **Kill hunger pangs.** Tighten your stomach muscles as firm as possible, and slowly count to 10. You'll help curb the flow of stomach acid that causes the hunger sensation.

4. **Set your eyes on the prizes.** Although losing weight may be your primary goal, it shouldn't be your only goal. Focusing only on how many pounds you lose and how fast you lose them may doom you to failure. "Many people become weight obsessed and become depressed if they don't lose enough weight. If you don't lose weight 'soon enough' or if you have some trouble, you could become discouraged and stop," says Nicholas Hall, Ph.D., director of the Institute for Health and Human Performance in Tampa, Florida. Set other health-related goals, such as lower cholesterol levels and blood pressure, reduced body fat percentage, and fewer sick days taken, that go along with weight loss. As you meet these goals, you'll be rewarded and keep on your quest to lose weight.

5. **Eat breakfast.** "Typically, men who skip breakfast eat more later, and then choose foods higher in fat and calories," says Franca Alphin, R.D., of the Duke University Diet and Fitness Center in Durham, North Carolina.

6. **Lick the salt habit.** If you're going to eat in a bar, find something that's low in salt, such as cut-up vegetables. If you crunch down those salty pretzels, corn chips, and nachos, you'll end up drinking more than you intended.

7. **Play a trick on yourself.** When you exercise strenuously, most of the calories you burn come from glycogen, a carbohydrate-based fuel stored in your muscles. Here are two ways to trick your body into using more energy from fat. First, start early. If you do aerobic exercise before breakfast, your body is more likely to be low in glycogen and burn fat instead, says Timothy J. Moore, Ph.D., a fitness consultant from Greenbelt, Maryland. Second, go long—really, really long. According to an article in the journal *Frontiers of Bioscience*, the longer you exercise at moderate intensity—55 to 75 percent of your maximum effort—the more fat your body uses.

8. **Graze often.** About 10 percent of your metabolism is devoted to digesting the food you eat. Your body actually uses up calories processing the calories you've just eaten. The more frequently you eat, the higher you can crank up this part of your metabolism. That's why it's important, if you're trying to lose weight, to eat many small meals each day. "Eat something every 3 hours or so, even if you're not totally hungry," says Jacqueline Berning, R.D., Ph.D., a nutritionist at the University of Colorado at Boulder. Skipping meals has the opposite effect—it shuts off this calorie-burning mechanism. And you're more likely to splurge if you skip a waistline-friendly turkey sandwich and an apple.

9. **Drink skim milk with meals.** The calcium may help reduce the amount of saturated fat your body absorbs by binding with it and flushing it through your system.

10. **Say yes to soups.** Eating vegetable and noodle soups before a normal meal can help you lose weight. The fiber causes food to move through your digestive system faster, and the water helps dissolve the fat. Add a potato to the soup, and you'll consume about 20 percent fewer calories over the course of the meal. Tomato soup has the same effect. You'll eat less during the meal, and you'll feel full longer.

11. **Run and eat.** If you know you'll be eating a high-fat breakfast, fit in a good workout the day before. The theory: Your muscles will absorb the new fat in your blood in order to replenish the amount you burned the day before.

12. **Turn out the lights.** Dim lights make you want to eat less than bright lights do. You can also reduce the amount you eat by using smaller, patternless dishes. You're programmed to eat more when you use large or patterned plates.

13. **Drink 8 pints of ice water a day.** Do this and you can drop a pound every 4 weeks. Your body expends 123 calories of heat daily to warm the water to 98.6°F.

14. **Learn to crunch.** Hard foods make hard bodies. Food that's digested slowly will kill your hunger, cut your glucose load, and turn off the hormones that make you hungry. Think raw vegetables and hard beans.

15. **Eat spicy food more often.** Spicy food will increase your metabolic rate significantly; when your face sweats from Chinese hot sauce, it's a sign that your body is working harder and burning more calories, even if you're just sitting in a restaurant.

16. **Take it easy.** Stress can make us do things that we really don't want to do—like eat an entire box of chocolate-covered doughnuts. Under any other circumstances, you wouldn't do such a thing. But stress creates a whacked-out connection between your mind and your stomach, with the former ordering the latter to consume everything in sight. When you feel the need to feast under stress, take a break for a quick breathing exercise, says Larry J. Feldman, Ph.D., director of the Pain and Stress Rehabilitation Center in New Castle, Delaware, and author of *Feeling Good Again*, a self-help book for dealing with stress. Inhale, and when your lungs feel naturally full, take in even more air until your lungs are completely full. Hold briefly, then exhale. Then push out even more air to a count of 10 until you have made your lungs as empty as possible. Start the process again by inhaling.

17. **Get some help from others.** Don't try to lose weight alone. Find a friend to come along for the ride, and you'll increase your odds of victory. "All these studies show that people who have the best success are those who have support," says G. Ken Goodrick, Ph.D., assistant professor of medicine at Baylor College of Medicine in Houston and coauthor of *Living without Dieting*.

18. **Press the "appetite balancing point."** You may reach for food when your body's vital energy is out of balance, which can be caused by stress or any number of things. Pressing the divot right above your upper lip restores balance and curbs your appetite. "It has a calming and centering effect," says Michael Reed Gach, Ph.D., founder of the Acupressure Institute in Berkeley, California, and author of *Acupressure's Potent Points*. Place your fingertip in the center of your upper lip, then move your finger about two-thirds of the way up between your lip and nose. Press firmly, pushing into your gums, and breathe deeply. Hold the point for about 2 minutes.

19. **Fly your way.** When traveling on an airplane, take matters into your own hands. In your carry-on luggage, pack a healthy snack, such as fruit, a bagel, or a one-serving box of cereal. Then you'll be able to wave off the beer nuts when the drink cart comes rolling around.

20. **Eat two apples a day.** Do this, and you'll lose 10 pounds in a year. The fiber in the apples promotes weight loss by helping to block your body's digestion of fat and protein.

5

DISEASE-PROOF

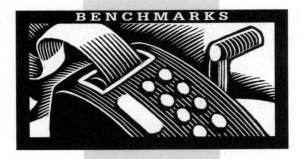

■ Percentage by which you reduce your risk of dying within the next 15 years by quitting smoking before age 50: 50

■ Percentage of hospital workers who wear used gloves to handle patients: 84

■ Average number of visits to the doctor per year for men: 2.7 (3.2 for women)

■ Life expectancy for boys born in the United States in 1998: 73.4 (80.1 for girls)

■ In 1940: 60.8 (65.2 for girls)

■ Percentage of men who had high blood pressure (over 140/90) from 1960 to 1962: 40

■ From 1988 to 1994: 25.3

■ Average cholesterol reading for men from 1960 to 1962: 217

■ From 1988 to 1994: 202

■ Amount of money for which Rolling Stones guitarist Keith Richards has insured his left (guitar-playing) hand: $1.6 million

■ Amount of money for which Bruce Springsteen has insured his voice: $5.6 million

■ Average number of people killed by lawn mowers each year: 75

■ Number of heart attacks on Wall Street the day the market dropped 513 points (in August 1998): 2

■ Number of heart attacks the next day, when the market rose 288 points: 3

■ Chance that a caller to the government's cancer-information hotline hears a busy signal or is put on hold until he hangs up: 1 in 3

■ Estimated number of Americans who regain consciousness during surgery each year: 40,000

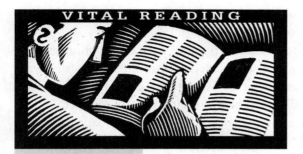

Touch Yourself All Over

Use your fingers for early detection of treatable health problems.

It's enough to chill the blood of any man, from the bravest fighter pilot to the most cowardly personal-injury attorney. The doctor's monotone request for you to bend over, followed by the snap of a latex glove and the squish of lubricant. You lower your gaze in embarrassed resignation as the fickle finger of fate checks the health of your prostate gland.

Although that particular test must be performed by a doctor, there are many exams you can do yourself to uncover health problems while they're most treatable. Here are tests for which the only fingers required are your own.

Roll. Whether you're asking for a big raise or telling your wife in no uncertain terms that you will be golfing every Saturday, you know the value of a healthy set of *cojones*. That's why you should be alert for testicular cancer, the most common form of cancer in men between the ages of 15 and 40.

As with all types of cancer, early detection is a key to survival. So at least once a month, perform this simple examination: Soap up in a warm shower to soften the scrotum, then gently roll each testicle between your thumb and forefinger. Better yet, ask your wife or girlfriend to help with the heavy lifting. Tell your assistant that each testicle should feel smooth and oval, kind of like an Easter egg without the shell. Double-check her findings yourself, being careful to note any hard areas or lumps. If you find an irregularity, call your doctor.

"It's especially important for young men—starting at age 16—to examine themselves monthly," says Richard Williams, M.D., professor and chairman of the department of urology at the University of Iowa in Iowa City. "An easy way to remember your self-exam is to tie it to some other monthly activity." Okay, then; mail in that car payment, and head for the shower.

Tap. If you have a headache and want to know whether it's sinus-related so that you can better treat the symptoms, tap your face lightly above your eyebrows, between your eyes and nose, and on your cheeks. If you feel a sharp pain when you tap, you probably do have a sinus headache.

"Nasal drainage, discolored nasal discharge, and nasal obstruction are even stronger signs that your headache is connected to the sinuses," says Howard Levine, M.D., director of nasal surgery at the Mount Sinai Nasal Center in Cleveland. Decongestants and painkillers can help alleviate sinus discomfort.

Poke. After parking a mile and a half from the beach, you load yourself up like a pack mule and haul folding chairs, a cooler, boogie boards, an umbrella, a couple of beach bags, and an inflatable tugboat toward the water. You slather sunscreen all over the kids and lay out the towels. Two hours later, when you finally slump into your chair and reach for a cold beer, you notice that your shoulders are a little bit sensitive.

To quickly assess whether you've been burned, use your finger to poke the area that has had the most exposure. If it blanches, the blood vessels have dilated—a sign of sun damage. If you find yourself believing that the blonde in the thong is checking you out, you're hallucinating—a more extreme indication that you've been in the sun too long.

"Pressing the skin is a good test for the average person," says Edward Bondi, M.D., professor of dermatology at the University of Pennsylvania in Philadelphia. "It can serve as a warning for those who aren't as careful as they should be." Unfortunately, some damage may already have occurred by the time you see red.

Little-known fact: A thin, white cotton T-shirt has a sun protection factor of 7. Dark blue denim? SPF 1,700.

Touch. Taking your pulse is an easy way to check the overall health of your heart, says Kenneth Ellenbogen, M.D., professor of medicine and cardiac arrhythmia specialist at Medical College of Virginia Hospitals in Richmond.

To take your pulse, place the first two fingers of one hand lightly on the inside of your opposite wrist, just below your thumb. Count the number of beats in 10 seconds and multiply that number by 6. The normal range while at rest is 60 to 100 beats per minute, but highly trained athletes can have rates in the forties.

"Taking your pulse can be a good way to determine whether you need to see a doctor," Dr. Ellenbogen says. "Significantly higher or lower rates, or irregularities, could indicate heart disease or some other problem."

If your heart rate changes significantly, or if you're concerned by an irregularity or a high heart rate, be sure to mention it to your doctor.

Probe. Unless you have the pain tolerance of G. Gordon Liddy, chances are, you won't be able to perform the standard groin hernia test on yourself. (You know the one: "Turn your head and cough.") But if you lie on your back and feel your groin and lower abdomen, you may be able to determine whether the pain you're feeling after moving your aunt's credenza to the basement is from a hernia or just a pulled muscle. You can also try to check for a hernia by pressing around your navel while standing up.

"Many hernias are self-diagnosed," says L. Keith Mason, M.D., a hernia specialist and surgeon in Shreveport, Louisiana. "If you feel a lump or bulge in your abdomen, by your navel, or in your groin, you should have it checked."

Prompt attention is essential, Dr. Mason notes, because a tear in your abdominal wall could grow larger or could crimp an intestine and cause a serious intestinal blockage.

Press. "You need to have your hearing checked," your girlfriend tells you after you inform her that, no, you don't remember her mentioning that you have an anniversary party to attend on Super Bowl Sunday.

If you have selective hearing that tunes out everything but ball scores and the dinner bell, that's one thing. But if you really do miss a lot, you may want to grab the phone and punch in (800) 222-3277, between 9:00 A.M. and 5:00 P.M. Eastern time. An operator will give you a local number you can call to take an automated Dial-a-Hearing Screening Test, which was developed by Occupational Hearing Service of Swarthmore, Pennsylvania. The 2-minute exam can tell you whether you should have your hearing checked by a professional.

"It's an easy but very effective screening test," says John Knox, an audiologist at the Medical College of Wisconsin in Milwaukee. "But you won't receive a diagnosis over the phone, so if you don't pass the test, you will need a complete hearing evaluation."

Push. Whether you're an avid runner packing in mileage in preparation for a big race or a beginner starting out on a walking program, chances are, you'll experience occasional pain in your lower legs and feet. If the pain becomes severe, you'll need to determine whether it's soft-tissue damage, such as shinsplints, or a stress fracture.

To do this, push with your fingers on the tender areas. "Whereas injuries such as shinsplints create pain over a broad area when you apply pressure, spot pain probably means a stress fracture," says Andrew Cosgarea, M.D., assistant professor of orthopedic surgery at Johns Hopkins University School of Medicine in Baltimore. Without the proper care, a stress fracture can become a complete break, which will mean more time recovering and less time training.

If rest and ice don't solve the problem within a couple of days, you should see a sports-medicine specialist, Dr. Cosgarea says.

Scratch. After you brush your teeth, use the nail of your index finger to scratch their surfaces, especially near the gum line. If you come up with a fingernail full of white gunk, you lose. That's plaque, the precursor to gum disease. It's also an indication that you don't know how to brush correctly or that your toothbrush is worn out. Ask the shapely hygienist at your dentist's office for a private lesson after your next appointment. "Plaque, which hardens into tartar, can cause your gums to lose their attachment to your teeth," says Andrew Zimmerman, D.D.S., of Clearfield, Pennsylvania. "This allows bacteria to lodge under the gums and cause disease."

Unless you're counting on some extra cash from the tooth fairy to fund your retirement, floss once a day and brush at least twice.

Compare. The length of your index finger compared with that of your ring finger may be a sign of fertility, according to a recent study by John Manning, Ph.D., of the University of Liverpool in England. In a test of 60 men at an infertility clinic, Dr. Manning found that men whose ring fingers are longer than their index fingers have higher testosterone levels.

Another handy finding from Dr. Manning's research: Men with asymmetrical hands—hands that are not basically mirror images of each other—produce fewer sperm. Twelve subjects who were producing almost no sperm had more than 1/8 of an inch difference between fingers on their two hands.

Feel. Swollen, tender lymph nodes under your ears and arms or in your groin are usually a sign that your body is fighting infection effectively. But tender glands that remain so for more than a few weeks, or swollen glands that are painless but persistent, may indicate a more serious problem, possibly even cancer, according to Robert Warren, M.D., associate professor of medicine at Georgetown University School of Medicine and clinical director of the Lombardi Cancer Center, both in Washington, D.C.

"If you have a runny nose and a sore throat and the glands in your neck swell, that's perfectly normal," Dr. Warren says. "The key is to notice if the swelling lasts beyond your cold, or if it exists when you have no other symptoms."

Back Insurance

Avoid future problems with these simple fixes.

Here's the thing about guys and backs: While most of us are smart enough not to deadlift heavy stuff like manhole covers or Oldsmobiles, we're not always that savvy about the sneakier threats to our backs.

"Most of us don't keep our backs in the right position as we perform day-to-day activities," says Russell Windsor, M.D., of the Hospital for Special Surgery in New York City. "Unfortunately, that can put a lot of stress on the muscles and disks."

In fact, every day we make moves that not only cause pain in our backs but also can cause damage over time. Here are some common activities that could have you calling for a doctor if you're not careful, along with tips on how to minimize the risks.

Shaving. We don't mean the nasty nicks you get from trying to remove back hair with your Atra. We're talking about the way you lean into the bathroom mirror as you scrape whiskers off your face. Bending like that, day after day, year after year, can stress your neck and lower back and create disk and muscle problems.

Train yourself to shave in the shower without a mirror. (You can quickly touch up the spots you've missed once you're out.) Not only is it better for your back, but you'll also get a closer shave. If you don't want to do that, buy an alligator-arm mirror so you don't have to lean in when you shave, advises Andrew Cole, M.D., of Northwest Spine and Sports Physicians.

Driving a hot car. We love your new 'Vette as much as you do, but you practically scrape your butt on the ground climbing in and out, and you're driving with your legs and arms extended—two great ways to wreak havoc on your upper- and lower-back muscles, says Helen Schilling, M.D., medical director for HealthSouth-Houston Rehabilitation Institute.

Slide the driver's seat as far forward as you comfortably can—remembering to stay at least 10 inches from the steering wheel if you have a driver-side airbag—and put a thin cushion between the small of your back and the seat. This will give you more lower-back support. When you're entering or exiting the car, put your knees together like a woman wearing a short skirt. This will keep you from twisting your lower and middle back (and cut down on catcalls from rowdy construction workers).

Sleeping on your stomach. We know, you're so bushed by the end of the day that you belly flop onto the bed and stay that way for 8 hours. Unfortunately, snoozing stomach-side-down can hyperextend your lower back and put pressure on your pelvic joints. Worse, if you prop up your head with pillows and turn it to the side, you're stressing your neck and upper-back muscles, too.

Roll over, Rover. Sleeping on your side with a pillow (or an attractive partner) between your legs will keep your pelvis from twisting and giving you a backache.

Crossing your legs as you sit. Doing your Dick Cavett impression again? Sorry, but crossing your legs—even just resting your ankle on your thigh—causes stress in your sacroiliac joints (where your hipbones join your spine).

If you can't break this habit completely, at least limit it to 5-minute stretches.

Reading too much. Actually, read all you want; just don't do it sitting at your desk with your head tilted down. This stresses your neck muscles, which weren't designed to keep your head—which weighs about as much as a bowling ball—from smacking on the desk.

Pull your chair in close to your desk, and concentrate on keeping your head in a vertical line with your shoulders. Better yet, buy a reading stand.

Putting your toddler in a car seat. Everybody knows that you shouldn't pick up heavy stuff by bending from the waist. But maneuvering even a moderate weight in the wrong way can be just as bad. "Disks tolerate forward-back and side-to-side motion fairly well," says Jeffrey Young, M.D., associate director of spine and sports rehabilitation at Beth Israel Medical Center in New York. But twisting your back, as you do when you stand outside the car and lift your kid into his car seat, makes the disks vulnerable to shearing.

Pick up the child, climb into the backseat, and then put Junior into his car seat.

Sitting at your desk all day. Sitting for too long tightens and shortens your hamstrings and the muscles in the fronts of your hips. How does this hurt your back? When you stand, these muscles tug on the ligaments around your pelvis, which can alter the natural curve in your lower back, Dr. Young says.

Keep your hamstrings and hip flexors loose by standing and moving around every hour. And stretch your legs under your desk at least that often.

Overworking your pecs at the gym. This is a typical problem among weight lifters, who often build up their chests while ignoring the muscles in their upper backs. ("Cadillacs in front, Volkswagens in the rear," is how Dr. Young puts it.) The result: an imbalance that can overload the trapezius, the rhomboids, and other back muscles.

Stay in balance by building your chest and back equally. "If you bench-press 150 pounds, you should be able to put the same weight on the rowing machine and do the same number of repetitions," says Dr. Young.

Wedging the phone between your head and shoulder. "Biomechanically ab-normal," says Dr. Cole. Scrunching up one side of your neck while stretching the other side can cause spasms in both the ropelike muscles attached to your skull and the large, flat muscles of your upper back.

Hold the phone in your hand. Or buy a headset.

Playing golf, especially if you're lousy. It may seem like a serene sport, but golf can cause rugbylike stress on your body. "When you start your swing, you shift your weight, and the spine becomes a whip," explains Dr. Windsor. "It's under maximum torque. If the power that travels from the club through the legs into the ball isn't uniform, or if you take a divot, there's a terrific amount of re-sistance." You can end up with muscle spasms, or even a herniated disk in your lower back.

Taking lessons to make your swing smoother is a good first step. Beyond that, you can take pressure off your spine by keeping your hip flexor muscles as flexible as possible. Try this exercise: Sit on the floor with your legs straight out in front of you. Bring your right knee toward your chest, then cross your right foot over your left leg and place it outside your left knee. This stretches the right hip flexor. Stretch it farther by grabbing your right leg and bringing it closer to your chest, or by pushing it farther out with your left leg. Repeat this exercise with your left leg to stretch the left hip flexor.

Prevent the Big C

Steps to keep cancer at bay.

Life is filled with things we can't control: the weather, the stock market, teenagers who wear their pants halfway down their butts.

But one phenomenon on which we really can exert some influence is cancer. Over the last several years, researchers have become increasingly convinced that it is what we do and don't do in our lives that helps determine our cancer risk.

"Only 5 to 10 percent of cancers are inherited," says Moshe Shike, M.D., director of the prevention and wellness program at Memorial Sloan-Kettering Cancer Center in New York City. "The rest are due to interactions with the environment."

If you don't believe it, just look at the latest statistics. After rising 7.8 percent between 1971 and 1990, cancer deaths in men have recently started falling—dipping 4.3 percent between 1991 and 1995. That's the first sustained decline since record keeping began in the 1930s, according to the National Cancer Institute (NCI). Although improvements in treatment and diagnosis are largely responsible for this decline, another major influence has been the increased emphasis on cancer prevention—in particular, urging people to stop smoking.

But passing up the Pall Malls is only the first step in reducing your cancer risk. In fact, you can take a number of other steps right now to significantly lower your odds. Here's the plan.

Talk to all those relatives you can't stand. The more of your close relatives who have cancer that can't be blamed on obvious environmental factors such as smoking, the greater your genetic predisposition to the disease probably is.

If you do have a troubling family history, though, don't panic. It simply means that you may have to begin cancer screenings at an earlier age. And even if you don't have a family history of cancer, regular screenings are a good idea.

Start with monthly self-exams for testicular cancer (gently roll each testicle between your thumb and forefinger, looking for lumps or areas of hardness). Then talk to your doctor about bumping up your screening schedule, which should at least include yearly checks for cancers of the mouth, prostate, skin, and colon. Screenings for the latter two are particularly beneficial because doctors can detect and remove precancerous growths before they do any serious damage.

Another strategy for those with shaky family histories is a relatively new defense known as chemoprevention—the use of drugs or of compounds that occur naturally in food to make preemptive strikes against diseases you're at risk for but haven't yet developed. Talk to your doctor to see if you might be a candidate.

Eat better than 77 percent of the population. One of the most important things you can do to cut your cancer risk is eat at least five servings of fruits and vegetables a day. A 14-year study found that the men whose daily diets were highest in fruits and vegetables had a 70 percent lower risk of digestive tract cancers. Yet, according to an NCI survey, a shockingly low number of Americans—only 23 percent—meet the five-a-day goal.

Here's the easiest way to reach your quota: Never eat a meal that doesn't contain a fruit or vegetable. It doesn't have to be much—some fruit on your cereal and a glass of orange juice at breakfast, a couple of thick slices of tomato on your sandwich at lunch, an apple for a snack, a nice salad with dinner—but it should be consistent.

And don't rely on supplements to make up any deficit. Although there's been a lot of hype about studies that have linked vitamins such as C, E, and folate and minerals such as selenium with the prevention of a range of cancers, there's little evidence that popping pills delivers the same benefits as eating foods that contain these cancer fighters.

Eat more chicken. Red meat can be the bad boy of an anticancer diet—appealing, yet potentially destructive. In one Harvard study of 48,000 men, those who ate beef, pork, or lamb as a main dish five or more times a week were 3.5 times as likely to get colon cancer as men who ate red meat less than once a month. Substituting chicken or fish more often may cut your cancer risk; one study of Californians found that people who ate about 1½ pounds a week of both had a 43 percent lower risk of developing precancerous colon polyps than people who ate roughly the same amount of red meat.

Start a new tradition for Labor Day. Hovering over a hot barbecue will always be a man's prerogative. But studies suggest that searing beef, pork, poultry, or fish at high temperatures triggers reactions in compounds they contain that can produce up to 17 potential carcinogens. The probable cancer causers, known as heterocyclic amines, are found in meat and in smoke, too. So far, evidence of their harm is test-tube-based and preliminary. Still, at your next backyard bash, it probably will pay to hedge your bets.

A study from Lawrence Livermore National Laboratory in California found that marinating chicken for 4 hours prior to 20 to 40 minutes of grilling eliminated most traces of heterocyclic amines. A good soak should work for beef, and it may work for pork and fish, too; any marinade will do.

Marinate ground beef and it turns to mush, so zap it instead. Livermore scientists found that microwaving meat for 2 minutes prior to cooking cuts heterocyclic amine content by 90 percent.

Put on a condom. Certain sexually transmitted viruses may play a role in some forms of cancer. For example, contracting the hepatitis B virus boosts liver cancer risk, and human papillomaviruses—the major cause of cervical cancer in women—have been linked to cancer of the penis. And don't forget about HIV—it can open the door to rare cancers such as Kaposi's sarcoma. A vaccine can protect you from hepatitis B infection, but condom use can help reduce the transmission of all three viruses.

Stop smuggling in those Cubans. We know the arguments: You stoke the occasional Presidente only after dinner or when you're out with the guys. And you don't inhale. Sorry, that doesn't get you off the hook. An NCI report concludes that, whether or not you inhale, smoking cigars will raise your risk of cancers of the mouth, larynx, esophagus, and lungs.

And whether it's cigars or cigarettes, the amount you smoke may not be a reliable gauge of your risk. "We see people who smoke two packs a day and don't get cancer, and half-a-pack smokers who do," says Therese Bevers, M.D., medical director of the cancer prevention center at the University of Texas M. D. Anderson Cancer Center in Houston. "Everyone's risks are different."

Bring home flowers tonight. Studies suggest that stress can depress the immune response (the body's defense against disease) and that men under stress tend to engage in behaviors that put their health at risk—such as smoking, drinking, and eating poorly. But Swedish researchers have found that emotional support during stressful times—major worries about a loved one, a financial crisis, work or legal troubles—may be a buffer. Men with strong support from family or friends who experienced three or more stressful events in a year had an 83 percent lower risk of death from cancer and other causes compared with similarly stressed-out guys who had little or no emotional support.

Work out more. Regular exercise has been shown to reduce risks for a number of cancers, including those of the prostate and colon. How much sweating is necessary to do the job? One Harvard study of nearly 48,000 middle-age male health professionals found that men who ran a total of 4.5 miles a week at a 10-minute-per-mile pace had about half the colon cancer risk of sedentary subjects. At the very least, says Dr. Shike, you should be following the government's exercise guidelines: 30 minutes of moderate activity on most days of the week.

Make an early tee time. Skin cancer rates have skyrocketed 162 percent since the mid-1970s, affecting men two to three times as much as women. The good news is that this is one of the easiest cancers to prevent. For starters, even on cloudy days, put on sunscreen before you go outside. (Choose one that has an SPF of at least 15 and that blocks ultraviolet A and B rays—exposure to both increases risk.) Though one report questioned the protective benefits of sunscreen, there's little doubt of their effectiveness: Many other studies have shown that sunscreens help shield skin from sun damage, and both the American Academy of Dermatology and the American Cancer Society continue to strongly advocate their use. After you slather on the sunscreen, cover up with tightly woven clothing and a wide-brimmed hat. And try to stay out of the sun between 10:00 A.M. and 4:00 P.M., when rays are strongest.

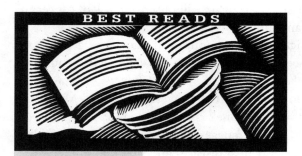

BEST READS

Start Living the Disease-Free Lifestyle Tonight

Most death is inflicted from within. The overwhelming majority—close to 75 percent—of deaths are caused by disease. Multiplying cancer cells will destroy whatever vital organ they occupy or spread to. Lung cancer, for example, will literally strangle you. Similarly, heart disease will stop your pulse. And any disease—most famously AIDS—can so tax your immune system that an opportunistic infection or some other pathological vulture can come in and finish the job. To keep disease at bay, you need to live a certain attainable lifestyle. Selene Yeager, Kelly Garrett, and the editors of Men's Health *Books outline how to adopt this lifestyle in this excerpt from* Death Defiers: Beat the Men-Killers and Live Life to the Max *(Rodale Press, 1998).*

Diseases don't just happen. Something has to go wrong. Most of the time, that something has to do with how you treat your body—that is, what you do with it and what you put into it.

In other words, fate is a minor factor in disease. *You* are a major one. If your behavior is in harmony with the way your biochemistry wants to work, you're living a disease-free lifestyle.

So let's get right to it: The major elements of a disease-free lifestyle are a healthy diet, regular physical activity, appropriate body weight, no smoking, controlled stress, and timely medical checkups.

Sense a little déjà vu? None of those six things are what the Pentagon folks would call classified information. We've all heard them since childhood, with overtones of discipline. But "good" behavior isn't the point. The issue's much simpler. Incorporate those six guidelines into your lifestyle, and you may prevent disease. Ignore them, and you may create disease.

The lifestyle link to disease prevention is so strong that it begs some questions.

Why don't we eat right? In other words, why so much animal fat (an across-the-board disease causer) and so few fresh fruits and vegetables (risk reducers for virtually everything)? Because, points out John Wurzelmann, M.D., clinical assistant professor of medicine at the University of North Carolina at Chapel Hill School of Medicine, "there really is such a thing as comfort food." Fat has a tendency to satisfy you far more than any mere vegetable would. "That's why you enjoy vegetables more when you put a fat dressing on them," he says.

Furthermore, says Moshe Shike, M.D., director of the prevention and wellness program at Memorial Sloan-Kettering Cancer Center in New York City, "it's a habit. You get used to eating hamburgers and french fries, and you don't think about the consequences."

Why don't we exercise? Because we don't need to, according to Walter M. Bortz II, M.D., clinical associate professor of medicine at Stanford University School of Medicine and author of *Dare to Be 100*. Of course, we *do* need to if we want to avoid heart disease, diabetes, and lots of cancers, because that's the way our bodies are designed. But it's not the way our everyday life is designed—not when pizzas can be delivered at the touch of a speed dial or home theaters can be controlled at the click of a remote. "In our culture, we don't have to move for anything," Dr. Bortz says. "We're the only species that doesn't have to move even to eat."

Why do we let ourselves get fat? Mostly because we eat too much. "There's no doubt that caloric consumption is too high," Dr. Wurzelmann says. "There are too many fat people in the United States." Obesity is a different risk factor than a lousy diet, but one easily follows from the other.

And inactivity leads to, and follows from, both. "If any other species had food supplied to it the way we do, it would get fat, too," Dr. Bortz says.

Why don't we quit smoking? It's not that a smoker doesn't care that more people die from tobacco use than from automobile accidents, drug abuse, AIDS, and alcohol combined. It's that he's probably addicted. "The nicotine receptors in the brain are very similar to the receptors for cocaine and heroin," says Thomas Glynn, Ph.D., director of cancer science and trends for the American Cancer Society. What's more, those receptors stay eager to receive years after you quit. One puff can get you back to a pack a day before you know it.

Why do we ignore stress? Probably because we're not too sure what it is. "People don't have a lot of knowledge about it and what to do about it," Dr. Shike says. "I think people understand that excess stress has a negative impact on their lives." Heart disease is one negative impact. Undermining the rest of your disease-free lifestyle is another. "Some people, when stressed, run to the refrigerator," Dr. Shike says. "Or they smoke."

Why do we avoid checkups? Denial, according to Dr. Shike, "is the feeling that 'it will never happen to me,' only to somebody else." In reality, all that is being denied is the possibility of early detection, which, for most men-stalking diseases, is the best bet for cure or containment.

Whose Lifestyle Is It Anyway?

Do you know what a disease-free lifestyle really is? It's taking control of your own health. You either seize the power or cede it to the bad guys.

That is precisely what a lot of people do. "They get born into this world and then just bumble their way through it," Dr. Bortz says. "They insulate themselves from the fact that what they do affects what becomes of them. And if something happens, they turn themselves over to a doctor and hope that he does something about it."

But by pursuing a disease-free lifestyle, you're doing something about it before it happens. That's a wiser strategy, Dr. Bortz maintains. It's also a major act of heroism, given that you're not exactly smothered with support from the prevailing culture.

Take, for example, the eat-right plank on your disease-free platform. You'll probably read time and again how much it helps to cut down on the animal fat in favor of fiber. But is there enough doctor's advice in the world to offset TV images of Michael Jordan telling you how wonderful it is to eat hamburgers?

"We're a cowboy culture," Dr. Wurzelmann says. "There's a deeply ingrained and continuously reinforced belief that our strength derives from eating cows. What it comes down to is that eating beef is seen as having a lot to do with masculinity."

But that's where taking control of your own lifestyle comes in. Here's how to do it.

Remember what it's all about. The best beginning for a disease-free lifestyle is understanding the end. "You have to know why you're doing it," says Ed Burke, Ph.D., vice president of the National Strength and Conditioning Association and coauthor of *Getting in Shape*. "If all you want is to lose 5 pounds to look good when you go to Jamaica on vacation, then don't bother." Instead, Dr. Burke says, think about having more energy always, about feeling stronger forever, about losing weight and keeping it off. "Your approach should be long-term," he says. "Make it part of your life."

Keep things underwhelming. All six disease-free lifestyle elements are essential. But if you suddenly get religion and resolve to change your diet, lose weight, start exercising, and quit smoking on day one, you're going to be overwhelmed. "You can fail miserably if you try to do too much at one time," Dr. Glynn says. "It should be a sequence of lifestyle changes rather than one big one."

The slow-but-sure approach works best for any individual lifestyle element, too. "You can't run a half-hour if you've never walked around the block," Dr. Bortz points out. "Take small steps of mastery."

Rewire yourself. For weight loss, gradual and steady progress isn't just easier. It's what works. You didn't gain the weight in 2 weeks, so you can't lose it healthfully in that amount of time either. You have to learn new behaviors. "Once you got fat, the eating center of your brain became fixed on that," Dr. Bortz says. "If you starve yourself and lose 20 pounds in 2 weeks, you haven't had time to rewire your brain."

Hence, you haven't accomplished much, and you're probably going to gain the weight back. "Short-term enthusiasm is wonderful, but until you get your behavior reprogrammed, your long-term results are going to be poor," Dr. Bortz says.

Get physical. In some circles, it's no longer considered correct to use the term *exercise*. The focus, if you please, is now on *physical activity*. "Exercise tends to be a negative term for many people," says Kerry Stewart, Ed.D., a clinical exercise physiologist and director of cardiac rehabilitation and prevention at Johns Hopkins Bayview Medical Center in Baltimore. "They think of exercise as pain or extremely hard work."

Buried somewhere in that semantic sideshow is a helpful message for the retooling of your lifestyle—namely, that while structured, moderate exercise is best, any kind of regular movement helps. "The major problem is not doing anything," Dr. Stewart says. "With physical activity as the goal, you can build activities into your lifestyle that aren't usually considered exercise—like a sport you think is fun or just mowing the lawn regularly."

Make exercise your cornerstone. The beauty of the disease-free lifestyle is that every element seems to boost every other. For example, reducing stress helps you quit smoking, which helps you exercise, which helps you lose weight. But exercise itself may be the sultan of synergy. "Start by exercising, and that will ignite all the other things," Dr. Burke says.

Exercise may work as your lifestyle cornerstone because it has been shown to increase what is known as self-efficacy. "That means that people who exercise have a higher degree of confidence in their ability to do things and they're more likely to do them," Dr. Stewart says. "People who are physically active tend to do other things as well to keep them healthy."

Keep it positive. If you equate a healthy diet with deprivation, you're not going to be very enthusiastic about it. So concentrate on what you should eat, not what you shouldn't, suggests Edward Giovannucci, M.D., Sc.D., assistant professor of medicine at Harvard Medical School. "Rather than obsessing about the fat content of your diet, focus on positive things like getting more whole grains and fruits and vegetables," he says. "Think more along the lines of balance. It's not that you can't eat any dairy products or beef. Just don't make them the focus of your diet."

Boosting Your Immunity

To remain disease-proof, you must possess a strong immune system. With a weak or impaired one, you greatly increase your chances of catching everything from the common cold to fatal diseases. A strong immune system is characterized by a number of things, all of which are discussed in this excerpt from Healing Power: Natural Methods for Achieving Whole-Body Health *(Rodale Press, 1999) by Bridget Doherty, Doug Hill, and the editors of* Men's Health *Books.*

Your immune system is smart. Throughout evolution, it has learned to detect the millions of outside invaders that try to find their way into your body. It knows what should be there, what shouldn't, and how to get rid of unwelcome visitors. The complex line of defense starts with your skin, the first barrier for attackers to cross. It has secondary defenses: nose hair, mucus, and saliva. If anything gets past all of that, your immune system turns to chemical warfare to destroy the invader once and for all.

Despite all its accumulated knowledge, your immune system is not fail-proof. Like any other complex machine, it needs to be taken care of to perform at its best. That's where you come in. By taking the right steps, you can ensure that your immune system is ready at all times to do its job.

Feeding the Army

There's no magic fruit or vegetable that will make you a virtual man of steel when it comes to your immunity. But when you stop to think about it, that's actually good news. Mother Nature gives us products that contain a wealth of substances to maintain a strong immune system. Every fruit and vegetable packs powerful yet different immunity-enhancing chemicals, nutrients, and a host of other things that science hasn't even discovered yet. Instead of relying on one or two select fruits, you can pick from all of them and know that you've just done something to help maintain a healthy immune system.

To use food to strengthen your immunity, you must eat a wide variety of fruits, vegetables, and whole grains, says Thomas Petro, Ph.D., associate professor of microbiology and immunology at the University of Nebraska Medical Center in Lincoln. By casting a wide net, you're bound to hit many of the nutrients found in food that build up your natural defense system. By sticking to only a select group, you're missing out on the many nutrients you need.

Unlike supplements, food delivers these immune-enhancing nutrients in the best package. We know from studies that people who eat fruits and vegetables have better immune systems. But many times a researcher will extract a particular vitamin or nutrient from a food, thinking that it's the key to the fruit or vegetable's power. When the tests come in, though, it often doesn't show the same beneficial results. It may be that only the natural form of the nutrient works. It may be that another nutrient present in the food is responsible. Or it could be that it isn't one nutrient but how all the nutrients work together that keeps an immune system healthy. "We simply don't know enough about them yet," says Susanna Cunningham-Rundles, Ph.D., associate professor of immunology at New York Hospital–Cornell Medical Center in New York City.

Your best bet is to eat at least five—and preferably closer to nine—servings of fruits and vegetables a day, eat whole grains, and cut down on fat. "For the guy seeking to keep his immune system strong and healthy, you have to start with the basics," says acupuncturist Victor S. Sierpina, M.D., assistant professor of family medicine at the University of Texas Medical Branch in Galveston.

Covering All the Bases

Although no one denies that the best way to get the nutrients you need is through food, there are a few stand-out vitamins and minerals. These few have proved to be integral to the functioning of the immune system. Without them, your defense system has a gaping hole in it.

Vitamin E. Take a supplement of 400 international units of vitamin E a day, advises Dr. Petro. Because it is found mainly in fat, it's hard to get the amount of vitamin E you need for a healthy immune system. If you are considering taking vitamin E in amounts above 200 international units, discuss this with your doctor first. One study using low-dose vitamin E supplements showed an increased risk of hemorrhagic stroke.

Vitamin E acts as an antioxidant, protecting your body from disease-causing molecules called free radicals. Studies have shown that extra vitamin E enhances the immune function in animals and people. "The most astonishing results we have seen are with vitamin E," Dr. Petro says. A study at Tufts University in Boston found that having older people supplement with vitamin E improved their immune systems.

Vitamin C. You should look for a supplement of 500 milligrams a day of vitamin C. "Vitamin C is a factor in normal immune cells," says Dennis D. Taub, Ph.D., acting chief of the laboratory of immunology at the National Institute on Aging. Numerous studies have shown that vitamin C is needed for a healthy immune system. Like vitamin E, vitamin C is an antioxidant and prevents disease by controlling free radicals. Some studies have even linked vitamin C to fighting off infections.

Zinc. Without zinc, many of the immune cells can't do their job. This trace mineral is critical for immune function. Yet a little goes a long way with zinc. Stick to the Daily Value of 15 milligrams, about what you will find in a multivitamin, says Chris D. Meletis, N.D., a naturopathic physician, dean of clinical education, chief medical officer, and professor of natural pharmacology and nutrition at the National College of Naturopathic Medicine in Portland, Oregon. Too much zinc actually suppresses your immune system because of the depletion of copper.

B vitamins. All three of the important B vitamins—B_6, B_{12}, and folic acid—play major roles in keeping your immune system up and running. You deplete your B vitamins during times of stress, says Dr. Sierpina. So it is important to get them either in a multivitamin or in a B-complex supplement. Look for the Daily Value of all three: 2 milligrams of vitamin B_6, 6 micrograms of B_{12}, and 400 micrograms of folic acid. Someone under a lot of stress should try to get even higher amounts of B vitamins, says Dr. Sierpina.

Passing the Stress Test

Nothing can shut down your immune system like stress. "Stress has incredible effects on the immune system. It is monstrous," Dr. Taub says. When your body goes into its fight-or-flight mode, it saps all the energy from your natural defense system, leaving you more open to all kinds of nasty things. So control stress, and you'll gain some control over your immune system's health. Here are some ways suggested by experts.

Listen to the music. The right music can aid you in your quest for calm in a stressed-out world, says Steven Halpern, Ph.D., president of Inner Peace Music in San Anselmo, California, and a composer. "It's like vitamins in the airwaves. You can enhance your immunity by choosing music that evokes your relaxation response," he says. There are several ways that you can use music to decrease your stress and help your immune system.

- Keep headphones in your office. Having instrumental, light music in the background creates a calming atmosphere in your office. If playing music in the background disturbs coworkers and you can work with headphones on, do so, Dr. Halpern says. If the music distracts you, use the headphones to take stress breaks. Instead of a coffee break, use those 5 to 10 minutes to take a music break. Put the headphones on and relax, he says.
- Move to the music. Call in the rock-'n'-roll doctor. Put on whatever music makes you get up and dance. Sing, play air guitar, or prance around the room to a song to which you can rock out. Do this for 10 minutes, and you'll get out some aggression and have some fun, Dr. Halpern says.
- Pick up sticks. You don't have to buy a drum. A pencil and your desk will do just fine. Rap on your desk. The physical act of making rhythmic music releases some pent-up frustration and tension, notes Dr. Halpern.

Take a breather. A simple breathing exercise can restore some peace to a crazed day, says Larry J. Feldman, Ph.D., director of the Pain and Stress Rehabilitation Center in New Castle, Delaware, and author of *Feeling Good Again*, a self-help book for dealing with stress. This breathing technique should help you relax; get some sleep, if need be; and provide control over tension: Inhale. When your lungs feel full, exhale naturally. After you have exhaled naturally, push out even more air for a count of 10. Start all over again by inhaling. Repeat the process five times, he says.

If you need to chill out some more, take a 2-minute break, then do the exercise five more times. To really control stress, practice this once or twice a day. By making it a habit, you'll stay calm during times of stress, Dr. Feldman says. If you are short on time, simply focus your attention on your breathing.

Count backward. When all you see is red, take a moment and start counting back from 40. With each number, take a full breath. In your mind, count each breath off as you exhale, saying the word *relax* after each number you count. By the time you reach zero, you should be in more control, Dr. Feldman says. Not only will this work in the heat of a stressful situation but also it will do wonders if you practice it once a day. "It will prevent you from getting all tense and stressed out. The more you do it, the better it will work. And in no time, you won't need to count back from 40," Dr. Feldman says. Practice enough, and you'll be able to get the same calming effect counting from 20, or even lower, he says.

Rub out stress. A good massage not only reduces stress but also has actually been shown to boost immunity on its own. A study at the University of Miami School of Medicine found that HIV-positive men who received daily massages for a month saw a jump in the number of their natural killer cells—cells that protect you from diseases. "When a person is touched and massaged in a therapeutic manner, the body's system is going to react," says Robert A. Edwards, a licensed massage therapist and director of the Somerset School of Massage Therapy in New Jersey. Do some at-home massage, or make an appointment with a qualified massage therapist.

Sign up for yoga. Yoga postures and breathing techniques, if practiced regularly, bring about a serenity that lingers with you throughout the day. "A yoga workout generally relieves stress," says Mara Carrico, a yoga instructor based in San Diego, creator of *The 10-Minute Yoga Work-In* audiocassette program, and author of *Yoga Journal's Yoga Basics*. Many yoga classes and workouts end with a meditation. Meditation helps you let go of stress and can add to the quality of your life by teaching you how to live each moment to the fullest, Carrico says.

Meet the Press

According to the Chinese technique of acupressure, all the stress you encounter creates an energy imbalance in your body. This imbalance then weakens your immune system. Several acupressure points are believed to get that energy back on track and bring back balance and a healthier immunity.

Lend an ear. Place your finger on the piece of cartilage that is in front of your ear canal. Put your thumb behind this piece of your ear cartilage and squeeze. For best results, pinch pressure hard enough so that you feel a hot stinging sensation. This point, called the adrenal point, stimulates hormone production to kick-start your immunity, says David Nickel, a doctor of Oriental medicine; a certified acupuncturist in Santa Monica, California; and author of *Acupressure for Athletes*. Squeeze the point for 5 seconds as you exhale through your mouth, then let up for 5 seconds as you inhale through your nose. Continue these 5-second intervals for about a minute.

Reach for your funny bone. An acupressure point in the elbow crease called the Crooked Pond is thought to correct weaknesses in the immune system. Bend your arm so that you form a crease inside your elbow. Place your thumb on the upper edge of the crease on the outside of your arm. Apply firm pressure into the joint and hold for 1 minute as you breathe deeply. Do this twice a day, says Michael Reed Gach, Ph.D., founder of the Acupressure Institute in Berkeley, California, and author of *Acupressure's Potent Points*.

"You should feel a slight pain, but it will be a good hurt," Dr. Gach says.

Unleash your energy. Get on your back with your knees bent to activate this point, which strengthens the immune system, Dr. Gach says. The point, called the Sea of Energy, is two finger-widths below the belly button, between the belly button and the pubic bone. Apply firm pressure down and in toward the vertebrae on your lower back. You know that you have the correct point if you feel the pressure deep inside, Dr. Gach says. Breathe deeply as you hold the point for 2 minutes.

Nature's Reinforcements

Several herbs are believed to have immune-boosting qualities. Now that herbs have experienced a renaissance of sorts, you should be able to find the following in drugstores, supermarkets, and health food stores.

Derail the cold bug. Echinacea acts as an immunostimulant. Simply put, it rallies your immune system. By doing so, it increases your body's resistance to bacterial invaders. Take it as a tea or tincture since there is some indication that it activates the immune system through mucosal absorption in the mouth. Take it at the first sign of a cold or flu. You can also use it if you have been exposed to someone with a cold, like that coworker who came in and sneezed all over your office, says Dr. Meletis. "It may help abort the cold from taking you over," he says.

To make a tea from echinacea, pour boiling water over 2 to 3 tablespoons of dried, fresh, or powdered herb and steep for 5 minutes. Drink three cups a day. Or take 30 drops of tincture three times a day. Double this dosage if you want to ease the symptoms 2 to 3 days after the onset of a cold, Dr. Meletis says. Do not use echinacea for more than 8 weeks at a time; if you have an autoimmune condition such as lupus, tuberculosis, or multiple sclerosis; or if you are allergic to chamomile, marigold, or other plants in the daisy family.

Ward off diseases with garlic. In olden times, some people claimed that garlic could cure "all diseases." That may be overstating it, but garlic is a talented herb/food when it comes to immunity. Garlic has been shown to lower cholesterol and thin the blood, which could help prevent heart attacks and strokes. It appears to block the growth of cancer cells. And it has been shown to kill at least 14 strains of bacteria taken from the noses and throats of children. The best way to get garlic is to toss about a clove a day in with your cooking, Dr. Meletis says. If you dislike the pungent aroma of fresh garlic, you can take enteric-coated capsules. Take one capsule containing 4,000 micrograms of allicin a day.

Go for an oil change. The essential oils thyme, peppermint, and pine increase your body's energy and boost your body's natural defense system, says Michael Scholes, president and founder of the Michael Scholes School of Aromatic Studies in Los Angeles. You can use each of the oils separately or mix a combination of them together, depending on your personal preference, he says. Try a massage with them heavily diluted in carrier oils such as canola, jojoba, or sweet almond. Using 10 to 12 drops of essential oil in an ounce of massage oil is just right. Any scent that makes you feel good reduces stress, which, in turn, can help your immune system, Scholes adds. Pick a few of your favorite essential oils and have them around to help you through stressful times. But be aware that some essential oils can cause skin irritation or may even be toxic. Check with a knowledgeable aromatherapist before experimenting with them.

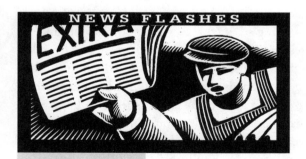

Low Vitamin Levels Can Result in Lead Retention

CAMBRIDGE, Mass.—Harvard researchers have discovered that if your vitamin C, vitamin D, and iron levels are low, your body may absorb and retain lead from sources such as drinking water and lead-based paints. Study coauthor Howard Hu, M.D., evaluated 747 men and found that those who took in a daily total of less than 179 international units (IU) of vitamin D, less than 109 milligrams of vitamin C, or less than 11 milligrams of iron had the most lead in their blood and bones. "Even low levels of lead have been linked to elevated blood pressure, kidney dysfunction, and anemia," says Dr. Hu. Skip the extra iron—it may contribute to heart disease—but boost your vitamin C intake to 250 milligrams per day and your vitamin D intake to 250 IU per day, Dr. Hu advises.

Simple Equation Predicts Heart Disease Risk

SYRACUSE, N.Y.—Grade-school subtraction could save your life. According to a study published in *Hypertension*, an easy equation can uncover your risk of heart disease. A study of nearly 20,000 French men found that you can calculate the stiffness of your arteries by subtracting the diastolic number (the lower number) of your blood-pressure reading from the systolic number. If the result is greater than 60, you need to consult your doctor. "As arteries stiffen, your systolic blood pressure increases and your diastolic pressure goes down, making this equation a simple way to predict heart disease," says the study coauthor, Harold Smulyan, M.D., of the State University of New York Health Science Center.

Ward Off Adult-Onset Diabetes with Carotenoids

ATLANTA—Research from the Centers for Disease Control and Prevention reveals that carotenoids—plant pigments related to vitamin A—may help prevent adult-onset diabetes. One study conducted by Earl Ford, M.D., measured the level of carotenoids in the blood of 1,665 people. He found that people with normal glucose levels had the highest carotenoid levels, and those with newly diagnosed diabetes had the lowest carotenoid levels. "Increasing your fruit and vegetable intake could help prevent the development of diabetes," says Dr. Ford. Carotenoids are abundant in sweet potatoes, tomatoes, cantaloupe, carrots, oranges, and broccoli.

High Calcium Intake Linked to Prostate Cancer

CAMBRIDGE, Mass.—You may be able to lower your prostate cancer risk by limiting your calcium intake and eating more fruit. Harvard researchers studied 47,000 men and found that those who consumed 2,000 milligrams of calcium a day were almost twice as likely to develop prostate cancer as those who consumed 1,000 milligrams (about three glasses of milk). And the men who ate the most fruit were 22 percent less likely to develop the disease than those who ate the least. According to one of the study authors, Edward Giovannucci, M.D., Sc.D., assistant professor of medicine at Harvard Medical School, too much calcium can lower your body's level of a vitamin D–related compound. The sugar found in fruit can raise it. "High levels of 1,25-dihydroxyvitamin D inhibit the growth of cancerous cells," he says.

Shorter, More Frequent Workouts May Be Best for Your Heart

BOSTON—According to researchers at Brigham and Women's Hospital, even a quick sweat can help keep your heart healthy. Their 12-year survey of 22,000 men found that exercising vigorously for 11 to 24 minutes twice a week reduced heart attack risk by 36 percent. Men who exercised for more than 24 minutes reaped no greater rewards—but those who did quick workouts five or more times per week cut their risk of heart attack by 46 percent. "Shorter, more frequent workouts may be better for your heart than longer, less frequent sessions," says Claudia Chae, M.D., a study research fellow.

Dairy Products May Cut Colon-Cancer Risk

NEW YORK CITY—According to a study published in the *American Journal of Clinical Nutrition*, dairy products may reduce your risk of colon cancer. Eighteen people who consumed 1,000 milligrams of calcium per day from dairy products stopped doing so for 1 week. When their stool samples were compared with samples from the previous week, there was a significant rise in cytotoxicity, a risk marker for colon cancer. "Calcium and phosphate probably eliminate bile acids, which increase the toxicity of feces," says Joseph Rafter, Ph.D., of the department of medical nutrition at the Karolinska Institute of Huddinge Hospital in Missouri. Aim for 1,000 milligrams of calcium per day from dairy products—about 8 ounces of nonfat yogurt plus 16 ounces of skim milk.

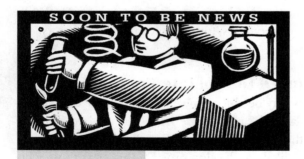

Bad Teeth Linked to Heart Trouble?

A study from the University of Minnesota in Minneapolis–St. Paul suggests that bacteria found in dental plaque may cause cardiac damage. When researchers injected rabbits with certain streptococcus bacteria present in plaque, the rabbits soon demonstrated faster heart and breathing rates and abnormal electrocardiograms. The bacteria seem to cause blood platelets to form dangerous clots in arteries, says Mark Herzberg, D.D.S., Ph.D., the study leader.

"We don't know if this occurs in people, but it's all the more reason to keep your teeth clean and see a dentist regularly," says Dr. Herzberg.

An End to Hearing Loss?

Head-bangers rejoice: A study at the Kresge Hearing Research Institute in Ann Arbor, Michigan, revealed that an antioxidant may prevent hearing loss. Researchers gave desferrioxamine (an antioxidant that removes excess iron from the blood) to mice, and found that it protected their hearing from sustained loud noises. "A loud noise triggers an overproduction of the free radicals that destroy the cells needed for hearing," says Jochen Schacht, Ph.D., the lead researcher. "Antioxidants prevent that damage."

Further studies are needed before a similar antioxidant treatment can be used on humans.

Toothpaste to Fight Viruses and Bacteria?

Researchers at Pace University in New York City discovered that zinc, aloe, and grapefruit extracts destroy viruses when added to toothpaste. When they mixed 0.1 percent of these purified extracts with several toothpastes, they found that each mixture killed every virus it was tested against. "Your mouth contains viruses and bacteria that can enter the bloodstream and travel to the heart," says Milton Schiffenbauer, Ph.D., the lead biologist. "We wanted to develop a system that destroys these microorganisms orally."

Dr. Schiffenbauer hopes that, after further studies, extracts like these will be added to all toothpastes and mouthwashes.

Faster Prostate Testing?

Your doctor will soon be able to screen for prostate cancer with a simple saliva test. With the Rapid Saliva Prostate Cancer Test, a doctor collects your saliva with a sponge and squeezes it onto a test strip. After 15 minutes, the strip will either remain white or display a pink line of an intensity that corresponds to your level of prostate-specific antigen (PSA). "If there's any pink, your doctor should follow up with a confirming PSA blood test," says Nicholas Levandoski, Ph.D., who conducted research for the test.

The new test should be widely available within 6 months.

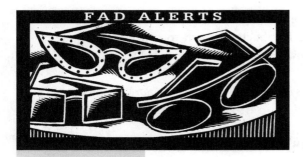

Waterless Hand Gels

 You pump some gas, then hit the drive-thru. As you tear into your burger, you realize that your hands are loaded with the germs that the previous 47 gas pumpers left on the handle. That's why such brands as Lysol, Softsoap, Dial, Purell, Germ-X, Suave, and Tommy Hilfiger have introduced waterless, antibacterial hand gels that you can use anywhere—no faucet required. Just rub a dime-size dollop on your hands, and 99 percent of disease-causing germs, most makers claim, will be dead within 15 seconds. Most of these gels cost between $2 and $4 for an 8-ounce bottle.

Though the gels don't remove visible grime, they instantly leave your hands feeling clean and dry and smelling clean enough for surgery. These products contain about 60 percent ethyl alcohol, a powerful disinfectant that hospitals have used for decades. "Cleaning your hands with rubbing alcohol would probably kill bacteria just as effectively, but there's a greater chance that it would irritate your skin," says Craig Eichler, M.D., a dermatologist at the Cleveland Clinic in Fort Lauderdale, Florida. The gels contain ingredients that stop the alcohol from drying out your skin.

One caveat: If you've ever sprouted a rash after using other hand products, stick with soap and water. "Some people are allergic to propylene glycol, a solvent used in several of these gels," says Karen S. Harkaway, M.D., a dermatologist in Mount Laurel, New Jersey.

Echinacea

 Echinacea is known as the cold-fighting herb. (Three species—*Echinacea purpurea*, *E. pallida*, and *E. angustifolia*—are available in the United States.) Taking 250 milligrams, standardized to contain 4 percent echinoside, every 6 hours for 2 days can help you shake cold symptoms faster, says Varro E. Tyler, Ph.D., distinguished professor emeritus of pharmacognosy at Purdue University in West Lafayette, Indiana.

But people misuse echinacea in one of two ways. Some drink a few tinctures and suck on a few lozenges every day, thinking they'll fend off colds. That's a waste of money—and taking echinacea for more than 2 months may cause immune system problems. A study of 302 people found that echinacea was no better than a placebo at preventing colds. Other people take echinacea only when they're hacking like an *ER* extra. The rhinovirus is well-established by then, and echinacea will be less effective. "You have to take it at the first sign of a cold," says Dr. Tyler. If you wait more than 3 days, it's probably too late.

L-Glutamine

 L-glutamine is an amino acid that your immune system cells use for fuel. Researchers propose that L-glutamine supplements can boost immunity and levels of growth hormone. Some vitamin companies imply that there's a link between elevated growth hormone and an increase in muscle mass.

In a study of 151 marathon runners at Oxford University in England, 72 of the athletes took 10 grams of L-glutamine before one or more races, and 79 took a placebo. After a week, almost twice as many men in the placebo group as in the L-glutamine group had cold symptoms.

Also, a tiny study at Louisiana State University in Baton Rouge showed that three men who took 2 grams of L-glutamine daily for 2 weeks had more plasma bicarbonate, a substance associated with a rise in growth hormone.

"Taking L-glutamine may help athletes who overtrain avoid infections," says Melvin Williams, Ph.D., an exercise physiologist at Old Dominion University in Norfolk, Virginia, and author of *The Ergogenics Edge*. But normal gym goers don't need it, and increasing your intake of one amino acid might cause imbalances with others.

As for bigger biceps, "research didn't measure any actual muscle growth," says Peter Lemon, Ph.D., chairman of exercise nutrition at the University of Western Ontario in Canada.

Dr. Williams says no claim could stand on that three-man study, "and some studies on growth-hormone supplementation show that it doesn't affect muscle growth in intense exercise." So don't bother.

Folic Acid

 Folic acid is a vitamin found in spinach, citrus fruits, beans, liver, and most breakfast cereals. Orange juice is an especially good source. Folic acid reduces the body's levels of homocysteine, an amino acid from protein-rich foods that appears to contribute to heart disease. "Homocysteine may combine with low-density lipoprotein ('bad') cholesterol to form plaque on artery walls," says Kilmer McCully, M.D., a pathologist at the Veterans Administration Medical Center in Providence, Rhode Island, and an expert on homocysteine.

In a study at the Medical College of Wisconsin in Milwaukee, 25 people drank about 20 ounces of orange juice (containing about 115 micrograms of folic acid) daily, and their homocysteine levels dropped by 11 percent within a month.

Drinking a few glasses of orange juice each day will give you half your recommended daily intake of folic acid. You can get the rest by eating five servings of fruits and vegetables, or a bowl of fortified cereal. Or you can take a multivitamin that contains 400 micrograms of folic acid. If you've had heart trouble or if heart disease runs in your family, ask your doctor whether you should take higher doses.

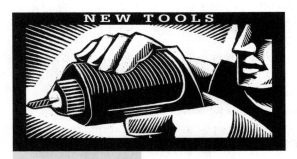

NEW TOOLS

Better Plaque Removal

Sonicare Toothbrush

Topped with toothpaste, any cheap, soft-bristled toothbrush will scrub away plaque. But if a high-tech brush can do a better job, why be primitive? The bristles on Optiva's Sonicare ($100) hum at 31,000 rpm, and the manufacturer claims that this creates a "sonic wave" that removes hidden bacteria as you gently touch each tooth. According to dentists and clinical studies, it works. "The sonic waves create bubbles that essentially jar the plaque loose without damaging your gums," says Dennis Mangan, Ph.D., of the National Institute of Dental and Craniofacial Research in Bethesda, Maryland.

Optiva's studies have shown that the Sonicare removes bacteria that cause gum disease better than a manual toothbrush can. But Kenneth Burrell, D.D.S., senior officer at the American Dental Association, points out that if you already brush conscientiously, you may not need this device.

Some rules: Use a feather-light touch, brush for a full 2 minutes, replace the head every 6 months (they're $15 a pair at most drugstores), and continue flossing. "Nothing can replace flossing," emphasizes Dr. Burrell.

More Accurate Prostate Cancer Diagnoses

Hybritech Free PSA Test

If your prostate-specific antigen (PSA) level is between 4 and 10 nanograms per milliliter, your doctor will probably perform a prostate biopsy. But there's a 75 percent chance that you don't have cancer. To reduce unnecessary biopsies, the FDA approved the Hybritech Free PSA test. The test determines how much PSA in your blood is free, or unbound to protein. If the count is at least 25 percent, it's unlikely that you have cancer. In a study of 773 men ages 50 to 75, the Free PSA test diagnosed 95 percent of the men with cancer. No other free-PSA test can make that claim. For more information, call (888) 880-0518.

Fewer Blood Clots

ProVex CV

A flavonoid supplement may be more effective than aspirin at preventing blood clots. For 1 week, 14 subjects took a daily dose of ProVex CV, a supplement containing extracts from grape skin, grape seed, *Ginkgo biloba*, bilberry, and the flavonoid quercetin. (Flavonoids found in red wine and grape juice seem to prevent blood platelets from clumping.) The supplement reduced the subjects' platelet activity by about 52 percent. "It may be especially useful for people who want the benefits of red wine but who can't or don't want to drink," says the lead researcher, John Folts, Ph.D., of the University of Wisconsin in Madison. Speak with your doctor if you're interested in taking ProVex CV.

Lower Stroke and Heart Attack Risk

Baycol

"We have definitive proof that taking just one cholesterol-reducing pill a day can reduce your risk of a heart attack or stroke by as much as 40 percent," says Roger Blumenthal, M.D., director of the Ciccarone Center for the Prevention of

Heart Disease at Johns Hopkins University in Baltimore. Unfortunately, only one-third of the 21 million Americans who need this type of medication are taking it.

Baycol is one of the latest in a class of cholesterol-reducing drugs known as statins. These drugs block the activity of an enzyme the liver uses to make cholesterol, causing the liver to remove more cholesterol from the blood. All statins can lower total cholesterol by at least 20 percent, but Baycol, according to Dr. Blumenthal, is "a little less expensive and a little more powerful than the other drugs in this class."

In a 24-week study of 934 patients, Baycol lowered low-density lipoprotein cholesterol (the "bad" kind of cholesterol) by 28 percent, and raised levels of high-density lipoprotein cholesterol (the "good" kind) by 10 percent. If you have high cholesterol (200 mg/dL of blood or greater) and other risk factors for heart disease, ask your doctor whether you should consider taking Baycol.

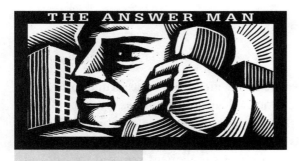

THE ANSWER MAN

Passing Along a Virus

Can I catch a cold by drinking from a water fountain after a sick person has used it?

—D. W., Anchorage

Yes, but probably not in the way you're thinking, says Travis Bomengen, M.D., a physician at the University of Wyoming Family Practice Clinic in Casper. "If you don't put your mouth on the faucet head, it's extremely unlikely that you'll come into contact with cold viruses," he says. It is possible, however, to pick up a cold virus by touching the water-fountain button: The sick guy wipes his nose, then pushes the button for a drink. Is there any way to avoid his germs? "Just wash your hands with soap and water fairly often, and avoid touching your face," says Dr. Bomengen.

Shading Those Eyes

My dad, who's 70, just had surgery to remove a cataract. Are there any preventive measures I can take to avoid cataract problems when I'm his age? (I'm 40 now.)
—C. N., Tracy, Calif.

The best preventive measure is to protect your eyes from the sun by wearing a wide-brimmed hat or sunglasses whenever you're outdoors, says Andrew S. Farber, M.D., spokesman for the American Academy of Ophthalmology. "Studies have shown that this significantly decreases your risk of cataracts," he says.

It's also important to take in enough vitamin C through your diet. A study at Tufts University in Boston found that people who took vitamin C supplements over a 10-year period were 77 percent less likely to develop cataracts than those who didn't take supplements. Try to get about 200 milligrams of vitamin C every day, suggests Paul Jacques, Sc.D., who authored the study. (Most multivitamins provide about 60 milligrams. If you're eating four or five servings of fruits or vegetables every day, you probably don't need a supplement.)

Finally, if you're a smoker, stop now. It increases your risk for cataracts, says Dr. Farber.

The Importance of Calcium

My wife takes calcium to prevent osteoporosis, but I've never heard anything about calcium requirements for guys. Do I need to worry about osteoporosis? And if so, how much calcium should I be taking every day?
—P. B., El Cajon, Calif.

Osteoporosis, a chronic condition marked by brittle bones and spontaneous fractures, is something men as well as women can develop, says Elizabeth Kunkel, R.D., Ph.D., professor of food science at Clemson University in South Carolina. "Men lose bone mass in their forties at about the same rate as women," she says, "but because men have more bone mass to begin with, problems with osteoporosis won't show up until relatively late in life." By the time you reach 80, osteoporosis is somewhat likely. It can result in spinal compression, which can mean a loss of height or a hunched-over appearance.

To decrease your chances of developing osteoporosis, you need to take in 1,000 milligrams of calcium a day—roughly the amount in two glasses of milk and two servings of broccoli. Other excellent calcium sources include cheese, yogurt, soybeans, and green leafy vegetables.

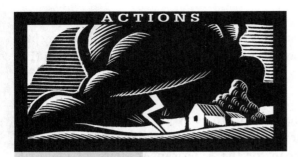

ACTIONS

When the topic is mortality, heart disease and cancer get most of the attention. And for good reason: No other cause of death, including accidents, comes close to either of them. But if heart disease and cancer alone account for slightly more than half of all deaths in the United States, that means that all the others account for only slightly less than half. Attacking anywhere from your brain to your bowel, the Grim Reaper's supporting cast can kill you just as dead as the big two. Or they can color the rest of your years varying shades of miserable. Here are some ways to ward off life's ailments, large and small.

1. **Zap back pain.** Seventy-five percent of all lower-back problems can be prevented by building your abdominal muscles. Aim for 12 to 15 crunches a day.

2. **Pull asthma's triggers.** Asthma attacks don't just happen. Something triggers them, and those triggers vary with the victim. They can be anything from dust to gases to allergies to viruses. The best way to take control of asthma, according to the American Lung Association, is to discover which conditions set off the attacks. Then avoid those conditions.

3. **Eat 30 percent less food.** Being at least 20 percent overweight for your height and build puts you at substantial risk of premature croaking. In fact, doctors at Duke University in Durham, North Carolina, estimate that there are probably 300,000 obesity-related deaths annually in this country. Dropping any number of pounds will improve your health, but if you're serious about making it to 90, you may want to start really cutting calories.

Normal, active guys in their thirties are supposed to eat a balanced diet containing about 2,500 total calories per day. However, researchers at the National Institute on Aging found that monkeys who consumed 30 percent fewer total daily calories (but maintained their levels of vitamins and other nutrients) appeared to age more slowly than monkeys whose calories weren't restricted.

4. **Get vaccinated against pneumonia.** Yes, there's a pneumonia vaccine. And though it won't fend off every type of pneumonia in existence, it will protect you from pneumococcal pneumonia, the most common bacterial kind. It's relatively cheap (about $25), it's covered by Medicare, it's side effect–free, and it will last you at least 10 years.

5. **Fight off the bugs.** According to an overview of studies on immune response, a dose of aerobic exercise raises your immune system's ability to recognize invading bacteria and viruses. Any form of moderate exercise done for 30 to 60 minutes is ideal, says David Nieman, Ph.D., a professor in the department of health and exercise science at Appalachian State University in Boone, North Carolina. It doesn't matter what form of exercise you do, says Dr. Nieman. "The things that matter are the intensity and duration." Dr. Nieman looked at 150 people who had walked regularly for 12 weeks. Those who had exercised moderately, he found, had half the number of colds and sore throats of the least active subjects. Don't overdo it, though: After 90 minutes at high intensity, your body releases stress hormones that push the odds of illness in the other direction.

6. **Die broke.** If you want to live a long and satisfying life, make it your goal to die broke. Although a sizable nest egg relieves stress (which, in turn, enhances health), this is only true to a certain age. According to Royda Crose, Ph.D., director of the center for gerontology at Ball State University in Muncie, Indiana, and author of *Why Women Live Longer Than Men . . . And What Men Can Learn from Them*, after the mortgage is burned and the kids' college bills are paid, it's far better to spend than to save.

"The drive to accumulate money is Depression-era thinking," Dr. Crose explains. "It's the old idea of leaving the farm to the kids so it will continue. But we don't live in that kind of society anymore. Instead of thinking of your legacy in terms of money, think of it as good memories generated by what you can do now by spending it."

7. **Exercise 3 hours a month.** You already know exercise is important, but it's worth emphasizing again, given a recent study. In a quest to finally separate the influences of heredity and exercise on longevity, researchers followed 16,000 twins for 19 years. They found that you can overcome genetic faults: Individuals who took brisk 30-minute walks just six times a month were 56 percent less likely to die than their more sedentary twin brothers or sisters.

8. **Change jobs.** For her book, Dr. Crose interviewed men age 80 and older, looking for clues to their longevity. "One of the things that surprised me," she says, "is that lots of them had really checkered work histories. They worked at something for a while, then they moved on to a succession of other things. Some of these men even took risks such as opening their own businesses."

Dr. Crose speculates that this kind of career-hopping extends life because it prevents men from making a common, fatal mistake: defining themselves by their jobs. "Men's identities are often so wrapped up in their work that when they retire, they lose their entire sense of self-worth," she says. "In fact, the highest suicide rate is among white men over age 65." Switching jobs and starting over teaches them to be more resilient, more flexible, and less afraid of new beginnings.

9. **Party on without fear of reprisal.** Saying no to that fifth beer is one option, but if it's too late, try this to avoid a hangover: Before you go to sleep, eat honey on crackers or toast.

10. **Be your own doctor.** This is how you earn the degree. Go to your computer, log on to the Internet, and type in the following address: www.yahoo.com. (Or pick your own favorite search engine.) Go to the health section, and in the "search" box that appears, type in whatever is ailing you—prostate, migraine, cholesterol, bashful bladder. . . . Then press the "enter" button and watch your personal medical library unfold. You'll find all the latest information, treatments, and journal articles on your screen. You'll also find more than a few outright quacks, so be careful. Still, when you're trying to overcome a health problem, it works better than watching *ER*.

Become an expert in your illness, and by sharing what you find, you'll force your doctor to be one, too. Self-education is key. Be your own advocate. It's your life.

11. **Shake off the Monday morning blues.** Avoid sleeping late on Sunday mornings. It throws off your body clock and makes it difficult to get up for work on Monday.

12. **Have more sex.** Nine hundred middle-age men in southern Wales were enlisted for an unusual research project to determine whether sexual activity affects longevity. Each man was given a comprehensive medical exam and, in the name of science, asked to record how often he ejaculated. After 10 years, the most sexually active men had a 50 percent lower mortality rate than the least sexually active men—prompting the theory that regular orgasms can protect men's health. So get busy.

To make sure you're able to free Willy well into your golden years, the most effective thing you can do is keep your cholesterol within recommended levels. According to Roger Kirby, M.D., a urologist at St. George's Hospital in London, one of the biggest erection facilitators is a chemical called nitric oxide. It's a vasodilator, which means it helps trigger bloodflow to the penis (and, thereby, harden it). Having lots of cholesterol in your circulatory system restricts bloodflow to the penis and inhibits nitric oxide production—which makes Willy flounder.

13. Drink less. Spend too much time toasting your health, and soon your friends will be toasting you . . . at your wake. In a 10-year study of 22,000 male doctors, Harvard researchers found that men who consumed between two and six drinks a week had nearly half the risk of death of men who downed two or more drinks a day. One explanation: Limiting alcohol may protect your heart.

14. Know the side effects of your medications. Some older patients may be the casualties of medication, not age. "You're especially at risk if you take multiple medications, see more than one physician, or have prescriptions filled at more than one pharmacy," says Ilene H. Zuckerman, Pharm.D., an associate professor of pharmacy at the University of Maryland in Baltimore.

Indeed, deaths from accidental poisonings by medication increased 250 percent from 1983 to 1993, according to researchers at the University of California, San Diego.

There's no reason for this to happen to you. "Many adverse drug effects are predictable and avoidable," says Dr. Zuckerman—if you keep your doctors and your pharmacist informed about all the prescription and over-the-counter drugs you're taking. Stick to one pharmacy, too, she says, so your medication history is in one place.

15. Keep blisters at bay. Apply a light coating of petroleum jelly to your heels and any other hot spots on your feet.

16. Crush kidney stones. "In our studies, dietary potassium has been more protective than any other nutrient," says Gary C. Curhan, M.D., director of the Partners Center for Kidney Stone Disease at Massachusetts General Hospital in Boston. Consuming 4,000 milligrams daily can cut your risk of kidney stones in half. Potatoes, cantaloupe, bananas, and lima beans are good sources.

17. Box out back strain. If you're picking a box up from the floor, squat with your feet shoulder-width apart, "surround" the box with your arms, keep your abs tight, and stand with your back straight. This gives your back an assist from your legs and butt muscles. Keep the box close to you. And when you turn, first point your feet in the direction you're turning, so you don't twist your back. Set the box down on something that's about as high as you're holding it.

18. Feed your vision. You probably already know that a diet rich in leafy green vegetables, such as spinach, can help protect your vision. New research shows that red, yellow, and orange fruits and vegetables are just as useful. Researchers at the University of Texas Medical Branch in Galveston recently found that corn, orange peppers, red grapes, kiwifruit, and squash are excellent sources of lutein and zeaxanthin, two antioxidants that may slow or prevent age-related vision loss. The study leader, Frederik van Kuijk, M.D., recommends eating at least five servings of fruits and vegetables a day.

19. **Read the tea leaves.** Drinking tea may lower your heart attack risk. Researchers from Brigham and Women's Hospital in Boston and Harvard Medical School compared 340 men and women who had suffered heart attacks with 340 who hadn't. Those who drank a cup or more of black tea per day had a 44 percent lower heart attack risk than those who didn't drink tea. The researchers aren't sure whether the lowered risk is due to the tea's high content of flavonoids (antioxidants that may reduce cellular damage to arteries) or whether tea drinkers simply tend to lead healthier lives.

20. **Tame your tongue.** Does talking fast raise blood pressure? Researchers measured the blood pressures and heart rates of 111 cardiac patients as they read the U.S. Constitution rapidly for 2 minutes, then slowly for 2 minutes. Rapid reading triggered a rise in the subjects' blood pressures and heart rates, according to the study. Never forget: You have the right to remain silent.

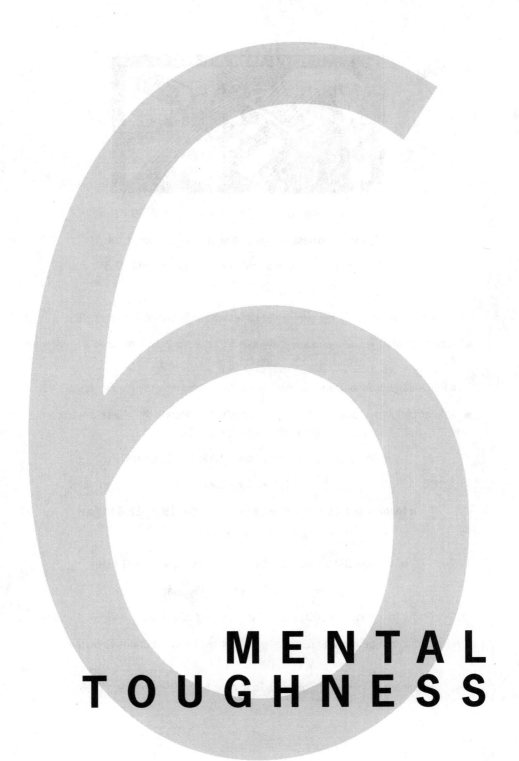

6

MENTAL TOUGHNESS

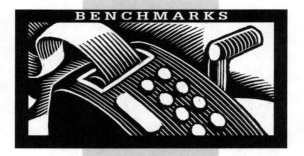

BENCHMARKS

- Age of the oldest person to learn to read: 99

- Age of the oldest person to coach college football: 84

- Average hours of sleep achieved per night in 1960: 7.5

- In 1999: 6.9

- Number of words per minute the fastest talker in the world can say: 637

- Percentage of Americans who say they wouldn't accept a job if it required a lie-detector test: 55

- Percentage of Americans who can't name "a country near the Pacific Ocean": 42

- Number of hours it took two men to win a contest to decode the federal government's data-scrambling system: 56

- Annual office visits for depression in 1995: 5.6 million

- In 1996: 6 million

- Number of prescriptions written for Prozac in 1995: 18.8 million

- In 1996: 20.7 million

- Average SAT scores for men in 1998: 509 verbal, 531 math

- For women: 502 verbal, 496 math

- According to a survey of 300 people, the least stressful day of the week: Thursday

- Percentage of people who consider president of the United States to be the most stressful job: 19

- Number of injuries attributed to road rage from 1990 to 1996: 12,610

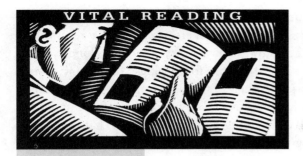

VITAL READING

Up and at 'Em

Use the power of your brain to start the day with gusto.

There are two kinds of mornings: good ones and bad ones. Sometimes you can't wait to get out of bed. You're up and out faster than Tipper Gore at a porno theater. But other times, even when you've gone to bed early, climbing out from beneath the covers seems more like digging your way out of a grave. Haven't you ever wondered why?

You may think that your morning malaise stems from something physical: drinking too many beers, staying up too late, taking the wrong woman to bed (she's still wearing the hair net). But more often than not, it's all in your head.

What rouses you from slumber is increased bloodflow to the brain triggered by stress hormones, says J. Christian Gillin, M.D., of the San Diego Veterans Affairs Medical Center. But this mechanism has to compete against another physiological drive—the one that pleads for more rest.

"It's a teeter-totter effect," says Timothy Roehrs, Ph.D., director of research at the sleep disorders and research center at Henry Ford Hospital in Detroit. "One drive is activating the sleep system, and one's activating the arousal system." The outcome of that battle can determine the course of your whole day.

The secret is to fuel your arousal system so it can beat the pants off your sleep system. "Sleepy people don't experience increased levels of blood to their brains right away," says Dr. Gillin. "They require about 20 minutes to shake the cobwebs off." But by creating positive stimuli—the kind of feel-good expectations that trigger hormones to wake the brain—you'll override the need to sleep, and you'll be able to jump out of bed like a man on fire. Here's your 7-day planner for great awakenings.

Monday. You need rewards. How about sex? It's the heavy artillery of morning motivators and the only trump card that beats the second most compelling reward for a hardworking guy: sleeping forever.

"If the biggest reward in your morning is sleeping in, you'll do it," says Joseph Rock, Psy.D., a Cleveland psychologist. Poor wakers need to find a reward that can compete with the thrill of the pillow. "Do whatever you like, as long as it gets you going," Dr. Rock says. "Have a meal you like for breakfast; have sex with your wife." Have sex with your wife over breakfast if that's what it takes. Just be sure to schedule something every day that'll motivate you to crawl out from under the comforter. Start one day a week with a doughnut for breakfast. That new box of Peanut Butter Crunch you bought on Saturday? Wait until Monday to open it. If you're a coffee hound, buy an automatic coffeemaker with a timer to lure your body out of bed and into the kitchen.

Or make the reward contingent on reaching a certain goal at work, says Michael Mercer, Ph.D., industrial psychologist and author of *Spontaneous Optimism*. "If all you have to look forward to is something general, such as working hard and not getting fired, it's going to be hard to get out of bed," says Dr. Mercer. Try something like this: Tell yourself that if you make 10 sales calls by the end of the day, you get to shoot hoops with the guys that night. If you don't make the 10 calls, you don't go. You'll be excited about the prospect of playing basketball, so you'll have a good reason to kick your butt out the door.

Tuesday. You need novelty. Ever have a relationship that started off with a nearly obsessive amount of sex and passion, only to have it deflate faster than a technology stock? Almost overnight, the wild thing becomes the same-old.

Routine can make it hard to climb into bed with a familiar lover. Why get up if your love life, your job, your clothes, your car, and the route you drive are dripping with sameness? Might as well sleep through it all. "When you keep doing the same thing, you fall into a rut or a comfort zone," says Dr. Mercer. "Every day, before you go to sleep, figure out something exciting to do the next day."

You don't need to buy a new car to look forward to driving to work. Why not have your old one detailed? Or buy new music for the tape player? Even a new shirt and tie, or a *laundered* shirt and tie, can help. "In the old days, women suffering from depression were advised to buy new hats," says Michael J. Salamon, Ph.D., a New York psychologist. It's not so much the hat, he says, as the new sense of confidence that comes with it. So go out and find a new woman with a new hat.

Wednesday. You need excitement and surprises. Your brain during sleep is like a customer-service number during the night shift: It never fully shuts down, but it's very selective in what it chooses to deal with. "Mothers of newborn babies readily wake up when their babies cry," says Dr. Roehrs, "but they may not wake up when a train or bus goes by." While you're sleeping, your brain is deciding what's an important stimulus and what's not. To psych your brain into wakefulness, you need to mimic the same rush you feel on the morning of a great road trip or a hot date. Here are some simple ideas.

- E-mail an old friend before you leave work at night, so you can't wait to check your incoming mail when you get to the office the next morning.
- Choose one morning when your hobby, not your job, will come first—an early hike, 30 minutes surfing the Web, a 15-minute dumbbell workout.
- Buy a CD after work, but don't listen to it until your morning shower.

Thursday. You need to eliminate obstacles. Your rough mornings may have more to do with mental roadblocks than with a lack of physical arousal. "Sometimes, not wanting to get up in the morning is the symptom of a bigger issue," says James F. Calhoun, Ph.D., professor of psychology at the University of Georgia in Athens. Maybe it's a dreadful job or a dissolving relationship. Research shows that anxiety can cause people to linger beneath the bedclothes after they wake up.

If the morning dread stems from your long list of prework chores (ironing, walking the dog, packing your lunch, putting gas in the car, and don't forget reading the McKenzie file), then launch a preemptive strike the night before. Take 20 minutes at the end of the workday to clear your desk, empty your in box (the McKenzie file goes to Johnson), and nail your errands so you can start your workday clean.

Friday. You need recess. Why did it seem easier to wake up early when you were in fifth grade than it does now? Third-period kickball, that's why. Even if the rest of the day consisted of diagramming sentences and reciting multiplication tables, there was always the allure of the big game.

Now you have to schedule your own big moments—and make sure they include other people. Interacting with others can be almost as exciting as the activity itself, says Dr. Salamon. Maybe a Friday-morning breakfast with the boys, or one day a week that your work group tries a new restaurant for lunch. If you have an hour for lunch, use it. Knowing that something fun is only 3 hours away—not 8 or 9—makes the morning rise easier.

Saturday. You need climate control. You'd think that the weekend would be incentive enough to wake up, but with Friday night being, well, Friday night, you can probably use some extra nudging. Maybe it's time to play around with your body temperature.

Turn up the heat. A drop in temperature is a signal to your body that the time has come to hibernate, says Rosalind Cartwright, Ph.D., a sleep expert at Rush–Presbyterian–St. Luke's Medical Center in Chicago. Warmth means it's time to wake up and crawl out of the burrow. Fool your body by attaching a timer to an electric blanket so the temperature increases at about the time your alarm sounds. (Make sure the timer and blanket are current-compatible, and don't forget to shut them off before you leave on vacation.)

Sunday. You need enlightenment. You've probably told your body that today is the day it gets to sleep in. That might not be the best idea. If you awaken at 6:00 A.M. every morning during the week but switch to 10:00 on the weekends, in effect you're setting your internal clock ahead 4 hours. For every hour you push it ahead, you'll need a day of getting up at the usual time to reset it. With that scenario, it may take until the following Friday to return to your normal weekday sleep schedule, says Mark J. Chambers, Ph.D., of the Sleep Clinic of Nevada in Las Vegas. Giving up those 4 hours of sloth needn't be a hardship. Here are a couple of tricks to help.

First, move your bed so that you're facing a window. Sunlight is a cue that tells your body that it's time to hunt that saber-tooth, says James Maas, Ph.D., professor of psychology at Cornell University in Ithaca, New York, and author of *Power Sleep*. Raise your window shade halfway before you go to bed to let in the morning light. About 30 minutes of light should be enough to rouse you.

Second, if you wake up in the middle of the night to go to the bathroom, don't turn the lights on. Even brief exposure to light will cause your body to stop producing the hormone melatonin, and that will disrupt your normal sleep cycle. Buy a night-light. And a good tile cleaner.

Sneaky Signs of Stress

Defuse these often-overlooked symptoms of too much pressure.

The usual pressure points are pretty easy to spot: We sweat like a cold beer on a warm day, we argue with our PCs, we snap at the wife and kids. But tension can bubble up in other ways, too. The next time you experience any of these five symptoms, it might be time to put your job on the examining table. "Treating these specific stress symptoms may give you temporary relief," says Reed Moskowitz, M.D., a stress expert at New York University Medical Center in New York City, "but unless you reduce your overall stress levels, the problems will likely return."

Killer heartburn. Stress makes your stomach produce more gastric acid, says Sheila Rodriguez-Stanley, Ph.D., of the Oklahoma Foundation for Digestive Research in Oklahoma City. Combining that with greasy, grab-and-go food can lead to severe heartburn. In some cases, acid may rise into your esophagus; that's called reflux.

Drink some water every half-hour. This will not only give you a regular stress break, it will also wash the stomach acid out of your esophagus and dilute it, temporarily soothing the burn. Cut the fast food; high-fat lunches might calm your nerves (digestion relaxes you), but they'll turn your gut into a volcano. Avoid foods that spur heartburn, such as coffee, tomato sauce, onions, chocolate, and peppermint. See a doctor if your heartburn persists for more than a week, or if it's accompanied by dizziness, sweating, or light-headedness.

Shaky hands. "Hand tremors can strike men who have built-up anger," says James Campbell Quick, Ph.D., editor of the *Journal of Occupational Health Psychology*. You can't tell your boss to stop taking credit for your work, so you involuntarily shake off the rage through your hands. Caffeine withdrawal or fatigue can also cause unsteadiness.

The best cure? Unload your problem on your boss. But if that sounds dangerous, let the aggression drain out of your fingers by squeezing, flexing, and then relaxing your hands for several minutes, advises Dr. Quick. If you feel the urge to strike something, as many hand tremblers do, he recommends keeping a punching bag at home. It'll make concrete walls less tempting. Strenuous exercise and an extra hour of sleep should also steady your hands and reduce your stress. If they don't, see a doctor.

Sudden dizziness. "Some men have a tendency to breathe too shallowly when they're tense, and this can make them feel light-headed," says Dr. Moskowitz.

Dizziness can signal that your blood pressure has dropped because you're anxious, adds Dr. Quick. Stay hydrated and keep your blood sugar levels steady, he says. Chug an 8-ounce glass of water every hour and eat a snack (such as an apple) every few hours.

If you have a dizzy spell, advises Dr. Moskowitz, sit down and try this breathing exercise: Inhale slowly and fully through your nose, drawing air deep into your lungs and holding it for a moment. Then slowly exhale through your nostrils. This will increase your oxygen intake and also give you a full feeling, which relaxes your nervous system.

See a doctor if dizziness strikes more than twice. It could mean heart trouble, says Dr. Quick.

Hives. Hives are itchy welts that can form on your skin when cells release histamine (a chemical that causes small blood vessels to dilate and fluid to accumulate near the surface). An allergy or irritation usually causes this response, but hormones released in times of stress can worsen it, says Doris June Day, M.D., dermatologist at New York University Medical Center.

Stress-induced hives even have a name: stress urticaria. This problem often has a simpler cause, though. Stressed men sometimes scratch themselves raw, says Jonathan Cook, M.D., a dermatologic surgeon with the University of Pennsylvania Health System in Philadelphia.

Don't rake your neck or claw at your chin when you're tense, advises Dr. Cook. Keep something in your hands so you won't start scratching yourself: a pen, a football, a wad of therapeutic clay, anything but a loaded firearm. Physicians often prescribe meditation and other relaxation practices to stop hives. If you start sprouting hives, rub them with a mentholated lotion (such as Sarna) or an ice cube wrapped in plastic to cool your skin.

Excessive spending. It's not a physical symptom, but spending too much money is an often-overlooked sign of stress. Spending cash gives some stressed-out men quick comfort, says Mack Lipkin, M.D., a stress expert at New York University. Doling out the green momentarily gives you the feeling of control. Unfortunately, this stress-busting pastime can invite calls from collection agencies.

If you feel a spending spree coming on, reach for a catalog instead of visiting the mall. "Catalog shopping enables you to feel like you're spending money, but it can delay the actual purchase until you're clear-headed," says Dr. Lipkin. It's also easier to cancel shipment on that CD system than to schlepp the thing back to the store.

No Need to Lose Your Mind

Ward off the effects of aging with these simple memory tricks.

Somewhere on this small planet, a man is looking for his lost eyeglasses. Naturally, they're resting on top of his head. Somewhere else is a poor guy who can't remember where he parked his car. Eventually he'll realize that—it being a nice day—he walked to work this morning. And perhaps right now, there you are: a smart man who can't seem to recall what he did with the remote. Then, finally, you figure out where you left it. (Odd. You took it to the bathroom with you.)

You're not losing your mind. Wait. Actually, you are. When your brain's nerve cells deteriorate, as everyone's do between the ages of 25 and 49, your memory powers also start to decline. But knowing that you have plenty of confused company is little consolation, since forgetfulness can have big consequences. It can make you look thoughtless (her birthday was yesterday), careless (her belated present, a teddy, is three sizes smaller than what she wears now), and stupid (her name is spelled wrong on the card). It can also be a massive time waster. The average man spends about 15 hours every year hunting for lost keys.

At this point in medical science, there's nothing available that will reverse this gradual decline in memory skills (to which the drugs you may have done in college were not a contributing factor). There are, however, numerous cheats you can use to cover up the fact that you no longer remember the first time you had sex, let alone the last time.

Pinch your nose. You walk out of the airport terminal, head to the parking garage, and whip out the keys. But you're not parked in row M—or in row N, O, or P. In fact, you can't even remember if your car is on level 2 or 3. True, walking in circles while muttering obscenities might burn calories, but it won't help you remember where you parked. Instead, try the following trick.

Close off one nostril by pressing the side of your nose. Your brain operates on a 90-minute schedule. The left hemisphere is dominant for 90 minutes, then the right takes over, says William Cone, Ph.D., author of *Stop Memory Loss!* Fooling with your nose's breathing cycle can change that rhythm. When your left nostril is open, the right hemisphere of your brain is dominant, and vice versa. Because the two sides store and process different types of information, it's possible that you'll find the memory of your parking space on the side of your brain that would normally be at rest. "You usually don't know where a particular piece of information is hiding. Try eight breaths through one nostril, then eight through the other," Dr. Cone says. If neither works, take your finger off your nose. People are starting to stare.

Train your brain. If you don't keep working your muscles, your body will turn flabby. It's the same with your mind. The more you work it, the more likely you'll remember things in the clutch: the name of your boss's wife, your PIN code, how many aces have been dealt. "Your brain is like a muscle. It has molecules that reward cells for doing a job. Learning something new tells the cells to increase production of these reward molecules, which gives you more brainpower to remember things," says Lawrence Katz, Ph.D., coauthor of *Keep Your Brain Alive*. So whenever you can, put your brain to work in ways that it's not used to.

Take different routes home from work. When you drive the same old streets, your brain goes on autopilot. Try traveling from points A to B in various ways, instead. This will teach your mind to think about directions and geography, which may come in handy when you're lost in that parking garage or can't remember which fork in the trail you took 2 miles back.

Cut off your senses. Most often, people use their sight to identify surrounding objects. You can challenge your mind by using your other senses in ways you normally wouldn't. Find the correct key for your front door by touch. Guess how much change you have in your hand just by feel. Identify a flavored coffee by smell or taste rather than by label.

Spend a Saturday wisely. Brainteasers don't have to be work. In your down-time, try playing Stratego—it's a great game for helping you remember where things are. To win, you have to recall which of your opponent's pieces he moved and which he didn't. Read complex, brain-engaging novels such as *One Hundred Years of Solitude* by Gabriel García Márquez or *Harlot's Ghost* by Norman Mailer, instead of the usual junk. Watch complicated movies like *The Game*, Bogie's *The Big Sleep*, or *The Usual Suspects*. They have more twists than a 1960s sock hop. Or spend a few hours in a museum or a library. Research suggests that browsing among art or books may slow the cognitive decline that comes with aging. Playing backgammon or sketching will work, too.

Feed your mind. Research has long shown that some vitamins and minerals improve memory. Load up on vitamins B, C, and E; beta-carotene; and the minerals calcium, magnesium, zinc, iron, selenium, chromium, and manganese. Here's a salad to remember: Top lettuce with carrots, chickpeas, kidney beans, broccoli, and some chicken or tuna.

Practice your speech in a suit. You know your presentation cold—every sentence, every slide, every lame joke. But come speech day, you forget to make points 6 through 10 and you can't remember the punch line to your best joke. Why? Because you practiced in your pajamas while eating a PB-and-J sandwich in front of the TV. You're more likely to recall something in the same atmosphere in which you learned it, says Helen Cassaday, Ph.D., a psychologist at the University of Nottingham in the United Kingdom. So you have two options for a successful speech: Practice in your work clothes, or wear pajamas to the office.

It's best to rehearse your presentation under conditions that approximate the real event. If the speech is first thing in the morning, don't practice after happy hour. Give it a run in the morning. Drink two cups of coffee beforehand if that's what you'd do at work. Stand behind a table to simulate a podium. Have your kids heckle you. Put on a suit. "Your brain responds to external stimuli. It will recall information that it learned under similar stimuli," Dr. Cassaday says.

Know when to say when. Besides the fact that they suck, there's another reason that you learn absolutely nothing from those 4-hour training seminars at work: brain overload. You simply can't remember everything you're supposed to—even if it's something fun, such as a golf, skiing, or guitar lesson. Researchers at Johns Hopkins University in Baltimore measured bloodflow in the brains of 16 people and concluded that if you learn two different tasks in one session, you're more likely to forget the first one. "It's better to follow the first learning session with 5 to 6 hours of routine activity that requires no new learning," says Henry Holcomb, Ph.D., the study author. So tell the golf instructor not to drill you on the art of chipping until you can consistently hit one off the tee.

Sticky Situations

Try these excuses the next time you get in a jam.

Compared with most guys who screw up their lives on a daily basis, politicians have it easy. They can be caught selling the office postage meter, lying on their résumés, and soliciting women of dubious pedigree at 4:00 A.M.—and before the ink is dry on the police report, an army of handlers is already at work, spinning the story like a Coke bottle at a junior-high make-out party.

The rest of us, sadly, have no such damage-control service. So we muddle through with our own lame, hastily devised excuses and pray for mercy. It's just not fair. A little assistance from the public relations department now and then could really make our lives easier.

That's why *Men's Health* magazine enlisted the best minds in Washington, D.C., to help come up with some excellent excuses—uh, explanations—for those times when you do find yourself in a bind. Use them wisely, and you may emerge from various predicaments to find that you're held in higher esteem than you were before—or at least without any permanent damage to your bridgework.

Your wife catches you staring at the coed in cutoffs washing her car. Turn your wandering eye into heartfelt feelings. "This one requires acting and quick reflexes," says Jonathan Kopp, a former White House staffer and opposition researcher for the Clinton/Gore campaign. When your wife catches you, keep staring. Stare as if you're catatonic, and respond only when she pokes you in the shoulder three times. Act startled—as if you've been awakened from a daydream—and say, "You know, I was just thinking about that wonderful weekend in the Poconos, and how much fun we had in that heart-shaped bathtub."

Your wife catches you staring again; this time it's the waitress in biking shorts. Simply say, "I'm just amazed by how much she reminds me of you, dear." Then add, "But I got a closer look, and you're far prettier." By telling your mate that the babe is a bust compared with her, you actually profit from leering (meaning you avoid the right cross that you so richly deserve).

Note: This tactic works only if there is some resemblance.

Your boss asks you why your project isn't finished. You could level with him about your tardiness, but then he'd want to horn in on your sponge baths with the interns. Rather than leave the impression that you're a bum, simply turn that old, unfinished project into a brand new one. "I'm glad you asked me about that project, because it has turned into something much bigger than before—something so much more involved—a real moneymaker! We need to talk about this. How about next Wednesday?" Then come up with a dumb idea that he's sure to hate—a solar-powered lazy Susan, or what have you. "He might fire you for laziness, but not for being wrongheaded," says MSNBC political analyst Jay Severin, a master strategist for more than 100 political campaigns. Assuming your job is intact, you've bought more time to complete the original project.

You forget your wedding anniversary. Women can't fathom why guys can recite dialogue from *Caddyshack* word for word yet can't recall the date that changed their lives forever. The answer: Men know their priorities. But how to handle such a mess without appearing thoughtless? Easy. Turn hopelessly romantic. When she confronts you with the question ("Do you know what today is?") and then drops the bombshell, respond calmly, "Dear, I always thought of our anniversary as the first time we met, at the bar on Capitol Hill on St. Patrick's Day."

"I used that one when I missed my first anniversary," says Chuck Conconi, veteran gossip columnist and editor-at-large for *Washingtonian* magazine. But remember that no sensible woman will allow this kind of spin to be repeated. Like a Spice Girl, the charm wears off the second time around.

You forget your wife's birthday. Never buy the "I don't mind" baloney. Instantaneously, she's calculating punishment, which will likely involve cryptic notes ("Mom's moving in," "Sold your golf clubs to pay for drapes," "Out for latte with Anne Heche"). You can, however, help prevent such retribution with a simple explanation: You actually bought her a wonderful gift; it just hasn't arrived yet. "Say something like, 'That diamond tennis bracelet you wanted is on order, and I'm picking it up next week,'" recommends political analyst Craig Shirley, who consulted on the Bush and Reagan campaigns. Add wistfully, "I wanted it to be a surprise." Then get your sorry butt down to the mall, pronto. Spend double what you would normally have spent—had you remembered—and under no circumstances convince yourself that she'd much rather have a walk-in humidor.

She wants to shop for linens, but the beer is chilled and the game is on. Look, you want to shop for linens, too. You've even had your eye on some Laura Ashley prints that make you tingle like a schoolgirl cycling on cobblestones. But you can't go anywhere for the next 4 hours. You have to endure this stupid game. Why? Your career depends on it. Here's the gist: "I need to watch what my boss watches. Tomorrow, when he and my coworkers talk about the game, I'd better be up to speed or I'll look stupid, and I can kiss that promotion goodbye. No promotion, no more money, no more Laura Ashley stuff. You should be grateful that I'm watching this game!" (Then pick up a yellow legal pad to show you'll be taking notes.) "I pull this whenever a hockey game is on," says Severin. This spin is so potent, however, that you might want to save it for something bigger than one game—like when you buy a satellite dish and install it in the herb garden.

You've given a speech, and you're asked a question that you either don't know how—or don't want—to answer. Clam up and you'll look either confused or evasive, or both. Instead, Severin says, answer the question you wish you'd been asked.

If you're asked about migratory waterfowl and you want to talk about taxes, say, "I'm really glad you asked that question about migratory waterfowl, because it brings us back to the vital question of taxes." Then make it a point never to look back at that person (that eliminates follow-up questions). Quickly scan the other side of the room and say, "Let's see if we can include some people over here." If there aren't any other people, consider getting out of speech making altogether.

Another tactic: Respond to the question in a very low voice so that the person can barely hear you, says Mike Murphy, a GOP political consultant. When the question is repeated, quietly repeat your answer and point helplessly at the nearby whirring helicopter blades. Then walk away. *Caution:* This tip works only if you have a helicopter.

The boss walks into your office and finds you playing Quake 2. It may look like you're wasting valuable work time—but no, you're doing research. "You know, the color schemes in this game are exactly what (largemouth bass, Little League coaches, Presbyterian ministers) will be looking for in our new line of (fishing lures, aluminum bats, candlesticks) next summer." "Here, you strip away any nefariousness and show that your intentions are constructive," says Severin. If your boss has half a brain, he'll know that you're yanking his chain. But he may respect you for coming up with something that ridiculous.

Note: This can also work when you're caught perusing X-rated Web sites. Provided, of course, that your pants are still on.

You hand in crummy work and your boss calls you on it. You could honestly explain why the work was so poor: You were working on more important stuff (removing the 300 copies of your résumé that jammed the copier). But that would only upset him—like he needs another excuse to make you wax his car.

Instead, immediately apologize for accidentally submitting the wrong draft and promise to present him with the right copy as soon as humanly possible. React with horror: "I must have printed out the wrong copy! I'll get you the final copy off my hard drive in the morning." Your boss might buy this, because even he's done that before. "That should buy you some time," says Kopp. You should use it to save your butt. (Or perhaps to get started on a cover letter.)

Another option: Use your gaffe to backstab an office rival. "Sorry about that, Mr. Burns. I think I printed out Joe's draft by mistake!"

You are woefully underdressed for a formal dinner party. It's not that you're a hopeless slob or can't afford fine duds, says Kopp. You just have so many more important things to do.

Liberal party: "Hey, I'm sorry I'm such a mess, but the Habitat for Humanity project ran a little longer than expected, and I didn't have a chance to go home and clean up."

Conservative party: "I'm sorry I'm late, but it took forever to gut and freeze the spotted owls I shot, and then my lousy chauffeur got stuck in traffic."

You tell the joke about the nun and the giraffe, and somebody finds it offensive. If the tasteless joke came from a respectable source, it's no longer your fault, says Severin. So tell the joke, and when the angry party glares at you, wait a beat, and say,

- "Can you believe that was actually printed in *Time* magazine? I am appalled!"
- "And a squirrel actually said that in a Disney movie! What is this world coming to?"
- "They let that go on C-Span! They ought to be ashamed of themselves!"

You're asked to contribute your thoughts in a meeting (while fantasizing about saving the company from financial ruin). No, you weren't daydreaming. You were lost in deep thought, contemplating a pressing issue from earlier in the meeting. "Quickly think of the last thing you remember being said in the meeting and who said it," says Shirley. Then say, "That's a great question—but I'd like to go back to the point Dick made earlier." This prevents you from being exposed as the mindless boob you probably are and instead gives the impression that you're a deliberate, careful boob.

The boss finds you stumbling into the office late, unshaven, and hungover. To the chief, it may look like your social life is out of control. Actually, it's not your social life but your work life that's led to your sorry condition. "See, you went out with those guys in sales last night to see what's behind those strange revenue projections," says Jack Felton, president of the Institute for Public Relations at the University of Florida in Gainesville. But because you can't keep up with their legendary drinking ("Those guys are out of control—disgusting animals!"), you nearly sacrificed your life and liver to protect the company's bottom line. If he buys it, not only do you look like you care about the company, but you also get to expense your bar bills. Cheers!

"What was your car doing parked in front of Lords of the Lap Dance?" Shirley suggests that, like all good spinmeisters, you shift the focus off your lurid perversions and place it squarely on the person making the charge. What was your Altima doing in front of a strip club? "Good question," you say. "But a better one is why you're so compelled to follow me around town. What were you doing

down there? If you had paid closer attention, you would have realized that I parked there because it was the closest space to Staples."

And next time, park your car in the underground parking lot.

"Why haven't you called?" If you don't care whether you hear from her again, why spin? Just say, "I would have phoned, but they only give me one call a day." But if you actually meant to call her and you plumb forgot, turn it into a simple misunderstanding.

- When she asks why you haven't called, respond emphatically, "I have! Here's the number right here, 555-6505!" When she says, "No, it's 6506," you're cool. Say, "I thought you were blowing me off with a wrong number! And now you think I'm an ass for not calling!" Within seconds, you'll have neutralized her, says Severin, and she might let you see what she learned in yoga class after all.
- Turn into Mr. Sensitive. "I've been dying to call you, but I didn't want to scare you off and appear overanxious. I should have acted on my instincts and called you, but I thought I had to play it cool. Now I feel like an idiot." Pull that one off, says Kopp, and you'll definitely win the women's vote in the next election.

You're a complete screwup at work. This is where your secretary comes in. "Blame her," says one consultant (who wishes to remain anonymous and, as such, remain on good terms with his receptionist). "If a client asks what happened to the invoice, say that your secretary slipped it into a copy of *Business Week*." The great thing is, you can blame her for everything. For instance:

- Why haven't you returned our calls? "You mean my secretary didn't tell you that I was out of town?"
- Why weren't you at the meeting? "My secretary put it down for next Tuesday!"
- Is that an empty vodka bottle in your wastebasket? "Oh, dear, my secretary's gone off the wagon again!"

You haven't read the book everyone's talking about at the party. Instead of betraying your profound ignorance, simply appear even more thoughtful than your geeky friends by admitting you didn't read the book, says Conconi. "I've seen so much publicity on this book that I'm afraid it's going to color my feelings if I read it now. So I'm going to wait until the hype settles down, and then I'll pick it up." Then stare off at the chandelier as you gently sip your port—and hope they don't bring up *Green Eggs and Ham* again.

Your girlfriend wants to get married, but you don't. A predicament. Right now, you're getting frequent sex, companionship, and an occasional well-cooked meal without going through any paperwork or bothersome blood tests. Appear to waffle about wedded bliss, however, and she may kick you out on your guitar amp. Here's what to do: Pretend you've thought about this a great deal, says Severin. And say, "I love you so much that I have taken the time to notice the tragic number of people who get married too early—half of whom end up leaving each other. I just want to be sure that when we do make that commitment, it's forever." She may buy it; she may not.

You need to fire a lousy, unstable employee. You'd have no problem cutting this guy loose, but the "Politicians Prefer Unarmed Peasants" bumper sticker on his El Camino is a little unnerving. So don't make it sound like the company is dumping him; simply spin it so that he's just too good for you, says Murphy. "We simply can't offer you an opportunity here where your talent can truly soar. And we don't want to hold you back—there's a whole world out there dying to use your gifts." Just in case, set up motion detectors outside your cubicle.

A worker asks for a raise that you can't give. Turn the tables on the sucker. "When I hear you ask for a raise, what I'm really hearing is you asking for more responsibility. So, why don't you tell me what you want to accomplish this year, and we'll make a list." Then make up an extremely long list, filled with goals so impossibly vague that they're begging to be misinterpreted (Goal #1: Evaluate core competence. Goal #2: Evaluate prototype for Goal #1. Goal #3: Rethink Goal #2.) After the list is made, say, "When these goals are met, you'll have your raise." So rather than giving in to the employee, you've actually gotten something out of him, instead. That's a spin to be proud of—even if it has guaranteed you a special place in hell.

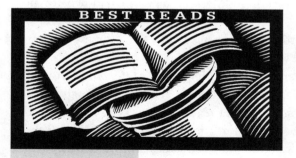

BEST READS

Why Most Men Are Emotionally Impotent

No doubt about it: Most American men are brought up to repress a wide range of emotions in the belief that strong men aren't expressive. Robert S. Ivker and Edward Zorensky tackle this issue head-on in this fascinating excerpt from Thriving:

The Complete Mind-Body Guide for Optimal Health and Fitness for Men
(*Crown Publishing, 1997*). *They take a look at why we're brought up this way and
the negative effects it has on our lives.*

Have you ever walked into a room and felt another person's rage without his
saying a word or moving a muscle? To what exactly were you responding? At
times like these, we say the air felt charged, that the tension was so thick you could
have cut it with a knife. Rage, like any emotion, consists of energy. Depending on
the emotion you are feeling, this emotional energy emanates from different parts
of the body, and we characterize it accordingly: "I have a gut feeling." "My heart
aches." "The words caught in my throat." "She gives me a headache." "Don't be
such a pain in the butt!" We use these expressions without thinking about them,
but they each describe a discomfort associated with a specific emotion localized
in a particular part of the body.

In connecting us to our bodies, our emotions ground us in the physical
world. They comprise an energetic structure of their own that I will refer to as
the emotional body, with a strong correspondence to the physical body. They give
us our bearings and balance. Together with our genetic history, the emotions
identify our uniqueness and put us in touch with what we really want and who
we really are. The problem is that most men tend to keep their emotions inside,
where they go unexpressed and ignored. A 1996 *Men's Health* magazine-CNN
survey entitled "How Men Deal with Stress" found unsurprisingly that the most
common source of stress for adult men was job-related. According to the survey
of the most common ways of dealing with this stress, 74 percent of men chose to
keep it inside, 50 percent got angry, and almost one-third (29 percent) used alcohol to relieve it.

Emotions such as fear or exhilaration are expressions of bioenergy that control our minds and bodies and affect our behavior far more than we know.
Their positive, loving expressions can boost our creativity, enhance physical
health, and help ensure intimate relationships. In their negative, fearful form,
emotions can help us to survive an immediate crisis. They are remnants of
fight-or-flight instincts that have enabled our species to evolve. In their pro-
tracted or habitual form, however, when we are long removed from a real or
present danger, these negative emotions can stunt personal growth, cause disease, and poison marriages.

Ignoring, denying, or repressing emotions almost always results in destructive energy. We all know individuals—even our own family members—who consistently embody unnecessary negative energy. These "sappers" are difficult to be
around. Their emotional energy is so constricted and so debilitating that they can

drain our own resources and leave us feeling exhausted and frustrated. Just as the health of the physical body requires a free flow of oxygen, blood, nutrients, and wastes, so the emotional body requires the unimpeded experience and expression of feelings of every type, no matter how joyful or painful.

Human experience alternates between two basic emotional poles—love and fear—both of which require our full attention for us to thrive. The energy associated with feelings of love or joy (trust, intimacy, approval, power, exhilaration, and peacefulness) is more expansive in character. The energy of fear or painful emotions tends to be more constrictive in nature; emotions such as anger, anxiety, depression, guilt, and shame are all expressions of fear. The polarity between love and fear—joy and pain—exists in a dynamic balance, and the trick to thriving is staying flexible and attentive enough to maintain that equilibrium.

At any given moment, we experience a combination of love and fear. For a variety of reasons, however, men in particular are reluctant to express both emotions. In our efforts to hide or ignore these feelings, we attempt to contain our experience of all emotions. We try so hard to control our emotions that we prevent ourselves from simply experiencing them. As a result, we often fail to receive emotional messages that are trying to tell us what we really care about.

I can't count the number of times I have asked male patients to describe their feelings about a painful crisis or conflict, only to have them respond with an extended rational analysis of how and why the situation developed: "I think it was unfair." "She should have done it this way." "She's wreaking havoc in my life." In describing these situations, men almost always exclude their feelings. This is partly because as boys, we were discouraged by parents, society, and especially our peers from expressing sadness, fear, and tenderness, feelings that were characterized as feminine. (On the other hand, girls were discouraged from expressing anger, aggressiveness, and curiosity because these external, outgoing emotions were considered more masculine.)

Men also use their brains to contain their feelings because no one ever gave us "permission" to have those emotions. Not only did many of us grow up feeling that we were "bad boys" if we expressed our fundamental feelings, such as fear or sadness, but many of us were shamed into believing that something was intrinsically wrong with us for having these feelings in the first place. As a result, we grew up with only a fragmentary sense of self-awareness shaped by internal statements that constantly challenged the reality of our emotions: "I shouldn't feel this way." "There's no reason to react this way." "I'm not going to let this (feeling) get to me."

The consequences of boys denying their feelings show up in some revealing statistics cited by psychotherapist Michael Gurian in his book *The Wonder of Boys.*

- Infant boys are cuddled, talked to, and breastfed for significantly shorter periods of time than girls.
- By the age of 9, most boys have learned to repress all primary feelings except anger.
- Emotionally depressed boys outnumber girls four to one.
- Learning-disabled boys outnumber girls two to one.
- Boys are six times as likely to be diagnosed with hyperactivity.
- Male infants suffer a 25 percent higher mortality rate.
- Boys are twice as likely to be victims of physical abuse.

Nothing shapes the emotional landscape of a young boy like a parent—especially a father. Never underestimate the power of a son's identification with his father, nor that father's continuing emotional impact throughout the life of the son. Parents take their cues about gender appropriateness from their own parents and from society at large, and they tend to pass on their insecurities in the form of judgments, reprimands, and disciplines that stifle healthy childhood emotions. Messages such as "big boys don't cry" or "there's nothing to be afraid of," especially coming from those on whom we depended most, had an overwhelming effect on how we prioritized and expressed emotion. As a consequence, we learned to reveal only those emotions that we knew were most acceptable, and we hid the rest. We were never able to benefit from what those other emotions were trying to communicate to us.

The fact was, most of us were victims of "unconscious" parenting. Our parents were not evil or malicious. Believe it or not, they probably loved us, but were unaware of our emotional needs, just as they had been of their own. Having grown up during the Depression and World War II, many of our parents were too preoccupied with survival to take time to understand their emotions. Our fathers, in particular, passed on this survivalist mind-set to us through the powerful and automatic impact of our identification with them.

In his book *Emotional Intelligence*, Daniel Goleman describes the "emotional contagion" that occurs between two individuals or groups of people by which they mirror the emotional state of the other. Goleman cites a dramatic example of emotional contagion that occurred during the Vietnam War. An American platoon and a unit of Vietcong were in a heavy firefight in the middle of a rice paddy, the two forces positioned on either side of a berm bisecting the rice paddy. According to an American soldier, David Bush, who witnessed the incident, suddenly out of nowhere a line of six monks walked across the berm, calmly poised between the two firing lines. No one fired at them, and the fighting entirely stopped. "I just didn't feel like I wanted to do this anymore, at least not that day," said Bush.

In questioning how this magical transmission of emotion occurs, Goleman suggests that the "most likely answer is that we unconsciously imitate the emotions we see displayed by someone else, through an out-of-awareness motor mimicry of that person's facial expression, gestures, tone of voice, and other nonverbal markers of emotion. Through this imitation, people recreate in themselves the mood of the other person—a low-key version of the Stanislavsky method, in which actors recall gestures, movements, and other expression of an emotion they have felt strongly in the past in order to evoke those feelings once again."

As infants and toddlers, this same identification occurs between child and parent hundreds of times a day and is especially magnified between parent and child of the same gender. During early childhood, we mimic every facet of that constant, powerful display of gesture and expression. Each frown or smile becomes fixed as part of a larger emotional pattern that strongly affects how we now behave as adults.

Most of us assume that we escaped the emotional influence of our parents when we moved out of their house. In fact, we did not escape as much as we might have thought. Like most men, we failed to complete this process of emotional self-determination in our late teens. Instead, we jumped into other responsibilities: education, a job, or a family of our own. In transposing our emotional energy into job performance, income level, and lifestyle, we took our attention away from understanding the pressures that had shaped our emotional life in the first place. We described these new responsibilities to ourselves as essential to our "functioning in the adult world." We committed our energy and discipline to performing as well as possible, but emotionally, we remained children, unconsciously avoiding the same old childhood insecurities. This has been particularly true of men, who typically were not encouraged to explore their emotions as fully as women.

Our popular culture only reinforces the emotional retardation of men. Consider the emotional content of most popular movies made for men—action movies. They feature a stoic, physically powerful hero who goes about blowing up cars or buildings and shooting villains, but expressing little, if any, emotion. Be it Gary Cooper, John Wayne, Steve McQueen, Clint Eastwood, or Bruce Willis, the American hero has always been a laconic figure who speaks more through action than words. His sense of understatement creates a dynamic inner tension that magnifies the force of his character. His pregnant pauses and long silences generate a vacuum that sucks up the audience's emotional energy. As men brought up on these models and fed a steady diet of competition and aggression, we were discouraged from showing insecurity or any weakness that might be used against us. Most of us didn't have to go to the movies to be exposed to men like this; they were living in our own homes.

As a consequence, the majority of us have learned to repress feelings of pain, fear, or sadness to the extent that we are unaware that we even have them. With its ubiquitous ads for beer, pain relievers, and antacids, contemporary American pop culture perpetuates the promise of a pain-free existence. Its ads primarily target men and teach us to suppress our daily stress quotient. Although they may be trying to deliver important emotional messages from the unconscious, the tension headache or the pain of an ulcer are unpopular in the workplace because they threaten productivity. It is no wonder that 80 percent of serious drug addicts are men, or that men are three times more likely to become alcoholics.

Relaxation Therapies

In today's hectic world, it can seem difficult to get away and relax. Truly relax. That doesn't mean plopping in front of the tube with a cold beer to watch a ballgame. What relaxing really means is outlined in this excerpt from The People's Medical Society Men's Health and Wellness Encyclopedia: Everything a Man Needs to Know for Good Health and Well-Being *(Macmillan, 1998) by Charles Inlander and the staff of the People's Medical Society. They follow that up with various relaxation techniques that don't take a lot of time and are easy to do. Try some to deal with the stress in your life.*

Relaxation is more than taking time away from the telephone, putting your feet up, and unwinding with a good book or movie. True, deep relaxation is a meditative state in which the mind is free of thoughts and worries; it's a state that can relieve stress and provide a number of emotional and physical health benefits.

In today's stressful world, relaxation is necessary to counter the negative aspects of stress. Whether you're dealing with a divorce, worrying about your job and financial future, or simply feeling tense because of a traffic jam, relaxation techniques can help restore your sense of balance and well-being and counteract the harmful toll stress takes on your body.

The Relaxation Response

Herbert Benson, M.D., is credited with introducing the concept of the relaxation response—the idea that practicing relaxation and meditation results in reduced tension, increased alpha (relaxed) brain waves, lower heart and breathing rates, slower metabolism, and decreased digestive acid secretion. This concept provides the basis for the use of relaxation techniques to improve health and reduce stress.

Dr. Benson's technique requires four basic elements.

1. A mental device or constant stimulus of some sort—such as a word, a sound, or a phrase repeated either silently or aloud. This is called a mantra.

2. A passive attitude that disregards any distracting thoughts. Any distraction is blocked out by the repetition of the mental device.

3. Decreased muscle tension by taking a comfortable position that requires minimal muscle work.

4. A quiet environment with few environmental distractions.

To practice the relaxation response, think about the four basic elements. Sit in a comfortable position and repeat your chosen mantra over and over again to drive out all distractions until you're thinking about nothing at all. This will take practice; don't become discouraged if you find it difficult at first. If thoughts come into your mind, acknowledge them and let them fade away. Meditate this way for 20 minutes every morning and evening.

Relaxation Techniques

There is a wide variety of ways in which to achieve the relaxation response, ranging from deep breathing and meditation to hydrotherapy and aromatherapy. Some relaxation therapies such as biofeedback and hypnosis are used in conjunction with medical treatments and are also known as complementary therapies.

Imagery. Imagery allows you to change your perception of a situation as a mental way to fight stress. It helps to promote deep relaxation, which causes a release of serotonin, a calming hormone that eases muscle tension and promotes healing. To practice imagery, stop what you are doing, close your eyes, and visualize a soothing scene—a beach with white sand and blue waters or the woods with birds singing and the scent of pine filling the air, for example. Spend 5 minutes or so examining and enjoying every detail of the picture. Feel the sting of the salt air or hear the birds sing. For a quick session of imagery, you might want to keep a pleasant picture or postcard in your wallet to look at in times of stress.

Progressive muscle relaxation. Muscle relaxation is a simple technique of contracting and relaxing the muscles in order from the feet to the head. It is best used when lying down so that the muscle groups can be isolated, tensed, and released one by one. As you are tensing and releasing the muscles, compare how they feel when they are flexed with when they are relaxed. Note any areas that are already tense and make a conscious effort to relax them. Progressive relaxation breaks tense-mind/tense-muscle syndrome by teaching recognition of physical stress. Practice allows you to relax at will.

It is possible to practice a simpler version of progressive relaxation while sitting at a desk. Raise your shoulders to your ears as tightly as possible, then release them, making sure they are low at the finish. This will reduce the stress that builds in your shoulder, shoulder blades, and neck during the day.

Deep breathing. This method focuses on slow, rhythmic breathing with deep inhalation and exhalation. To practice deep breathing, stand or sit straight and close your eyes for 5 minutes. Slowly take in a deep breath to the count of five. As you take in the air, let your abdomen and ribs expand up and out. Imagine the air entering every part of your body, into your head, your shoulders, your arms, your torso, and then your legs. When you exhale, imagine the air leaving through your toes. Deep breathing increases the volume of oxygen in the system and refreshes cells. It is often used in combination with other strategies.

Meditation. Meditation involves focusing on one object and ignoring external stimuli to promote relaxation. In fact, it was this ancient Eastern technique that was the inspiration for Dr. Benson's relaxation response. With meditation, oxygen consumption decreases; heartbeat, breathing, and metabolism slow; and blood pressure drops. To practice meditation, sit or lie comfortably with your eyes closed. Quietly repeat a chosen word, sound, or phrase continuously, concentrating on it to prevent distraction. Breathe deeply, as described above. Practice for 10 to 20 minutes twice a day or whenever stressed. Classes on meditation may be available at your local YMCA or through the Yellow Pages.

Mindfulness. Mindfulness is simply focusing on the tangibles around you in order to relieve stressful thoughts. It serves to calm the mind and distract it from anxiety-producing thoughts about the past or the future. To practice mindfulness, focus on the objects, colors, and sensations around you. Look at the color of the walls or the texture of the carpet, for example, or concentrate on the sound of the traffic or the clock ticking. Mindfulness is often used to maximize the relaxing effects of other strategies.

Aromatherapy. In aromatherapy, fragrant oils extracted from plants and flowers are used to promote relaxation. Fragrances can be imparted through scented candles, perfumes, skin lotions, or massage oils applied to the skin or added to warm bath water. Common scents used for relaxation include marjoram, lavender, geranium, chamomile, sandalwood, lily of the valley, roses, and apple spice. The smells prompt the signal portion of the brain that controls emotions and memories, triggering a release of calming hormones and increasing relaxing brain waves. There are many books available on the details of aromatherapy, and courses or workshops may be available in your area. Check the Yellow Pages.

Hydrotherapy. Hydrotherapy uses water to change body temperature and promote relaxation. It includes swimming, bathing, or showering or use of a whirlpool or sauna. Warm water promotes the release of calming brain chemicals and stimulates healing throughout the body by increasing bloodflow. Warm or hot water dilates blood vessels while cold constricts them. Both help improve circulation, enhancing relaxation. In addition, buoyancy takes pressure off taut muscles. Hydrotherapy is also widely used as a means of physical therapy.

Warm water promotes sleep, and hot water relieves muscle tension. Herbs and aromatherapy oils may also be added to the water (in what's called hydrochemical therapy) to aid relaxation.

Music therapy. This therapy focuses on the power of music to relax and soothe. It can be used alone or in combination with other strategies. Soothing music can help block negative and stressful thoughts. As a result, blood pressure drops, heart and breathing rates slow, and calming brain chemicals are released. Muscle tension decreases.

Listen to flowing or relaxing music—perhaps using headphones—with your eyes closed. New Age music, jazz, classical music, and recordings of natural sounds such as birds or waterfalls are available and may be good choices for music. Music with one beat per second is preferable because it mimics the body's natural rhythms.

Self-hypnosis. Self-hypnosis involves a set of specific mental commands a person gives to himself in order to enter a light hypnotic trance, a state of concentration similar to sleep in which the body can regenerate and energize itself more easily. Aside from relaxation, it can also be used in treating conditions such as nicotine addiction.

Self-hypnosis should never be attempted without the advice of a professional hypnotist. To practice, close your eyes and repeat the series of commands—for example, "My arms and legs are heavy"—until you believe that command has been achieved. With practice, self-hypnosis can be induced with only a few commands.

Biofeedback. Biofeedback is a method of consciously controlling involuntary body functions through concentration; it's taught using electronic monitoring of the body's responses. Biofeedback can result in slowing of breathing and heart rate, a change in body temperature, and a release in muscle tension. Once the method is learned, an individual can control such responses whenever necessary. Biofeedback monitors are available commercially, and you can find training at specialist centers, which are found in most cities.

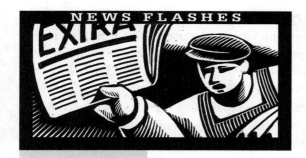

Stress at Work Can Cut Sperm Count

CALGARY, Alberta—After analyzing sperm samples from 1,469 men ages 20 to 69, researchers at the University of Calgary found that chronic, day-to-day work stress can drastically cut sperm count. Men who reported the most daily work-related stress had one-third less sperm in their ejaculate than the most relaxed subjects. Stress causes hormonal imbalances and changes in blood pressure and body temperature. Any of these may harm sperm, says study author Philip Bigelow, Ph.D. Worse, the sperm that the stressed-out men produced were sluggish swimmers. "Fortunately," says Dr. Bigelow, "if you reduce your stress level, your sperm levels should return to normal."

Talking about Stress Raises Blood Pressure

PARIS—A French study published in the *American Journal of Hypertension* found that talking about stress can significantly raise your blood pressure. Researchers tested the blood pressures of 50 hypertensive people as they sat silently, read, or talked about the stress in their lives. Chatting caused systolic pressures (the top number) to jump by an average of 17 millimeters of mercury and diastolic pressures to jump by 13 millimeters of mercury. Reading also caused a slight rise in blood pressure. To avoid skewing your vitals, sit like a brass Buddha until that armband comes off.

Optimism Breeds Disease Fighters

LEXINGTON, Ky.—A study of 50 first-year law students showed that having a positive outlook might increase the number of disease-fighting T cells in your system. At the semester's start, researchers gave students a blood test and psychological exam. By midsemester, the 25 students who were most pessimistic had lost about 3 percent of their T cells, but the 25 optimists had gained 13 percent. "Your attitude may affect one or more levels of defense in the immune system," says Suzanne Segerstrom, Ph.D., lead researcher from the University of Kentucky. Faking won't help, she says; you probably have to be truly happy to produce any changes.

Visualization Builds Strength

MANCHESTER, England—If you visualize yourself doing free throws, your gullible brain will think you're practicing, and your on-court shot will improve. But a study from Manchester Metropolitan University has found that visualization can actually build muscle, too.

In the study, six men contracted their pinkie fingers as hard as they could for 20 minutes a day, twice a week. Another six men only imagined doing the exercise. A final group of six did nothing. After a month, the first bunch had become 33 percent stronger and the last group remained unchanged, as expected. But the men who only visualized the exercise had actually become 16 percent stronger.

"This principle will work for any muscle group," says Dave Collins, Ph.D., professor of sports psychology at Manchester, "and it's especially useful for people who have injuries and can't exercise."

Stress Reduces Brain Tissue

MONTREAL—When researchers in Montreal sent 60 people through a maze, the 20 with higher levels of cortisol, a stress hormone, had more trouble finding the way out. A brain scan revealed that each actually had a smaller hippocampus, which controls memory.

"Several brain disorders are associated with high levels of cortisol, including depression and memory loss," says study coauthor Bruce McEwen, M.D., a neuroscientist at Rockefeller University in New York. "Over time, elevated stress hormones may be linked to the acceleration of senility." Pumping more cortisol could also cause you to gain belly fat, he says.

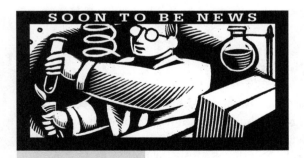

SOON TO BE NEWS

An End to Addictions?

Men struggling to give up cigarettes, alcohol, or even cocaine may soon have a valuable new weapon to use in their fight. An epilepsy drug could be the key to stopping many addictions. Gamma-vinyl-GABA (GVG) works by increasing the amount of a neurotransmitter that reduces the buildup of dopamine, a brain chemical that is elevated by drugs such as cocaine and nicotine. Animals addicted to nicotine and cocaine completely avoided these drugs after they were given GVG. "It appears to completely eliminate cravings associated with addiction," says researcher Stephen L. Dewey, Ph.D., of Brookhaven National Laboratory in Upton, New York.

GVG is currently awaiting FDA approval.

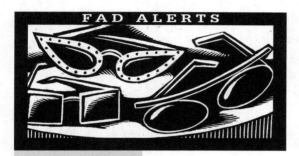

FAD ALERTS

Ginkgo

Ginkgo biloba, an extract taken from the leaves of the ginkgo tree, is a top seller, thanks to its reported ability to increase brainpower. Studies have found that it seems to sharpen memory and concentration in people with cognitive disorders, such as Alzheimer's disease.

But ginkgo, according to Varro E. Tyler, Ph.D., distinguished professor emeritus of pharmacognosy at Purdue University in West Lafayette, Indiana, has one nasty and little-known side effect: It reduces the blood's ability to clot. If people who take aspirin or other anticlotting drugs (often called blood thinners) begin taking *Ginkgo biloba*, the combination may cause internal bleeding in the brain, eyes, or other organs.

As the number of people taking ginkgo continues to increase, physicians expect to see more such interactions, says Richard J. Ko, Pharm.D., Ph.D., a food and drug scientist for the California Department of Health Services in Sacramento.

"People don't realize that if you're using an herb, you're using a chemical," says Mary Ann O'Hara, M.D., of the University of Washington in Seattle, author of a recent review of medicinal herbs. That chemical may react badly with other chemicals you've already put in your system.

Kava Kava

 Kava kava (*Piper methysticum*), a member of the pepper family, has been touted recently as a safe, natural sedative—an herbal alternative to Valium. Pyrones, chemical compounds in the root extract, seem to act as muscle relaxants and often produce a sedating effect within 2 hours.

But you'd better not be driving on the interstate when the kava funk hits. Kava kava depresses your central nervous system, and its side effects include loss of coordination, sluggish motor reflexes, and dilated pupils. One herb reference warns that kava kava can increase the risk of suicide among depressed people.

If you feel that you need medication—herbal or otherwise—to relieve anxiety, you need to see a doctor first. If your doctor gives you the nod, try kava kava extract for 90 days, and consult the doctor a second time before opening another bottle. And never mix kava kava with tranquilizers or other psychoactive drugs; the combination could make you foggier than Ronald Reagan giving a deposition.

Ginseng

 Improved stamina, increased libido, less fatigue. What claim hasn't been pinned on ginseng (*Panax ginseng* and *P. quinquefolius*)? Everything or nothing may be true; most U.S. studies have yielded inconclusive results, and how ginseng works is unknown. But a few studies have suggested that ginseng may safely enhance mood. And Commission E, the agency that regulates herbal medicines in Germany, lists ginseng as a safe energy and memory stimulant. These factors have helped make it a top-selling herb.

As with any popular herbal supplement, however, you have no way of knowing what's in the bottle. "Quality control is one of the biggest problems in the herbal industry," says Varro E. Tyler, Ph.D., distinguished professor emeritus of pharmacognosy at Purdue University in West Lafayette, Indiana. Because ginseng supplements are hot sellers and because genuine ginseng is expensive, this remedy, like ginkgo and St. John's wort, is a favorite target of hucksters who sell bogus herbs. It's an easy scam, since we have to trust herbal manufacturers that the bottle's contents match the label. When experts have analyzed selected ginseng supplements, they've found that many contained few or no active ingredients.

To increase your chances of getting authentic ginseng, find a product that includes 100 to 125 milligrams of ginseng extract standardized to contain 4 percent to 7 percent ginsenosides (the key component of ginseng). If this is on the label, the odds are better that you've found a reputable manufacturer.

St. John's Wort

 Studies have shown that St. John's wort (*Hypericum perforatum*) can fight depression, possibly by affecting your brain's levels of serotonin and other neurotransmitters. But for most people, this effect takes at least 6 weeks to kick in. Popping a St. John's wort tablet on a gloomy day or drinking a $5 St. John's wort concoction at some nouveau café is worthless. Any lift in mood will be the result of the placebo effect.

See a doctor before you take St. John's wort to self-treat depression. If your doctor okays the herb, look for a product that contains a standardized dose (300 milligrams of 0.3 percent) of hypericin, the red pigment that is present in the plant.

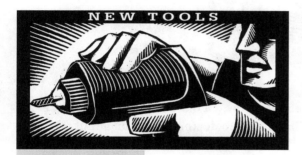

NEW TOOLS

Stay Alert

Caffeine Gum

If you're tired of drinking your caffeine, try chewing it. A new gum called Stay Alert contains 50 milligrams of caffeine per stick and is available in drugstores for a little less than a buck a pack. The gum is no Bubblicious—the caffeine adds a bitter flavor to the gum. Also, though a stick or two might keep you awake during a long meeting, gum junkies with a pack-a-day habit shouldn't make Stay Alert their regular brand. "I wouldn't exceed 300 milligrams of caffeine per day," says Beth Bussey, R.D., a nutritionist at the University of Alabama in Tuscaloosa.

Wider Knowledge

Instant Genius Audiotapes

If reading scores of weighty tomes is too much work, here's an even shorter shortcut to erudition. Billed as "the cheat sheets of culture," the Instant Genius audiotape series will let you bone up on the finer points of modern art, philosophy, etiquette, the stock market, and other topics as you make your morning drive. The tape on wine, for example, describes the basic types of reds and whites in a no-nonsense way and gives tips on ordering in a restaurant. The tapes, which run about 60 minutes each and cost $12 apiece, are available at bookstores or on the Web at www.instantgenius.com.

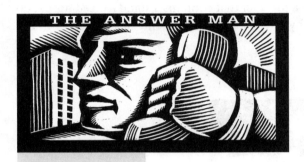

Hard-Luck Fan

Every year, my beloved Cubs get knocked out of the play-offs; and every year, I feel depressed about it. Should I see a doctor to find out about taking an antidepressant?
—**K. S., Chicago**

"If you're really upset over the Cubs or any other team losing, it's probably just a transient feeling that will pass in a few days," says Richard Balon, M.D., professor of psychiatry at Wayne State University in Detroit. If being a sports fan is a big part of your life, Dr. Balon says, start worrying when you don't care about your team losing or when you can't get excited about the pennant race.

Don't feel that you have to decide for yourself whether there's a problem. According to Michael Liebowitz, M.D., professor of clinical psychiatry at Columbia University in New York City, there may come a time when you should see a professional for help. "When your mood becomes a source of distress, when you're feeling troubled by it, or when it begins to have some real impact on your life, that's when you are approaching the functional definition of depression."

Fidgety Flier

I am extremely claustrophobic, so being trapped in a plane for hours at a time makes me squirm. Drinking doesn't seem to help me relax. Mayday!
—**W. S., North Kingston, R.I.**

Maybe you should figure out exactly what it is about flying that causes your cabin fever. Is it the inability to see outdoors? Lack of control in what could be a dangerous situation? Those in-flight magazines? One way to help conquer your problem, says Robert Taylor Segraves, M.D., a psychiatrist at Metro Health Medical Center in Cleveland, is to see a psychiatrist. He might give you "homework" assignments in which you place yourself in close situations for longer and longer periods of time, or have you imagine yourself in progressively smaller and smaller spaces. If your claustrophobia is bad enough to cause panic attacks, your doctor may also prescribe antianxiety or antidepressant medications to take the edge off.

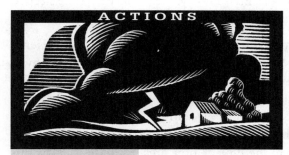

ACTIONS

Blame the millennium for the stress epidemic in our society. Arriving at the year 2000, you could say that we are in the midst of a social, cultural, and technological sea change. The last 50 years have been a time of unprecedented growth and transformation. Into the twenty-first century, we can expect the same—but even more so. To ensure that you're ready to meet the challenge, follow these 20 tips.

1. Get happy. When your manager assigns you to work the weekend trade show in the Quad Cities, head over to the gym for some strength training. Then return to the office, smile at her, and book your flight. A study of 39 men and women at the University of Richmond in Virginia demonstrated that strength training can sweeten a foul mood. The subjects rated their own moods, warmed up for 5 to 10 minutes, then performed four sets of bench presses and squats. Afterward, the same mood test recorded less tension, depression, and anger.

In a separate study at the University of New Orleans, 42 subjects reported similar results after a 50-minute step class.

A 20-minute workout may be enough to trigger a better mood, and the effect can last for several hours. "You can experience the psychological benefits of exercise in a single bout of 10 to 20 minutes, whether you're in shape or not," says

Robert W. McGowan, Ph.D., chairman of the University of Richmond department of health and sports science.

2. **Stay up all night.** Nature wants you to be unconscious at 1:00 A.M., but for 3.2 million Americans, that's lunchtime. These three tips can prevent the stupor that comes from working the night shift.

1. Take a cool shower before bed. A steamy one will raise your body temperature, triggering wakefulness.
2. Post your sleeping schedule. And no one—except firefighters—should disturb you.
3. Create "night" to sleep. Sunlight rouses you, so darken your bedroom and keep it cool, says Phyllis Zee, M.D., Ph.D., a neurologist at Northwestern University in Evanston, Illinois. Elvis Presley, a legendary daytime sleeper, supposedly used aluminum foil to cover his windows.

3. **Calm down.** Do you pop a cork more often than a wine steward? Here's one way to channel your anger: Slow down. "When you're angry, you're physically aroused," says Christopher Peterson, Ph.D., psychology professor at the University of Michigan in Ann Arbor. To corral the response, breathe through your nose. Inhale for four counts and exhale for four counts.

Try doing a specific task, such as tensing and relaxing your muscles, says Cary Rothstein, Ph.D., a psychologist in the Philadelphia area. Exercises such as this can help distract you.

4. **Look on the bright side.** A study at the University of Florida in Gainesville suggests that improving your outlook can improve your game. Researchers told three groups of tennis players that their performances were below average. Players in the first group were then told that they could control their success on the court, the second group was told that they lacked ability, and the third group was told nothing. After 3 weeks, the first group scored significantly better in performance tests and felt less anger and frustration. According to the lead researcher, Robert Singer, Ph.D., instead of saying, "I suck," tell yourself, "I can do better." Then consider the ways that you can improve your game.

5. **Make a cucumber sandwich.** The next time you need a fast snack, put some unpeeled cucumber slices and watercress on two pieces of bread, and top them with fat-free sour cream or mayonnaise. Not only does this sandwich contain more than one-third of your recommended daily dose of vitamin A (which you need to maintain your vision), but smelling the cucumber will also improve your mood, reduce your anxiety level, and cause your pulse to drop, says Alan R.

Hirsch, M.D., neurological director of the Smell and Taste Treatment and Research Foundation in Chicago and author of *Scentsational Sex.*

6. **Close your eyes.** Few of us can get away with taking a nap at work, but here's something almost as good: Leaning back in your chair, closing your eyes, and relaxing your body for a couple of minutes has almost the same effect as a quick snooze, says James Maas, Ph.D., professor of psychology at Cornell University in Ithaca, New York, and author of *Power Sleep.* You'll strengthen your attention to detail and improve your ability to make decisions—without the risk of unsightly drooling.

7. **Do a puzzle.** Researchers at the University of South Florida in Tampa have found that people with a genetic predisposition for Alzheimer's may be able to prevent or slow development of the disease by constantly challenging their brains. Scientists think the added mental development causes a change in brain tissue, which either slows the disease's progress or helps the brain compensate for its symptoms.

8. **Read the comics.** At last, medical justification for "Dilbert." "There have been more than 40 years of study on the physiology of laughter," says Joel Goodman, Ed.D., director of The Humor Project in Saratoga Springs, New York. "Today, we know that humor not only improves your respiration and circulation, it also helps to increase your blood's oxygen level, reduce stress, and improve your immune system's function."

9. **Handle a tight deadline.** Here's one way to handle stress when you're on the clock for a project: Find out when they really need it. Hard as it may be to believe, the boss who gave you that tight deadline may not really need the report when he says he does. Or maybe his boss gave him a phony deadline. "A lot of deadlines are really just bogus requests that filter down from on high," says Peter Wylie, Ph.D., Ed.D., an industrial psychologist and consultant in Washington, D.C. Dr. Wylie suggests that rather than blindly buying into someone else's sense of emergency, you should sit down with your manager to discuss, calmly and realistically, what all the fuss is about and how you can work together to accomplish the job. A lot of times, you can score an extension before you even start.

10. **Color me mellow.** Research has shown that the colors of walls and other interior surfaces can have a decided impact on mood. You can put that knowledge to work in your own surroundings, says Cam Busch, R.N., a certified art therapist in Chattanooga, Tennessee. Incorporate softer colors—lighter blues, greens, mauves, and eggshell white—in places where you're stressed. Use brighter colors in rooms where you want to be more upbeat and energetic. Red and orange, for example, are known as stimulating colors.

11. **Deal with midlife stress.** Most men reach their stress peaks during their late thirties to early forties, says Allen Elkin, Ph.D., director of the Stress Management and Counseling Center in New York City. "Younger men expect pressure, and they cope," he says. "But middle-age men are less optimistic; they're beginning to realize the path to success is rockier than they thought." Fortunately, the later decades of life are marked by steadily easing pressure. Careers become established, families stabilize, and money worries ease. By age 65, stress is relatively low again.

Here's a trick that Dr. Elkin uses to stay calm. When a stressful situation arises, he asks himself how important it is. Then he rates it on a scale of zero to 10. "If it's not a 9 or a 10, I realize I don't have to be that worried," he says. "It helps keep things in perspective." This simple technique is especially useful for middle-age guys trapped on that decade-long stress plateau, because it gives them a sense of control. Another way to use this technique is to assign numerical values to the major parts of your life, such as work, marriage, and family; this can help you better apportion your time.

12. **Sleep like a baby.** Few older men experience difficulty falling asleep, but many wake up often during the night. Wakefulness can be caused by anxiety, a physical illness (such as arthritis), certain drugs, or the need to visit the bathroom more frequently. (Or maybe it's the sharp blows to your head from your wife, because you're snoring so loudly.) All these things result in a lower sleep efficiency, the proportion of time in bed you actually spend asleep. Young adults' sleep efficiency is generally about 95 percent. By age 70, though, it's down to approximately 77 percent.

Adequate sleep is an essential part of physical and psychological health. Surprisingly, the amount of sleep you need (typically 7 to 9 hours per day) remains constant throughout your life. Although older men may sleep less at night, they generally compensate by napping during the day.

To increase your sleep efficiency, follow these recommendations from the National Sleep Foundation: (1) avoid stimulants such as caffeine, nicotine, and alcohol in the late afternoon and evening; (2) don't exercise within 3 hours of bedtime; (3) establish a regular go-to-bed routine; (4) don't watch television, read, or eat in the sack (beds are for sleeping and sex); and (5) if you don't fall asleep within 30 minutes, get up and do something relaxing until you do feel sleepy.

13. **Keep your buds.** Men in their teens and early twenties have the most friends, according to Dru Sherrod, Ph.D., a social psychologist in Los Angeles.

That's because male friendships are typically formed through shared activities, and these ages are when we're most likely to be doing things with other guys. When men become occupied with the demands of career and family, the opportunities for shared male activity decrease, and friendships dwindle.

Having friends is good for your health. Among nursing home residents, those with the most friends typically respond better to medication, recover faster from personal loss or illness, and live longer.

Dr. Sherrod says you need to do three things as you grow older: (1) create situations from which new friendships can grow, such as golf outings or poker nights; (2) make friends outside of work, so you won't lose them if you change jobs; and (3) instead of talking about what's happening in the world, discuss what's happening in your life. "Admit that you need a friend," says Dr. Sherrod, "and don't be afraid to open up to him."

14. **Know your triggers.** All of us have emotional triggers that can set off our negative thinking patterns. Learning what they are will help us keep our emotional safety switches on. "It pays to become a detective of your own behavior," says Carla Perez, M.D., a psychiatrist in San Francisco who has written extensively on controlling compulsive behavior. "You have to know what the enemy is before you can go after it. Pay attention to what sets you off."

15. **Liven things up.** If you can't always get out and enjoy the spectacle of nature, bring some of it to where you are. Being around plants, flowers, and trees is therapeutic, says Busch. That's why more and more hospitals are adding "healing gardens," both indoors and out, for the benefit of their patients and their staff. Putting some greenery in your office or home can stimulate a nurturing spirit and make you feel more at ease.

16. **Avoid a heart attack.** Before you fire the office slacker, consider this: You're twice as likely to have a heart attack the week after you kick his sorry butt onto the cold pavement. Researchers at Beth Israel Deaconess Medical Center in Boston studied 791 heart attack patients and found that a statistically significant 95 had fired someone, faced a deadline, or—unbelievably—landed a promotion in the previous week. It's no coincidence: "The exhaustion that comes after prolonged stress can contribute to a heart attack," says Murray Mittleman, M.D., the study author. And you're still at risk days after the event, not just on D day itself.

"It's especially dangerous if you're hit with a second stressor, such as a fight at home," says Joseph Loizzo, M.D., a stress expert at Columbia-Presbyterian Medical Center in New York City. Fortunately, you can usually predict these three major hurdles at work. Try to schedule a vacation for the week after you hit a deadline or hang pictures in a bigger office.

17. **Shop for sounds.** What kind of music works best for meditation? "Look for music that slows down your heart rate," says Steven Halpern, Ph.D., president of Inner Peace Music in San Anselmo, California, and a composer. "If you play slow music, your heartbeat will slow down. Fast music will speed it up. The phenomenon known as rhythm entertainment is an involuntary response to an external rhythmic stimulus. Your heartbeat literally will march to the beat of a different drummer."

18. **Stock up on laughs.** If you wait for something funny to happen to lift your spirits and lengthen your life, you may be frowning a long time. In these serious times, you have to be proactive about soliciting joyfulness, says Lee Berk, Dr.P.H., clinical preventive-care clinician and assistant research professor of pathology and laboratory medicine at Loma Linda University School of Medicine in California.

He suggests keeping a well-stocked arsenal of laugh makers on hand, such as joke books, comedy videos, funny films, and *Mad* magazine.

19. **Remain alert at the wheel.** The next time you decide to cross time zones in a bucket seat, make sure that you don't take an unscheduled nap at 65 miles per hour. Here are two ways to avoid road fatigue: Keep your head level. "Adjusting your seat correctly will stop a stiff neck," says Phil Berg, who drove 7,344 miles in 115 hours during the 1997 Trans-America Challenge. If you're looking up, your seat back is too far forward; if you feel like you're looking down, your seat back is reclining too much.

Stay clear, too. Stray reflections and glare from dirty glass cause fatigue, says Berg. Clean all the windows and apply a water repellent, such as Rain-X.

20. **Pause and listen.** Don't listen only to your reasoning mind. Listen to your inner urges, nudges, leanings, and voices. And give yourself permission to act on them, says Krista Kurth, Ph.D., a management consultant in Potomac, Maryland, who specializes in spirituality in the workplace. Also, make time to just put the world on "pause," Dr. Kurth says. "We get very caught up with all the events of our lives. And in order to have an intimate connection with some transcendent reality, we have to take time to stop and listen."

7

CURES

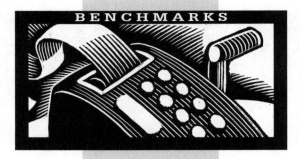

■ Number of people hospitalized each year due to the effects of prescription drugs:
1.5 million

■ Number of prescriptions written in 1997: 2.5 billion

■ Number of Americans who have someone else's heart: 300

■ Gallons of suntan lotion and oil used by Americans in 1 year: 1.3 million

■ Ratio of physicians to inhabitants of the United States: 1 to 549

■ Ratio of prison inmates to inhabitants of the United States: 1 to 497

■ Percentage of Americans who think science and technology may destroy the human race:
74

■ Percentage of visits to doctors' offices that last less than 11 minutes: 45

■ Chance that an impotence drug up for approval by the FDA lists yawning as a side effect:
1 in 3

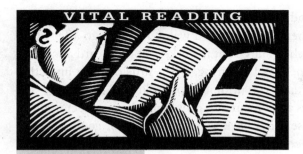

VITAL READING

Prescriptions for Life's Little Problems

Send these pains packing in half the time.

Ailments such as headaches, sore wrists, zits, and smelly feet may not be serious enough to merit a trip to the doctor, but they can be irritating enough to ruin your entire day.

There's plenty you can do to lessen your discomfort from even the tiniest of tormentors. And you can do it fast. Here are some simple ways to help you feel better twice as soon.

Cold Sores

Cold sores are caused by a herpes virus, which can live quietly deep in your nerves. The virus lives so quietly, in fact, that your body can't detect and attack it. Given the right conditions—including such commonplace things as sunshine, stress, cold weather, and fatigue—the bug takes a trip to your lip. You'll usually feel a tingling sensation about 12 hours before a cold sore develops, so you'll have a window of opportunity to head off its effects. Here are some pointers to help.

Cream it. Doctors have found that the prescription cream Denavir can keep a cold sore at bay or shorten its life, but only if you start using the stuff when you feel the tingle. "It speeds up the healing by about a day," says Stephen K. Tyring, M.D., Ph.D., professor of dermatology at the University of Texas Medical School at Galveston.

Cool it. Applying ice or a cold used tea bag to the sore can bring relief from itching and burning. Use it for 10 minutes four or five times a day.

Sack the snacks. Chocolate, oats, nuts, and gelatin are rich in an amino acid called arginine that helps cold sores thrive. Instead, eat yogurt, cheese, fish, chicken, milk, and other foods rich in lysine, a chemical that many experts think cues the immune system to attack the virus.

Try the pink stuff. Somebody figured out that since Pepto-Bismol fights the viruses that cause diarrhea when you drink bad water, it might go after other viruses, too. "There's no research to show that it works, but I've heard a number of people say that it helps them," says Dr. Tyring. Dab a little on your lip with a cotton swab and (this is important) rub until it stops looking like lipstick.

Stop the cycle. If cold sores are a recurring problem, ask your doctor about Valtrex or Famvir. Though these drugs have been tested only for genital herpes, many doctors will prescribe them to men with recurring cold sores. "In my experience, 95 percent of the patients who take either drug on a daily basis say it prevents most, if not all, of their outbreaks," says Dr. Tyring.

Definitely don't engage in oral activity with someone else, from kissing on down. Not only can the herpes virus jump from one set of lips to another, but it can also take up residence in any genital area it contacts. That's a gift she might never forget.

Burns

Freeze it. Put a bag of frozen vegetables on the burn as soon as you can. Smaller vegetables, such as peas and corn, work best because you can mold them around the burn. Or use ice cubes wrapped in a clean handkerchief or a thin towel. (Applying ice directly to the skin is dangerous.) "The ice helps to constrict blood vessels, reducing swelling and inflammation," says David Power, M.D., assistant professor of family medicine at the University of Minnesota Medical School in Minneapolis. Keep the area cool for 15 minutes.

Apply aloe gel. This natural gel promotes the healing of wounds, burns, and frostbite. In a study from Thailand, doctors found that aloe healed burns 4 days sooner than petroleum jelly did. If you have an aloe plant, just cut off a leaf and spread the juice on the wound.

Drink lots. "With a burn, you're losing moisture because your skin is basically drying out," says Dr. Power. Drinking an extra glass or two of water or juice each day will help you stay hydrated while you heal.

Consider seeing a doctor. It's a good idea to take your burn to a doctor if it's on your face, hands, or genitals, or if you have any question about its severity, says Jerold Z. Kaplan, M.D., medical director of the Alta Bates Hospital Burn Center in California. And definitely see the doctor if the burnt area covers more than 10 percent of your body (the palm of your hand, not counting the fingers, is 1 percent), or if it becomes infected—one sign of which is redness extending beyond the burn itself.

Don't pick at blisters. A blister is a kind of sterile covering. Destroying it leaves you open to infection. It will disappear once the skin underneath has begun to heal.

Stiff Neck

Rest a stiff neck in the early stages, but move it as soon as it starts to free itself.

Take long, hot showers. Let the water play on the back of your neck, says Brian Casazza, M.D., of the spine and sports care division at the University of Virginia Musculoskeletal Center in Charlottesville.

Look over your shoulder. If you move your neck gently four or five times a day, it's like pouring lotion on it. Turn your head carefully from side to side. Look over your right shoulder for a count of five, then do the same over your left shoulder. Repeat three times. If the movement causes pain, try again tomorrow.

Wrap up. If you have to curl up in an awkward position to stay warm at night, your stiff neck will come back. Keep your bedroom warm enough that you can stretch out. If you watch TV or read in bed, make sure your head isn't bent forward, back, or to the side.

Up against the wall. One good move to help relieve a stiff neck is to stand against a wall, says Dr. Casazza. Tuck your chin in, keep your shoulders down and back, and press your lower back against the wall.

Don't roll your head. Trying to "uncrick" your neck by rolling your head in a circle is likely to make it hurt, and it may do more harm than good.

Pimples

If you can tell that a monster is growing on your face, apply an ice pack. It will halt the inflammation. Here are a couple of other tips.

Call in the big guns. If you get a pimple that you just can't afford to live with, see a dermatologist. "He can treat you by injecting an anti-inflammatory steroid directly into the pimple," says Michael Kaminer, M.D., chief of cosmetic surgery at Harvard Medical School. If you're facing a full-blown outbreak, he can prescribe a corticosteroid. Either way, your skin should clear up in 2 to 3 days.

Don't squeeze. "Squeezing causes a buildup of pressure in the gland, which can cause it to rupture. That can lead to infection," says John F. Romano, M.D., clinical assistant professor of dermatology at New York Hospital–Cornell Medical Center in New York City. If the rupture occurs close to the surface of the skin, figure on a week before it disappears. If the rupture is deeper, you could develop a red lump that will leave a scar.

Headache

You want the pain to stop, and you're willing to open as many childproof bottles as it takes.

Stay active. "In the early stages, any kind of exercise, including sexual activity, can help abort an impending headache or migraine," says Roger Cady, M.D., medical director of the Headache Care Center in Springfield, Missouri. Not only does sex relieve stress, which is a factor in nearly all headaches, but it also triggers the production of endorphins, the body's natural painkillers.

Have a strong cup of coffee. The caffeine will help you absorb aspirin more quickly, says Egilius Spierings, M.D., a neurologist and headache specialist at Brigham and Women's Hospital in Boston.

Take a guided tour. Headache? What headache? Guided imagery is an effective way of getting rid of a headache, according to Dr. Cady. Try this exercise.

Close your eyes. Imagine yourself lying on a beach with the sun warming you through. (So don't pick Golden Gate Park in February.) Feel the waves rushing over you. As the water retreats, let it pull the tension from your body. When you're completely relaxed, visualize your headache as an object with size and texture. Turn it into a liquid and let it pour out through your fingertips. Don't scoff until you've tried it.

Get tested for the headache bacterium. Didn't know there was a headache bacterium? It's *H. pylori*—the same villain that causes ulcers. A recent study found that out of 200 headache sufferers, 40 percent tested positive for *H. pylori*. When researchers gave these people antibiotics to get rid of the bug, 86 percent said they suffered fewer or less intense headaches.

Put on the pressure. "Try using the pressure points on the back of your neck and upper back," says Dr. Spierings. "Feel for a tender point. That's usually the point to target." Apply steady pressure for several minutes. Massaging your head and the back of your neck is also good, but do it gently. Applying a cold compress may also help relieve the pain.

Don't stay in bed. Many headaches, especially migraines, are triggered in part by an upset of your internal clock, Dr. Cady says.

Joint and Muscle Pain

Most joint injuries are related to sports. Among golfers, tendinitis is as common as excuses for missed putts. Another good road to joint pain is putting together "some assembly required" furniture. No wonder you can't move your wrist the day after driving 200 screws into your new bookcases. You'll know that the problem is a tendon or a muscle if you feel a chronic, dull, throbbing pain that radiates down the extremity.

Ice it. Put an ice pack on the joint immediately, and leave it there for 15 minutes. Do this every 2 hours while you're still feeling pain. The ice will help reduce the swelling. Elevating the injured limb above the level of your heart—preferably above your head—will also help.

Rest it. "Rest the joint for several days before attempting to resume the activity," says David H. Janda, M.D., director of the Institute for Preventive Sports Medicine in Ann Arbor, Michigan. Your tee shots may suffer, but they won't suffer as much as you will if you don't give your injury time to heal.

Relieve it. Ibuprofen or aspirin will reduce the swelling and ease the pain. But take the oral form, since ibuprofen gel may not penetrate enough to work its full magic on joint injuries.

Exercise it. Gentle stretching 24 to 48 hours after a minor injury can help deliver fresh blood to the injured site, blasting out lactic acid and reducing swelling. "After the pain dissipates, start gentle stretching exercises with the affected joint, and then gradually resume your activities," says Dr. Janda. The best stretches work the tendon in the opposite direction of whatever you did to injure it. If your wrist is complaining about too many savage forehands, for instance, bend it backward gently for 2 to 3 minutes.

If your joint pain doesn't dissipate within a week, see a doctor or orthopedic surgeon.

Don't stress it. Avoid stress on your injury until the pain is gone. In other words, if you have tennis elbow, don't play tennis.

The Value of a Second Opinion

There are times when you should definitely get one.

Some things in life shouldn't depend on just one person's opinion. Like when you take the car in for a simple tune-up and the mechanic starts using dramatic words like "complete" and "overhaul."

Or when your other mechanic—the family doctor—delivers a scary diagnosis, one involving lots of drugs or post-op suffering. At times like these, you want to know all the available options. You want a fresh pair of eyes on the problem. You want a second opinion.

Here, then, are health concerns that might warrant a second look. Seek out another expert if your doctor suggests any of them.

"You have high blood pressure." A high reading or two in the doctor's office doesn't necessarily mean you have hypertension, says Thomas G. Pickering, M.D., Ph.D., a cardiologist at New York Hospital–Cornell Medical Center and author of *Good News about High Blood Pressure*. He says that men are susceptible to a phenomenon called white-coat hypertension. "Essentially, you get so worked up about your blood pressure that by the time you reach the doctor's office, your increased stress level causes a temporary rise in blood pressure." Ask the doctor to teach you how to monitor your own blood pressure. Or ask for an ambulatory monitor, which will measure your blood pressure during your normal activities.

Where to go for a second opinion: A physician who specializes in hypertension can help you make the call. Find one in your area by contacting the American Society of Hypertension at (212) 644-0650. Or go to the Hypertension Network at www.bloodpressure.com for a nationwide registry of more than 1,500 physicians who specialize in hypertension.

"Your borderline prostate test reading is nothing to worry about." Regular screenings are the best way to diagnose prostate cancer early. The American Urological Association recommends an annual digital-rectal exam for men 40 and over, and annual prostate-specific antigen (PSA) screenings beginning at age 50. (If you're African-American or if you have a history of prostate cancer in your family, start this test at 40, too.)

But your family doctor may not be the best person to interpret PSA test results. "Family doctors tend to like cut-and-dried, absolute tests. But PSA test results aren't necessarily cut-and-dried," says Judd Moul, M.D., director of the Center for Prostate Disease Research at the Uniformed Services University of the Health Sciences in Bethesda, Maryland. Typically, a PSA score of zero to 4 puts you in a low-risk category for developing cancer (your score should be less than 2.5 if you're under 50). A score of 4 to 10 puts you in a higher-risk category and warrants further testing.

"The problem with the scoring system is that many general practitioners see that number 4 as a magic cutoff point. If you had a score of 3.99, many general practitioners would say you were okay. But that may not be the case," says William Catalona, M.D., chief of urologic surgery at Washington University School of Medicine in St. Louis.

Where to go for a second opinion: A board-certified urologist can properly interpret your annual PSA results. To find a urologist—or a doctor with any specialty—go to the American Medical Association's Internet physician-referral service, at www.ama-assn.org/aps/amahg.htm.

"Your bad back requires bed rest." A week on the sofa with the remote and a bottle of muscle relaxants may sound inviting to you, but it won't necessarily help your back.

"A lot of doctors still believe that you should lie immobile in bed when you have a back injury. But if you lie down for too long—more than a few days—your muscles will get weaker and make the problem worse," says John Cianca, M.D., assistant professor of physical medicine and rehabilitation at Baylor College of Medicine in Houston. To cure the pain for good, find a doctor who can examine your biomechanics (the way you move and perform physical activities) and correct any imbalances.

Where to go for a second opinion: A specialist in physical medicine and rehabilitation is a good choice for help with back pain. Other possibilities include osteopathic doctors and chiropractors, who have training in biomechanics and physical medicine.

"Your blown knee needs immediate surgery." Tearing the anterior cruciate ligament (ACL) is a common hazard among men who like soccer, skiing, tennis, or any sport that requires cutting and pivoting. But if your doctor says you have only a few days or weeks to repair the knee before the damage becomes permanent, find someone more up-to-date.

"It used to be that you had only a short time to repair ACL damage. Not anymore. With today's reconstruction techniques, you can have the surgery at any time," says Andrew Cosgarea, M.D., assistant professor of orthopedic surgery at Johns Hopkins University School of Medicine in Baltimore. And depending on your age, your activity level, and the severity of the tear, you may not need surgery at all. With a few weeks of rehabilitation, you might be able to return to your normal routine with a torn ACL. (If you want to completely regain your former soccer-field prowess, though, you'll probably need reconstruction.)

Where to go for a second opinion: Look for an orthopedic surgeon with experience in sports medicine.

"Your kidney stones require an operation." As anxious as you might be to remove all that agonizing gravel rolling around in your plumbing, take a moment to consider another option. Eighty percent of all kidney stones are small enough to pass through your system naturally, though painfully, says Gerhard Fuchs, M.D., professor of urology at the University of California, Los Angeles, School of Medicine. Furthermore, 75 percent of patients who are likely candidates for traditional open surgery may not need it, thanks to a minimally invasive procedure known as lithotripsy. Using a device that generates sonic shock waves, urologists such as Dr. Fuchs (who pioneered lithotripsy in the United States) can blast the stones down to smaller, passable sizes, without making a single incision.

Where to go for a second opinion: Look for an endourologist. This type of specialist will have the most experience dealing with kidney stones.

"Your hemorrhoids can only be treated with surgery." Hemorrhoids are varicose veins in the wrong neighborhood. When you strain to move your bowels, veins bulge from the delicate tissue inside your rectum. Laborious straining can cause the veins to protrude outside the rectum, where they may cause irritation, inflammation, and occasional bleeding. But if your doctor says that you need surgery for the problem, you need to investigate further.

"Surgery is the last resort for hemorrhoids," says Peter McNally, D.O., spokesman for the American College of Gastroenterology. The reason is that hemorrhoid surgery can damage the delicate tissue in your rectum. "That tissue is sensitive enough to tell you whether you're about to pass a solid, a liquid, or a gas. That's information you want to have," he says.

When you go for a second opinion, ask about having the offending veins banded. In this procedure, a doctor literally wraps tiny rubber bands around the hemorrhoids, cutting off bloodflow. "Eventually, the tissue dies and falls off. No more hemorrhoids," says Dr. McNally.

Where to go for a second opinion: A colorectal surgeon who practices the banding procedure can tell you if you're a candidate.

"Your leg pain is caused by shinsplints." If the pain is confined to one spot on one leg, or if your leg hurts even when you're sitting still, shinsplints aren't your problem. What you probably have is a stress fracture, a tiny break brought on by training too hard or doing the same activity repeatedly. Stress fractures usually affect the leg, but you can sometimes get them in your foot or hip.

"Stress fractures can be tricky to diagnose; they don't show up on x-rays," says Dr. Cianca. "Your regular doctor might miss them." But a specialist knows the specific signs and will be more inclined than your family doctor to order a bone scan, an imaging test that can detect whether you have a stress fracture.

Where to go for a second opinion: Orthopedists and sports medicine specialists are on the alert for stress fractures.

"You should have cosmetic surgery." If you really want liposuction or some other type of cosmetic surgery, you don't just need a second opinion—you need to do a thorough job of shopping around, says Paul Schnur, M.D., president of the American Society of Plastic and Reconstructive Surgeons (ASPRS). "It's a discretionary procedure, not an emergency, so you need to spend time talking to different doctors. Learn what each one's expertise is, and choose one who makes you feel comfortable," he says.

Where to go for a second opinion: Make sure the doctors you're considering are certified by the American Board of Plastic Surgery. Ask specifically if they have privileges to perform plastic surgery at any local hospitals. Surgeons have to pass a rigorous evaluation to get these privileges, and not everyone earns them. Or call the ASPRS at (800) 635-0635. It'll give you the names of five board-certified plastic surgeons in your area.

Take the Pressure Off

Make these simple changes and live longer.

The problem with high blood pressure: It makes you stupid, then you die. A British study showed that 20 men and women with hypertension needed 37 minutes to finish a math test that healthy controls banged out in 10. Stress made the difference; it's hard to concentrate when the blood vessels in your head are throbbing like a bass drum. Those 20 people won't be bungling arithmetic much past their fifties, though. Even slightly high blood pressure—say, a reading around 135/85 mmHg (millimeters of mercury)—can cut years off your life span.

If you have hypertension, losing weight and getting regular exercise can lower your blood pressure by 15 to 20 points, says Irene Gavras, M.D., of Boston University. You'll cut your risk of heart attack and stroke by 40 percent, and you might avoid having to take blood pressure medications, some of which can cause impotence.

But some simpler changes can also help. Consistently doing things that lower your pressure for brief periods—or that prevent surges in blood pressure—can help reduce your overall risk of developing hypertension, says Thomas G. Pickering, M.D., Ph.D., a cardiologist at New York Hospital–Cornell Medical Center and author of *Good News about High Blood Pressure*. It's simple: The closer your blood pressure stays to 120/80 mmHg, and the longer it stays there, the lower your risk of having a heart attack or stroke caused by high blood pressure. So try these strategies.

Eat your wife's breakfast. Have cantaloupe and yogurt; they're high in potassium, a mineral that helps control blood pressure. A study review involving 2,600 subjects found that taking 2,000 milligrams of potassium daily—you can get that amount by eating a baked potato, a large banana, and 8 ounces of milk—reduced blood pressure by up to four points in 5 weeks.

Drink more orange juice. In a British study of 541 adults, those who had the highest blood levels of vitamin C also had the lowest blood pressures. Researchers believe that vitamin C helps blood vessels dilate. You can get your Recommended Dietary Allowance of 60 milligrams of vitamin C by eating broccoli, peppers, and citrus fruits.

Avoid extra stress in the morning. Men usually have heart attacks in the morning, and one reason is that your blood pressure stays elevated by at least 15 points until about 11:00 A.M. Try to avoid regular causes of stress—such as people who infuriate you—in the morning, says Daniel Jones, M.D., professor of medicine in the division of hypertension at the University of Mississippi in Jackson. Schedule those gripe-filled weekly staff meetings after lunch, and straighten your desk every night so you won't face a disaster site the next morning.

Cut down on coffee. People had a two- to three-point rise in blood pressure during the workday after they took caffeine pills that equaled a cup of coffee at breakfast and a cup at lunch, according to a study at Duke University in Durham, North Carolina. "Caffeine raises blood pressure by constricting blood vessels," says James D. Lane, Ph.D., associate research professor in psychiatry and behavioral sciences at Duke. If you won't give up java, keep it to a cup a day.

Throw garlic in the pasta. Eating a clove or two of garlic each day is one of the easiest ways to lower your blood pressure. A study review of 415 people with hypertension found that eating 600 to 900 milligrams of garlic powder cut blood pressure by an average of 11 points. The results were quick, too; the drop often came within 3 months. Garlic helps the body maintain adequate levels of an enzyme that prevents hypertension.

Let her talk herself out. Arguments with your wife can cause your blood pressure to skyrocket—no surprise there. But a study reported in *Health Psychology* found that although men maintained normal blood pressures as they listened and talked calmly, they experienced sharp increases in blood pressure when they began yelling, knowing that their persuasive skills were being judged. The bottom line is, let her do the yelling and screaming. And keep the investments in your name.

Answer to one boss at a time. Avoiding job stress helps control blood pressure. In a 3-year study of 195 men, reducing work stress lowered blood pressure by 10 points in hypertensive men and by 5 points in men with normal blood pressures. A common source of frustration is trying to please several supervisors, says study leader Peter Schnall, M.D., of the University of California, Irvine. "Clarify exactly whom you answer to," he advises.

Eat more salmon. When overweight study subjects ate 4 ounces of fish every day, their blood pressure levels dropped by six points within 4 months—even if they didn't lose weight. The protein and omega-3 fatty acids in fish help keep arteries elastic, says study author Trevor A. Mori, Ph.D., of the University of Western Australia in Nedlands. The fish eaters who also lost about 12 pounds lowered their blood pressures by 13 points.

Lay off the dinner rolls. The processed wheat in white bread causes a surge of insulin, which triggers a blood pressure rise for several hours. A study of 400 people at Tulane University in New Orleans found that people with the highest blood insulin levels were three times more likely to have high blood pressure.

Have a cup of ice cream. This gives you 150 to 200 milligrams of calcium. A Japanese study found that hypertensive people who took a 1-gram calcium supplement daily for 8 weeks reduced their average resting blood pressures by one or two points. Calcium seems to help artery walls stay flexible. Drinking a few glasses of milk each day will help, too.

Get outside at lunch. A German study found that taking in just 10 minutes of sunlight lowered blood pressure in 18 hypertensive patients by six points. The ultraviolet B radiation in sunlight helps the body make vitamin D_3, a nutrient that seems to interact with calcium to control blood pressure.

Work in a quiet place. Austrian researchers monitored 118 workers and found that working in a noisy place—such as a bustling factory—caused a consistent four-point rise in blood pressure. This happened even if the noise lasted only for short periods. So shut your office door, or drown out distracting sounds with a white-noise machine or a radio tuned between stations.

Do something really boring. A 3-month study of 100 people found that those who meditated for 20 minutes daily lowered their average resting blood pressures by 11 points after 12 weeks. If you don't go in for meditation, buy a fish tank. Watching tropical fish may lower blood pressure.

Have one dill pickle, not three. One large dill pickle contains 1,700 milligrams of sodium, more than two-thirds of your daily limit. It's still unclear if eating a lot of salt puts men at risk for high blood pressure; your doctor can monitor the effect sodium has on you. But studies have found that about half of all men with high blood pressure see a drop when they reduce their sodium intakes, so it can't hurt to keep yours below 2,400 milligrams per day. Physicians think that sodium may cause hypertension by adding fluid to your blood and by constricting artery walls.

Snack on almonds and pumpkin seeds. They're rich in magnesium. A study of 60 people with high blood pressure found that taking 480 milligrams of magnesium per day lowered their blood pressures by an average of four points. Researchers think magnesium may work as a muscle relaxant. You can get your normal daily allotment of 420 milligrams from 2½ ounces of dried pumpkin seeds. Halibut, wheat germ, spinach, and some fortified cereals are also good sources.

How High Is Too High?

If hypertension runs in your family, you should check your blood pressure monthly with a home testing kit. The stethoscope-and-arm-cuff models work best; they're sold in drugstores for $20. The top number is the systolic pressure—

the arterial pressure during a heartbeat. The bottom number is the diastolic pressure, or the pressure between beats.

Reading (mmHg): 120/80 to 139/89

Diagnosis: Normal to slightly high

Common treatment: That's a good reading. Check it at least once a year to make sure it doesn't rise—or fall. Low blood pressure is much more rare, but it could be the culprit if you have frequent headaches or fainting spells.

Reading: 140/90 to 159/99

Diagnosis: Moderately high

Common treatment: Your doctor will probably prescribe exercise and a low-fat, low-salt diet for 3 months. If that doesn't lower your blood pressure, you may need blood pressure medication.

Reading: 160/100 to 179/109

Diagnosis: Very high

Common treatment: You'll probably need a daily drug for the rest of your life. Your doctor may want to see you monthly for at least the first year.

Reading: 180/110 or above

Diagnosis: Dangerously high

Common treatment: This doubles your risk of a having a heart attack and quadruples your risk of suffering a stroke. You'll need medication and serious lifestyle changes, maybe including a new job.

BEST READS

A Menopause for Men

For years, the word menopause *was always associated with women. Men had their "midlife crises." In the past few years, several books have been written claiming that men do indeed go through menopause, and like women, it is hormonally driven. Eugene Shippen, M.D., and William Fryer expound on the topic of male menopause and what can be done to treat it in this excerpt from* The Testosterone Syndrome: The Critical Factor for Energy, Health, and Sexuality—Reversing the Male Menopause *(M. Evans and Company, 1998).*

A menopause for men? You'd better believe it. Men are in no way immune to midlife changes. They, too, suffer those transforming physical experiences that—when we see them in women—we call, with definitive finality, the change of life. It's the big change—the one that means you're no longer young.

Of course, we all change constantly as the years tick by. We get used to it. The alterations in our physical identities seem familiar, expected, even comfortable. But then suddenly, at some point in our lives, we are genuinely startled. Changes occur that we hadn't bargained for. Aging no longer looks benign. Pain, weariness, the fraying of desire, the dark shadow of depression all proclaim that a toll is being taken on our bodies and our spirits. By and large, the tollgates of change are hormonal. For some, the price of entry will be very high indeed.

Surely it makes sense to ask whether we can't reverse some part of this process of aging. Would it surprise you to know we can?

Allow me to define a word, without which the rest of this chapter is meaningless. Hormone. A hormone is a chemical substance produced in one part or organ of the body that starts or runs the activity of an organ or a group of cells in another part of the body. Testosterone, estrogen, insulin, adrenaline, cortisone—these are a few of the hormones found in most people's vocabularies and at least vaguely understood. Hormones can also be converted from one hormonal substance into another out in the tissues of the body. This is a newer concept, and it is referred to as intracrinology.

In the last few years, the popular anti-aging literature has given many people a familiarity with such hormones as DHEA, growth hormone, and melatonin. They are genuinely important substances, and perhaps some of you are already familiar with the idea that the levels of hormones can affect our actual (as opposed to chronological) rate of aging.

Every cell in the body is programmed by hormonal messengers. Hormones tune our systems—or untune them. We are hormonal creatures to at least as great an extent as we are oxygen-breathing creatures or blood-circulating creatures. We could not live a day or hardly even an hour without properly balanced hormonal input. Balance is the crucial word. Too much of the more important hormones would burn us out metabolically at a fantastic rate. Too little, and our systems begin to slowly shut down.

Think back to when you were young. If you were like most people, you reached your physical peak in your late teens or early twenties. It was a time of rambunctious energy that resisted every effort to squander it away. Late nights, too much work and too much play, and, for many of us, far too much eating and drinking—all this produced very little in the way of untoward effects. For many 20-year-olds, burning the candle at both ends is not a danger; it's an art form. Pushing past every reasonable limit, we recharged our cellular batteries as fast as we drained them. How were our organ systems and, indeed, every cell in our bodies able to keep up with the brutal pace? Hormones! We were in hormone heaven.

The optimal function of every cell requires optimal hormonal input—and we had it. Logically, therefore, any decline in hormonal activity from youthful norms will result in suboptimal cellular activity. Does that seem reasonable?

We know that it is. There are many reasons hormones change, including illness, stress, the autoimmune destruction of our glands, and, of course, the natural decline of aging. Any doctor who has carefully charted the hormonal changes of his patients knows that significant, long-term hormonal decline leads irresistibly toward illness, fatigue, malaise, and further aging.

And any doctor who looks for hormonal decline will find hormonal decline. Most of the major hormone systems drop significantly and steadily from year to year and decade to decade. It is one of the most important parts of the steady downward spiral into old age and debility.

Yet, incredibly, these major hormones can—so far as I know, without exception—be safely and efficiently replaced in men's and women's bodies. The result of that replacement is rapid improvement in physical function. More often than not, there is also a marked recovery in psychological attitude and mental alertness. This is a fact not widely known to laypeople and still stoutly resisted by some members of the medical profession.

The major controversy among physicians is whether gradual hormonal decline is a normal, healthy part of aging or a pathologic, diseaselike state. To me, this controversy sets up a false dichotomy. Hormonal decline is, of course, normal, but so is heart disease. They are also—and equally—disease states and will, in the end, prove fatal to any human being who allows either one to run its course unhindered.

Fortunately, the notion of hormone replacement is already well-established in one corner of medical practice. I'm referring, of course, to estrogen-replacement therapy for postmenopausal women. Some would suggest that this is quite different from giving testosterone to a man. Women have a menopause. Men obviously do not.

But didn't we just say that wasn't true? You're absolutely right!

Men Are Different from Women

Habitual knee-jerk reactions often go by the name of thought, and many people "think" that there is no male menopause. Why do they think this? Because an assumption is made that if a man had a menopause, it would conform to the pattern experienced by women. And, in women, menopause is anything but quiet. The cymbals clash, the hot flashes rush in, hormone levels drop like a barometer in a hurricane. In fact, for a significant percentage of women, menopause virtually is a 2- or 3-year hurricane that they profoundly wish would go away.

If this is menopause, I will gladly confess that not too many men experience anything like it. No man loses 90 percent of his sex hormones in a couple of years except as the result of severe and unusual illness.

Nonetheless, men do have a menopause. It creeps in upon them stealthily, until, at last, they reach a point where they can't help noticing their muscles shrinking, their energy withering, their self-confidence crumbling, and their virility taking a tumble. By then, most men recognize reluctantly that their quality of life is shrinking like a pizza pie under sustained attack by a carload of high-school kids. Men enter a gray zone, a time they neither understand nor wish to talk about.

The male menopause is one of the most dynamic and significant events a man ever experiences, but it does not announce itself boldly. In fact, the time that elapses between the first hesitant signals of the male change of life and its full, ugly flowering can easily be 10 to 15 years.

Just as there are many symptoms of the menopause, whether male or female, so are there many causes. But the root causes are hormonal. Women's estrogen and progesterone levels fall sharply at menopause. Men's testosterone levels fall steadily decade by decade. But all men are different. There are rare males whose testosterone levels stay at or near youthful heights right into old age. And, typically, the result of such unusual elevations is health.

I have measured the testosterone levels of many hundreds of men, and I have never seen an older male in excellent mental and physical health whose testosterone levels were not well within the normal range. And the healthiest, most vital individuals are always in the high normal ranges.

Does this mean that testosterone is the secret of male vitality? It is one of the secrets. But one of the most compelling and revolutionary insights in this book revolves around the relationship of the male sex to the female hormone. Testosterone does not rule the roost in lordly isolation. Estrogen can make or mar the overall functioning of the average man's body.

The fundamental metabolic fact that every doctor is aware of, though few give it much thought, is this: Estrogen is not simply a female hormone, nor is testosterone only a male hormone. The human body is far more mysterious and complex than that. Each sex has highly significant quantities of the opposite sex's major sex hormone in their bodies. Both men and women, therefore, require differing, but individually optimal, quantities of both estrogen and testosterone to activate their sexuality.

And, once we look at men and reflect on the role estrogen plays in their lives, we are going to find out why many otherwise good scientists have neglected testosterone-replacement therapy. We are going to learn that the most common method of delivering testosterone—the testosterone injection—is radically flawed. And we are going to see why some scientists have suggested, on the basis of carefully done, competent research, that the male hormone is not as good as it's cracked up to be, not effective in treating impotence, not right for most men, not appropriate for handling the male menopause, and so on. Their research was sound, but unfortunately it ignored the essential testosterone/estrogen relationship. Instead, they have studied their male patients solely on the basis of their testosterone.

When I first began treating menopausal men with the male hormone, I made the same mistake. I observed with fascination and delight the excellent improvements some men made as their testosterone levels rose. But I was sorely puzzled by the hormone's ineffectiveness in other men. It took time to understand the hormonal refinements that were at work. It took experience to realize that there is a window of optimal function for every hormone in the human body. Above all, it took measurement of estrogen levels to realize that estrogen can be as crucial as testosterone to the hormonal health of a middle-age man.

The Importance of the Male Menopause

It would be impossible to overemphasize the devastating effects that menopause has on millions of men and women. Doctors know because people come and sit in our offices and tell us secrets that they wouldn't even whisper to their spouses. And once you've listened for a while to people telling you that their sex lives are crumbling, their energy is shattered, their health is growing shakier by the year—and one soon finds out that they're right on that point—one feels a very real compulsion to do something about it.

Is all this unpleasant change the menopause? A whole lot of it is. Heart disease, high blood pressure, diabetes, arthritis, osteoporosis—indeed, most of the major risk factors for dying—are all intimately related to hormonal changes. To a surprising degree, many of these dreadful conditions reverse themselves when a proper balancing of the hormones in the body is combined with sensible diet.

That hormone balancing can be achieved either by various natural boosting techniques or by actual hormone replacement.

To say that the menopause is natural seems like a trivial distinction in the face of these calamities. Death is natural and inevitable, too, but many of us would like to postpone it. Moreover, I think I speak for most people when I say we would like to keep our youthful vigor throughout our lives, right up to the end. The real purpose of this book is to help make that possible.

What Happens in the Male Menopause

In men, the menopause—or andropause, as some would call it, because the male hormones are properly called androgens—is a more unpredictable process than in women. This is not only because of the gradual nature of its timing but also because the order in which symptoms appear varies from man to man, based on lifestyle and genetic inheritance. What many men first notice is a loss of sexual desire. That, however, can simply reflect the tremendous significance that many men give to sex.

I think that more often the first sign, perhaps passing unnoticed, is a subtle downward shift in strength and energy. In some men, a depressive change in personality quite apparent to wives and friends is the first indication.

Whatever comes first, the eventual effect of the male menopause is an erosion of the underpinnings of our personal strengths, whatever they may be. Loss of athletic ability, loss of dynamic executive capabilities, loss of self-confidence, eagerness, aggressive energy—a sense of loss magnified and multiplied by the total unexpectedness of what we're undergoing. This is change, indeed. The sharp edges of youth are replaced by the well-traveled roads of habit and lethargy.

I don't know how many men have come to me and said things like, "Objectives go, confidence goes, fear comes in. I don't have the desire to do things for myself anymore. Sometimes I don't even want to go out the door in the morning. The world is gray."

Very typically, men will put these changes down to overwork, stress, the vaguely understood concept of a midlife crisis. By and large, these explanations are pap. The changes that men feel are hormonal, are real, and can be understood first and changed second. They can be measured, too.

There isn't anything all that difficult about treating the male menopause and beating it. Complicated, yes, but not difficult. And the rewards are vast. Better life, longer life, brighter, younger, more vital life. Not to mention a remarkable decrease in the risk of major diseases that jut up like rocks in the road of longevity.

This book is one piece of a hormone revolution that is happening all around us now. Laypeople and a portion of the medical profession have woken up to the fact that hormones contain the juice of youth, and without their presence in optimal quantities, vital, vigorous life is nearly impossible.

Testosterone is far more than just a sex hormone. Testosterone travels to every part of the human body. There are receptors for it from your brain to your toes. Testosterone is vitally involved in the making of protein, which, in turn, forms muscle. Testosterone is a key player in the manufacture of bone. Testosterone improves oxygen uptake throughout the body, vitalizing all tissues. Testosterone helps control blood sugar, helps regulate cholesterol, helps maintain a powerful immune system. Testosterone appears to help in mental concentration and improves mood. Testosterone is most likely one of the key components in protecting your brain against Alzheimer's disease.

The "male hormone" is dynamite. Don't leave home without it.

10 Common Surgeries and Procedures

Doctors in our society are still, for the most part, seen as all-knowing healers who shouldn't be questioned. But that attitude is changing as people take greater charge of the medical care of their bodies. This informative excerpt from Men's Health for Dummies *(IDG Books Worldwide, 1999) by Charles Inlander and the People's Medical Society will arm you with information and questions to ask should you have to face the surgeon's knife.*

At some point in your life, you may need surgery or have to undergo a diagnostic procedure. And chances are good that the surgery or procedure will be one of the ones listed in this chapter. So as a savvy health-care consumer, it's in your best interest to know what's what about the following procedures and surgeries.

Before you agree to any surgery or procedure, ask your health-care practitioner a few questions.

• Why do I need this surgery/procedure?
• Why this particular type of surgery/procedure? In the case of a procedure, does it provide general or specific information? If it provides general information, ask what the next step will be.
• How reliable is the surgery/procedure?
• Is the procedure invasive or noninvasive? If it is invasive, what are the risks involved? Can a noninvasive procedure provide similar information?
• What possible risks does the surgery/procedure have?
• Does the surgery/procedure require any special preparation?
• How much does it cost?
• Are any alternatives available if I refuse this surgery/procedure?

All surgeries and procedures carry possible risks such as infection, human error, and anesthesia mishaps. Be sure to discuss the risks with your doctor before submitting to any surgery or procedure.

Arteriography. Arteriography is a diagnostic procedure that uses contrast dye and x-rays to evaluate the condition of the arteries in your abdomen, chest, arms, or legs. Special arteriographic procedures for the arteries in the brain (cerebral arteriography), lungs (pulmonary arteriography), and heart (coronary arteriography) are also done. Arteriography can determine abnormalities of bloodflow, including blood clots, aneurysms, and ruptured blood vessels.

The procedure, done under local anesthesia, is performed in the x-ray suite of a hospital. A radiologist inserts a special needle—called an arterial needle—in an artery. He or she then inserts a catheter (a fine tube) through the special needle and threads the catheter to the section of your body to be examined. The contrast dye is then injected and x-rays are taken. Rare but possible complications include allergic reaction to the contrast material, infection, damage to an artery, or loosening of a piece of clotted blood.

Cardiac catheterization. This diagnostic procedure determines the location and condition of blocked arteries that supply the heart, defects of the heart, severity of damage to heart function, and how well your heart pumps blood through your body. The principal problem that cardiac catheterization helps to diagnose is the narrowing of the coronary arteries caused by plaque (a complex mass of cells, cholesterol, and other organic matter).

Cardiac catheterization is performed under local anesthesia. A cardiac surgeon, radiologist, or cardiologist injects a special needle into an artery or vein of your arm or groin and then passes a catheter through the needle into the vessel. Next, he or she threads the catheter to an artery or heart chamber. When the catheter is in the right position, a contrast dye is injected and x-rays are taken. During the procedure, the doctor may give you a nitroglycerin tablet to help dilate the blood vessels, or you may be given an injection to help constrict the coronary arteries. After all imaging is done, the doctor withdraws the catheter. Rare but possible complications include allergic reaction to the dye, renal failure, blood clot, and circulatory collapse (cessation of effective bloodflow).

Aortocoronary bypass. Aortocoronary bypass, commonly known as coronary artery bypass graft (CABG), is surgery in which blocked coronary arteries are replaced with transplanted veins or arteries from your leg. CABG, which is performed in the hospital and under general anesthesia, takes between 2 to 4 hours to complete.

While your heart is stopped, circulation is taken over by a heart-lung machine, which ensures adequate bloodflow. Rare but possible complications include infection, stroke, failure of the breastbone to heal, and death.

Appendectomy. Appendectomy is surgery in which a surgeon removes an inflamed appendix from your body. Before the surgery, your doctor will prescribe antibiotics for you to help reduce the infection and limit tissue damage in your abdomen. The surgery is usually performed in the hospital under general or spinal anesthesia. The surgeon makes an incision in your lower-right abdomen and then cuts the appendix away from your body. Possible complications include infection and reaction to anesthetic drugs.

Bronchoscopy. Bronchoscopy, also known as endoscopic lung biopsy, is a diagnostic procedure generally performed under general anesthesia in which a small piece of lung tissue is removed for microscopic examination using a bronchoscope (a tubelike fiber-optic viewing scope). In this procedure—done in a hospital, outpatient surgery clinic, or well-equipped doctor's office—a surgeon or pulmonologist inserts the bronchoscope in your mouth, past the trachea, and into your bronchi (large airways). If the surgeon sees a suspicious area (such as a tumor), he or she will remove a piece of tissue using the cutting instrument in the bronchoscope. Rare but possible complications include bleeding, air in the chest cavity, and the breakage of brushes that are used for obtaining surface tissue samples.

Computerized axial tomography. Also known as CAT scan, computerized axial tomography is a diagnostic procedure used to determine a variety of conditions. For example, a CAT scan of the kidneys can confirm tumors, stones, infection, obstruction, and other diseases and conditions of the kidneys. In a CAT scan, a technician takes a series of cross-sectional x-rays and then uses a computer to construct highly detailed images of the inside of your body.

Diagnostic ultrasound. Ultrasound imaging, a diagnostic procedure, uses sound waves to show images of your internal organs, such as the liver, spleen, or pancreas. An ultrasound technician applies a lubricant gel to your skin over the area that needs to be examined and passes a transducer—a device that records the sound waves—over the lubricated area. An image of the area is captured on a monitor.

Endoscopy of the large bowel. This diagnostic procedure—done under light or heavy sedation and on an inpatient or outpatient basis in a hospital or outpatient surgery clinic—uses a colonoscope (a tubelike fiber-optic viewing scope) to check for benign or malignant tumors of the colon, bowel obstruction, inflammatory bowel disease, colitis, and foreign objects. A colon-rectal surgeon or gastroenterologist inserts the colonoscope through your rectum and snakes the device through your colon, looking for polyps and other lesions. Suspicious tissue is taken for microscopic examination. Rare but possible complications include bleeding, infection, and perforation of the colon wall.

Transurethral resection of the prostate. Transurethral resection of the prostate (TURP) is surgery in which a urologist removes a portion of your prostate gland that is partially or completely blocking the urethra. In TURP—done in a hospital under general anesthesia—the urologist inserts a cystoscope (a tubelike fiber-optic viewing scope) into your penis to examine the inside of your bladder for tumors and signs of infection. Once the urologist locates the portion of the prostate gland that is blocking your urethra, he or she cuts the diseased or malignant tissue with a cutting device called an electrosurgical loop. The urologist may put an irrigation catheter (which has tubes for inserting and draining irrigation solution) into your bladder for a day or so until the irrigation fluid is clear of blood clots and tissue fragments. Possible complications include infection and a puncture of the bladder by the cystoscope. After the surgery, possible side effects include erection problems, retrograde ejaculation, and sterility.

Respiratory therapy. Respiratory therapy is any procedure that improves or maintains your respiratory system. One example of respiratory therapy is mechanical ventilation. Respiratory therapy can be done at a hospital, at a clinic, or in the privacy of your home.

Mechanical ventilation uses a ventilator (mechanical breathing machine) and is used when you cannot breathe on your own or when your breaths are not strong enough to deliver air to your lungs. Possible conditions that can make it difficult for you to breathe on your own include blood clots in the lung, infections, or diseases such as adult respiratory distress syndrome.

Possible complications of mechanical ventilation include irregular heartbeat, collapsed lung, infection, and decreased cardiac output.

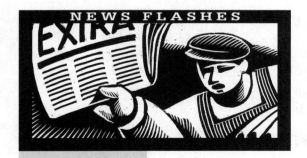

Procedure Offers Permanent Relief for Severe Heartburn

DALLAS—Most of the 60 million Americans who suffer from heartburn can control it with medication. But people with gastroesophageal reflux disease—a severe, chronic form of heartburn—should consider a new surgical option. Physicians at the University of Texas Southwestern Medical Center are using a minimally invasive surgery in which they wrap part of the stomach around the lower esophagus to stop the acid from rising. The surgery, called the laparoscopic toupet procedure, can offer permanent relief, and the only side effect is temporary esophageal pain. "It requires only five small incisions," says Daniel B. Jones, M.D., assistant professor of surgery at the medical center. Some patients may go home as soon as the day after surgery.

Cortisone Can Remedy Some Hair Loss

VANCOUVER, Canada—If you find a hairless patch on your beard, pubic area, armpit, or scalp, and it doesn't resemble normal male-pattern hair loss, it may be alopecia areata, a disease that affects an estimated 2 million men in the United States alone. It occurs when lymphocytes—a type of white blood cell—mysteriously attack hair follicles in a localized spot; but that's all researchers really know. "Alopecia areata takes a totally unpredictable course," says Jerry Shapiro, M.D., director of the hair research and treatment center at the University of British Columbia. The patch may fill in after a few months, and the condition may never recur. The worst case? Alopecia areata can progress and affect larger areas, says Dr. Shapiro. Luckily, that's rare. See a dermatologist if you sprout an odd bald spot, such as a dime-size spot on the side of your head. A cortisone shot may help stop the lymphocytes from attacking your follicles, and you'll likely see regrowth in about 2 months.

Golf Swing Can Hinder Knee Rehabilitation

CLEVELAND—According to a Cleveland Clinic study, playing golf too soon after knee surgery could put you at risk for further injury. After evaluating the golf swings of 13 healthy men, researchers noted that regardless of the subject's skill, weight, or shoe type (spiked or nonspiked), each swing had the same impact as running in a straight line and suddenly making a 90-degree turn. "Golf could easily be considered the silent contact sport," says Mark Grabiner, Ph.D., the study coauthor. Once your knees are completely rehabilitated, take half-swings for a few days before you actually tee off.

Herniated-Disk Surgery Is Now an Outpatient Procedure

HOUSTON—Thanks to microsurgery, repairing a herniated disk is now a 1-hour outpatient procedure. Using a surgical microscope, a physician makes a 1-inch incision just below the disk and then removes the portions that are herniated and degenerated. The success rate of a microdiskectomy is 90 percent, and recovery takes less time than with traditional herniated-disk surgery. "We're basically taking the minimally invasive techniques of brain surgery and applying them to the spine," says David S. Baskin, M.D., professor of neurosurgery at

Baylor College of Medicine. Most major medical centers have a surgeon trained in this technique.

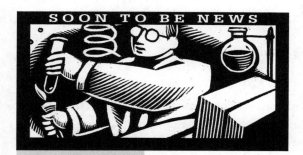

SOON TO BE NEWS

Faster Diagnosis of Heart Attacks?

It can take hours for doctors to determine what's causing your chest pain. But soon, a new combination of tests will accurately diagnose in-progress heart attacks in minutes. By measuring the blood levels of troponinT (a protein released during heart damage) and performing echocardiograms on 100 patients with chest pain, physicians in the University of Pennsylvania Health Care System in Philadelphia diagnosed men who were having heart attacks—and those who weren't—with almost 90 percent accuracy.

"With this combination, emergency room doctors can treat patients hours earlier and help prevent unnecessary hospitalizations," says Emile R. Mohler III, M.D., director of vascular medicine for the Health Care System.

The Real Risk Factor for Heart Disease?

A type of blood fat other than cholesterol may be the real risk factor for heart disease. Researchers at the University of Texas Southwestern Medical Center in Dallas analyzed the blood of 63 men who had heart problems but normal cholesterol levels, and of 23 men who were healthy but had high cholesterol levels. The men with heart problems had 33 percent more remnantlike particles (RLP) in their blood. RLP is created when triglycerides are broken down. "Most heart-attack victims have normal cholesterol levels, so RLP could be another important cause of heart disease," says study coauthor Ishwarlal Jialal, M.D.

RLP is treatable, and a test is awaiting FDA approval.

Vaccine for Ulcers?

Need some news that hits you in the pit of your stomach? A vaccine for *Helicobacter pylori*, the bacterium that causes peptic ulcers, is in the works. Researchers at the University of New South Wales in Australia found that mice given the enzyme catalase produced antibodies that protected them from *H. pylori*. The big scientific pothole: The mice received catalase combined with a cholera toxin that won't work for humans. "We may be able to use a modified toxin to make a vaccine that's effective and safe for people," says Stuart L. Hazell, Ph.D., a microbiologist and member of the research team. "This vaccine may be useful as a treatment for existing ulcers as well."

The vaccine may be available within 4 years.

Breathable Insulin?

Many of the 7.5 million men with diabetes would love to trash their hypodermics. Aside from components like wearable infusion pumps, there have been few alternatives to needles in the last 80 years. Now, Inhale Therapeutic Systems and Pfizer are testing a new insulin inhaler. The device converts insulin powder into vapor and delivers it to the lower lungs, where it's absorbed into the bloodstream faster than it could be from an injection. "That's important because right now, diabetics need to inject insulin 30 to 60 minutes before a meal for it to be absorbed properly. With this vapor, it will be easier for people with diabetes to quickly coordinate their insulin doses with their meals," says John Patton, Ph.D., Inhale's vice president of research. The inhaled insulin also seems to mimic the body's own natural hormone more closely than injected insulin, says Dr. Patton.

The inhaler may be available within the next few years.

Better Home Tests?

These home tests should hit pharmacies soon.

Prostate-specific antigen (PSA): The EZ-PSA by Biomerica, a finger-prick blood test, will detect PSA levels that put you at high risk for prostate cancer. It's available in Europe now and, with FDA approval, the EZ-PSA should be available in the United States within 2 years.

HIV urine test: Think of the home HIV-testing process minus the bloodletting. Send the Calypte Biomedical Corporation a urine sample and then call a toll-free number for the verdict and counseling, if you need it. The FDA has approved the process for doctors' offices and labs, so we could see the drugstore kit this year.

High-density lipoprotein cholesterol: A finger-prick blood test from Technical Chemicals and Products will tell you whether your total and high-density lipoprotein ("good") cholesterol fall within normal, medium-risk, or high-risk ranges. If the FDA gives its blessing, the test should be available this year.

Painless Monitoring of Glucose Levels?

Researchers at Massachusetts Institute of Technology (MIT) in Cambridge are using ultrasound to help measure glucose without needles or blood samples. They have discovered that low-frequency ultrasound can make skin permeable enough for interstitial fluid—the fluid between skin cells—to be drawn out with a vacuum pump. The fluid contains glucose levels similar to those in blood. "Diabetes patients should draw blood four times a day, but most manage only two times because of the pain," says MIT researcher Samir Mitragotri, Ph.D. Without regular glucose monitoring, deadly drops or spikes in blood sugar can occur.

An ultrasound device could be developed for home use in 3 to 5 years, according to Dr. Mitragotri.

Earlier Detection of Tumors?

A new imaging process can detect the earliest stages of tumor growth. Standard magnetic resonance imaging (MRI) can identify large tumors by revealing high concentrations of water in the body. But now researchers at Princeton University have developed a modified MRI that also scans for changes in the concentration of oxygen—a warning sign of early tumor growth. Since even small tissue changes affect oxygen concentration, "it's more useful in detecting tumors that are just beginning to develop," says the lead researcher, Warren S. Warren, Ph.D.

Human testing of the modified MRI is under way, and the new process should be widely available within 2 years.

More Time to Treat Strokes?

Typically, clot-dissolving drugs must be given within 3 hours of a stroke. But a new drug doubles the time doctors have to prevent stroke-induced brain damage. In a study presented at the American Heart Association's annual stroke conference, patients given prourokinase within 6 hours of their strokes had a 40 percent chance of recovering with little or no brain damage, compared with a 25 percent chance for patients given the anticoagulant heparin. "Prourokinase works quickly because it goes directly into the clot. Other drugs have to travel through the entire body before they start dissolving clots," says Anthony Furlan, M.D., the study author.

The drug has been submitted for FDA approval.

Relief from Arthritis?

Research from Louisiana State University in Baton Rouge shows that an herb may be able to relieve arthritis symptoms. In a laboratory study, isolated human cells exposed to an extract of the cat's claw vine fought off damaging free radicals and inflammation-causing toxins. Cat's claw also has the ability to prevent the activation of NF-KB, a protein that triggers inflammation. "Peruvian shamans have used cat's claw for thousands of years to successfully treat rheumatism, gastritis, and other inflammatory diseases," says Mark J. S. Miller, Ph.D., coauthor of the study.

Cat's claw formulations are already available in health food stores; clinical trials are under way to determine the most effective dosage.

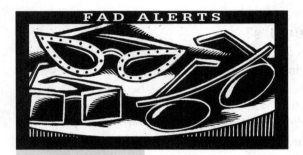

FAD ALERTS

Capsaicin

Most people know that chili peppers (capsicum plants) contain a substance called capsaicin. Like most muscle rubs, capsaicin causes a general irritation on your skin that produces a mild burning sensation and masks other pain. It may also block the transmission of pain signals to the brain. What's puzzling is that so many people gladly pay $5 for a tube of capsaicin "sports balm." Do this: Invest 50 cents in a hot pepper, break it open, and rub the inside on your sore muscles. (Test a small area first so you know you won't develop a skin reaction, and don't rub your eyes or touch your face until you've washed your hands thoroughly.) Bet it gives you the same relief as the brand-name stuff. You can mix pepper shavings into an inexpensive hand lotion, too.

Comfrey

You can buy comfrey (*Symphytum officinale*) in a topical gel form that you apply to minor cuts to fight infection and speed healing. It contains allantoin, a chemical that's known to help skin repair itself. But you can also buy comfrey in tablets, teas, and formulas that some people believe can treat stomach ulcers—although the herb has never been shown to do a thing to fight them. In fact, it contains toxic alkaloids that can destroy liver cells, and ingesting it can be dangerous. Some researchers believe that these alkaloids can be absorbed through the skin. They recommend staying away from comfrey in any form.

Eyesight Elixirs

 The products include Preventive Nutrition Ocular Formula, TwinLab OcuGuard Plus with Lutein, and Futurebiotics BrightEyes. They cost anywhere from $20 to $47 for a month's supply, and their main ingredients are beta-carotene, vitamin C, vitamin E, and zinc.

If you're Mr. Magoo, these supplements won't suddenly give you 20/20 eyesight. But reports suggest that the antioxidants they contain may help protect you against some eye diseases as you grow older, says Stephanie Marioneaux, M.D., an ophthalmologist in Chesapeake, Virginia. Taking vitamins C and E can cut your risk of cataracts significantly, and carotenoids such as lutein and zeaxanthin may reduce your risk of age-related macular degeneration—the leading cause of blindness in Americans over 65.

Are they worth buying? No. Vitamins C and E and carotenoids can help protect your eyes, but there's no proof that doses greater than the Recommended Dietary Allowances (RDAs) increase the benefit, so why pay extra for them? Eating more foods rich in carotenoids—oranges, green leafy vegetables, corn, red and orange peppers—and taking an inexpensive multivitamin that contains 100 percent of the RDAs for C and E should work just as well.

Prostate Pills

 The pills include One a Day Prostate Health, Centrum Herbals Saw Palmetto, Quanterra Prostate, and Celestial Seasonings Prostate Health. They cost anywhere from $17 to $26 for a month's supply, and their main ingredients are saw palmetto and zinc.

Saw palmetto and zinc have proven beneficial in treating an enlarged prostate, a condition common in men over 50 that causes pain and frequent urination. In fact, a recent analysis of 18 studies found that saw palmetto was as effective in treating the condition as Proscar, a popular prescription drug.

Are they worth buying? Yes. "More than 90 percent of my patients with enlarged prostates can be successfully treated with the right natural remedies," says Steven Margolis, M.D., clinical instructor of alternative medicine at Wayne State University in Detroit and at William Beaumont Hospital in Troy, Michigan. But talk to your doctor first: If you have a prostate cancer screening, the supplement may skew the results.

Milk Thistle

Milk thistle *(Silybum marianum)* is a prickly purple herb that contains silymarin, a compound that many researchers believe helps repair liver damage. Sixty 250-milligram capsules run about $20.

A study published in the *Journal of Hepatology* found that patients with cirrhosis of the liver who took 420 milligrams of silymarin daily for 2 years had a higher survival rate than patients who took a placebo.

Silymarin apparently binds to the surface of liver cells so toxins can't enter, according to John Pinto, Ph.D., director of the nutrition research lab at Memorial Sloan-Kettering Cancer Center in New York City. It also increases your body's ability to make glutathione, a compound that stimulates the regeneration of liver cells.

If your liver has been damaged by a disease such as hepatitis C, or if you take a tranquilizer that may stress your liver, such as Thorazine or Haldol, ask your doctor whether taking milk thistle would help you.

You have to take milk thistle for weeks, however, before the silymarin can build up a protective effect, says Ken Flora, M.D., hepatologist at Oregon Health Sciences University in Portland. Also, no research has shown that milk thistle is valuable if your liver is healthy.

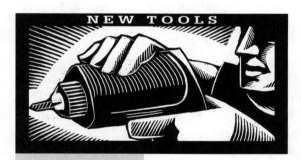

NEW TOOLS

An End to Gum Disease

Periostat

About 67 million American adults have gum disease, which is why many middle-age guys sport hockey smiles. Dentists have long treated chronic cases by repeatedly scraping the bacteria from beneath infected gums, but now a pill can also help stop the disease from returning.

Periostat is a low-dose antibiotic that counteracts collagenase, an enzyme that responds to gum bacteria by attacking the bone that anchors your teeth. "Patients with advanced disease still need scaling and root planing to remove the under-lying infection that's damaging the gums," says Robert Schoor, D.D.S., president of the American Academy of Periodontology. "But afterward, Periostat can help maintain bone levels."

In a 9-month study of 190 patients at five U.S. universities, subjects who took Periostat preserved 50 percent more gum tissue than a control group. Periostat has no known side effects, but it's a lifetime deal: You must take it twice a day to maintain your gum tissue. (A month's worth of Periostat costs $45.) And it's not a preventive measure; your dentist will prescribe Periostat only if brushing and flossing can't control your gum disease.

Stopping Heartburn

Prevacid

Over-the-counter heartburn remedies, including Zantac 75, Pepcid AC, and Tagamet HB, can treat an occasional flare-up, like the kind that comes after you eat a bucket of hot wings. But as many as 11 million American men suffer from chronic acid reflux—a disorder in which stomach acid leaks into the esophagus, causing severe heartburn and possibly increasing the risk of throat cancer. These men need a prescription drug to stop the burning.

Prevacid, the latest gastric-acid inhibitor approved by the FDA, works by in-terfering with a digestive enzyme that produces excess stomach acid. "It decreases acid secretion by about 90 percent," says Mel Wilcox, M.D., associate professor of medicine at the University of Alabama in Birmingham.

A study of 565 heartburn patients at Royal Berkshire Hospital in England found that those taking Prevacid experienced significantly greater relief after 3 days than those taking the decade-old drug Prilosec (omeprazole), an acid-reflux drug in the same class. A 30-day prescription of Prevacid costs $107 on average.

Broader Flu Treatment

Relenza

The flu vaccination you wisely have every autumn is effective for about 70 percent of takers. If you find yourself in the unlucky 30 percent, a new drug could blunt the symptoms and help you recover a few days sooner. The two drugs currently used to treat the flu—Flumadine (rimantadine) and Symmetrel (amantadine)—fight only the type A influenza virus, but Relenza attacks both type A and type B viruses, says Arnold S. Monto, M.D., professor of epidemi-ology at the University of Michigan in Ann Arbor. "It's also the first treatment demonstrated to prevent dangerous complications, such as pneumonia," he notes. Another reason for the drug's effectiveness is that it's an inhaled powder. "Most of the drug sits in the respiratory tract, where it can best treat the infection," says Dr. Monto.

Greater Mobility for Rheumatoid Arthritis Patients

Arava

About 600,000 U.S. men have rheumatoid arthritis, a progressive, debilitating disease that attacks the joints and can shorten the victim's life by as much as 18 years. One widely used drug, methotrexate, suppresses the immune system's attack on the joints, but it can leave the body susceptible to infection.

"Arava alters the way the immune system works without compromising its ability to fight off infections," says Lee S. Simon, M.D., associate professor of medicine at Harvard Medical School. "It's also the first drug that has been clearly shown to inhibit the progression of rheumatoid arthritis." In a study of 482 patients, those taking Arava had gained significantly more mobility after a year than patients taking methotrexate, and their arthritis had progressed at only half the rate. A month's worth of Arava costs $240.

More Effective Glaucoma Treatment

Xalatan

Glaucoma results from an increase in fluid pressure inside your eyeball. Ten million Americans, including some men as young as 20, have this elevated pressure, which can damage the optic nerve and eventually cause blindness.

Unfortunately, some medicated eyedrops that slow glaucoma (such as timolol) can in rare cases cause depression, hair loss, slowed heart rate, or even impotence. A new eyedrop called Xalatan may darken the iris and thicken eyelashes, but it doesn't cause the more troubling side effects. What's more, "Xalatan can be even more effective at reducing fluid pressure inside the eye than other drops," says Andrew Iwach, M.D., professor of ophthalmology at the University of California, San Francisco. A study found that the ocular pressure of 223 glaucoma patients decreased by an additional 8 percent when they switched from timolol to Xalatan, which costs $50 for about a 4-month supply.

"It's critical to catch glaucoma early," says Dr. Iwach. Physicians can't restore any vision already lost to glaucoma. Visit an ophthalmologist annually, and have him check your optic nerves and give you a glaucoma test.

Better Clearing of Stuffy Noses

Steroidal Nasal Sprays

If you suffer from hay fever or allergic rhinitis, try steroidal nasal sprays, not antihistamines, to treat a stuffy nose. David A. Stempel, M.D., an allergist at the Virginia Mason Medical Center in Seattle, evaluated 13 studies on the effectiveness of antihistamines versus nasal steroid sprays, and he found that the sprays were better at clearing nasal congestion. Sprays also cost less. "One problem is that people are never shown how to use the sprays properly," says Dr. Stempel. Here's how: Lean forward, insert the spray bottle into your nose, aim toward your ear, and squirt.

Faster Migraine Relief

Migranal

If you're prone to migraine headaches, you probably know about dihydroergotamine mesylate, or DHE. This drug can alter your serotonin levels to alleviate the pain. But taking DHE has long meant a trip to the doctor's office for an injection. Not anymore. Novartis Pharmaceuticals has developed Migranal, an effective prescription DHE nasal spray. When R. Michael Gallagher, D.O., of the National Headache Foundation, tested Migranal in 310 migraine sufferers, headaches disappeared in half of the subjects within an hour. And when the Denver Broncos' Terrell Davis left a recent Super Bowl with a migraine, a few snorts of Migranal allowed him to return and score two more touchdowns against the Packers. Ask your doctor about a prescription.

Less Invasive Back-Pain Relief

PENS

In a study published in the *Journal of the American Medical Association*, researchers found that a new nonsurgical therapy can reduce back pain by nearly 50 percent. Researchers compared percutaneous electrical nerve stimulation (PENS)—an acupuncture-like procedure using an electric current—with exercise therapy and TENS (electrical nerve stimulation using pads, not needles). Pain levels in 60 patients dropped by 46 percent after PENS, compared with an 11 percent drop after TENS and only a 2 percent drop after exercise therapy. William Craig, M.D., who developed PENS and is clinical assistant professor of anesthesiology and pain management at the University of Texas Southwestern Medical Center at Dallas, says that it works by blocking pain signals to the brain. There are currently 1,500 doctors in the United States who are trained to use PENS; four half-hour treatments over the course of 4 weeks should do the trick.

Stronger Weapon against Prostate Cancer

3-D Conformal Radiation

A prostate cancer treatment called 3-D conformal radiation, which arranges external radiation beams in the shape of the tumor, may soon become physicians' weapon of choice. Researchers at Fox Chase Cancer Center in Philadelphia studied 700 men and found that 88 percent of those treated with high-dose 3-D conformal radiation had been cured 5 years later, compared with 79 percent of those who received standard doses of external-beam radiation. The new procedure also produced lower rates of side effects, such as impotence and incontinence, than traditional procedures.

The new treatment "allows us to use a high dose of radiation while protecting normal tissue better than we were ever able to in the past," according to the lead researcher, Gerald Hanks, M.D., chairman of radiation oncology at Fox Chase Cancer Center. For more details, click on www.sms.siemens.com. (Siemens is one manufacturer of the conformal radiation system.)

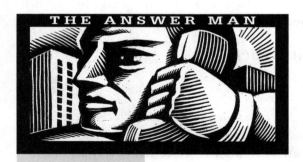

THE ANSWER MAN

Too Much Court Time

My elbow has been hurting like hell lately and I don't know why. I'm wondering if I have tennis elbow, but I don't know what it is or how to get rid of it.
—L. K., New Orleans

"Tennis elbow is the equivalent of a heart attack in your elbow tendon," says Robert Nirschl, M.D., an orthopedic surgeon at the Nirschl Sports Medicine Clinic in Arlington, Virginia. It's normally an overuse problem in which the tendon is mechanically injured, becomes stressed, loses its vitality, and eventually fails. The unhealthy tendon tissue can be painful.

If the pain is coming from the outside of your elbow, it's probably tennis elbow. "The only way to improve the tissue is through rehabilitative resistance exercises," says Dr. Nirschl. That means working the forearm muscle groups that attach to the bone of your elbow.

The following five rehabilitative exercises work these muscles. Do all of them with your arm bent and your elbow at your side. Perform each exercise 5 to 10 times, up to 5 times a day.

1. Wrist extension: Spread your fingers as wide as you can, then close them.
2. Wrist flexion: With your hand palm-down and loosely closed, bend your wrist so that your hand points toward the ceiling, then toward the floor.
3. Radial deviation: With your palm down, bend your wrist so that your hand points to the inside (toward your thumb).
4. Ulnar deviation: With your palm down, bend your wrist so that your hand points to the outside.
5. Rotate your forearm from a pronated position (palm down) to a supinated one (palm up).

Your elbow also needs a rest from abusive activity, including sports. And realize that using drugs for short-term pain reduction isn't going to solve your problem. "People mistakenly equate pain relief with cure," says Dr. Nirschl. "Drugs may give you comfort, but they don't fix the problem."

Oily Problem

I just moved from Denver (dry) to Houston (humid), and now my skin is so oily it's disgusting. What can I do?
—S. N., Houston

"Climate changes like this can have a big impact on your skin condition," says Nancy Silverberg, M.D., assistant clinical professor of dermatology at the University of California, Irvine. Depending on how severe the oiliness is, the solution may be as simple as washing your skin with a gentle soap three or four times a day. If you need it, an over-the-counter product called Seban (available at most drugstores) can also help. This product not only removes oil that's on your skin but also inhibits its return for a few hours.

Fading Vision

I've been wearing contact lenses for years. But now that I'm in my forties, my close vision is starting to go, too. Do I have any options other than old-guy glasses?
—C. L., Athens, Ga.

One option is to buy a pair of no-line bifocals, says Calvin Roberts, M.D., professor of ophthalmology at Cornell University Medical College in New York City. These look like regular glasses but gradually change from long-distance viewing at the top of the lenses to close-up viewing at the bottom. "Because the lenses change gradually, you get better intermediate vision than with traditional bifocals, which don't have a middle range," he says.

If you're determined to stick with contacts, you have two choices. First, you can get a different prescription for each eye—one for distance, one for close up. "This drives some people nuts, but others adjust quickly," says Dr. Roberts. Or, for roughly the same price as regular contacts, you can get bifocal contacts (hard or soft) that work exactly like no-line bifocals. "The technology has improved dramatically in the last few years, and patients can adjust to bifocal contacts within days," he says. In fact, Dr. Roberts says, disposable bifocal contacts should be available soon.

Pop Those Blisters

When I was a kid, my coaches always told me to lance blisters so they'd heal faster. Is that a good idea?
—A. T., Winston-Salem, N.C.

They may not have been able to teach you how to bunt, but your coaches knew blisters, says Douglas Richie Jr., D.P.M., a sports podiatrist in Seal Beach, California. "Studies have found that lancing a blister within the first 3 hours is much more effective than leaving it alone or removing it entirely," he says. In other words, pop it, but don't tear away the top layer of skin.

To lance a blister the right way, clean a needle with rubbing alcohol and make two punctures at opposite ends of the blister's perimeter, Dr. Richie recommends. "A single puncture is likely to clog and prevent all the fluid from draining," he says. Check the blister about 8 hours later to make sure it has drained. If it hasn't, repeat the procedure.

Cold Rush

When I eat ice cream or have a cold, slushy drink, the inside of my head is often paralyzed with pain. How come?
—F. K., Wheeling, W.Va.

You're referring to the phenomenon known as brain freeze or ice-cream headache, which can be as painful as a migraine. But it's harmless and brief. "It's a basic nerve reaction to the sudden introduction of a cold stimulus to the mouth," says Elliot Grossman, M.D., a neurologist in Florham Park, New Jersey.

The quickest way to relieve the pain is to press your tongue to the top of your mouth. The heat from your tongue should do the trick.

A warm drink also helps. To avoid future brain blizzards, take smaller bites or sips and more time between them.

Itchy Feet

I picked up a mean case of athlete's foot at the gym and it won't go away, even though I've tried every drugstore cure there is. Can a doctor offer me something more effective?
—C. D., Annapolis, Md.

Some over-the-counter cures are little more than talcum powder. Talc will keep your feet dry, but it won't control the spread of fungus. A doctor can prescribe an antifungal cream or powder, and in extremely persistent cases a dermatologist can prescribe an oral antifungal medication, such as Lamisil, Mentax, or Spectazole. These prescription medications are worth looking into, says Rebat M. Halder, M.D., a dermatologist at Howard University in Washington, D.C.

You should also check with a dermatologist to make certain you actually have athlete's foot, says Dr. Halder. "Eczema can cause a similar rash on the foot. You don't get that at the gym, and it doesn't respond to antifungals."

To avoid picking up athlete's foot in the first place, dry your feet thoroughly after you shower. Moisture, heat, and humidity allow the fungus to grow.

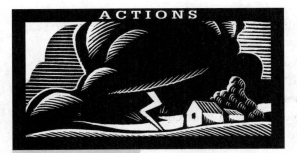

ACTIONS

Every day, men are plagued by serious and not-so-serious ailments. Instead of ignoring them in the hope that they'll go away, it's best to treat them and see a doctor, if necessary. Here are pointers for handling many of the pains that hound us.

1. **Inspect your mattress.** For a quick way to relieve back pain, strip the sheets off your bed and inspect the surface of your mattress, searching for signs of worn fabric. The more you find, the worse your mattress springs are and the greater your risk of back trouble. The Better Sleep Council, based in Alexandria, Virginia, also recommends asking yourself these questions to gauge your mattress's worthiness: Are you sleeping less soundly than you were a year ago? Do you wake up feeling stiff and sore, even after a good night's sleep? If you answer yes to either question, you need a new mattress.

2. **Practice breathing.** Practice breathing? You bet. In an Italian study, heart patients who were given respiratory training were able to cut their respiration rates from 13.4 breaths per minute to 6 breaths per minute. As a result, they increased their resting blood oxygen levels, which in turn enabled them to exercise longer with fewer breathing problems. To improve your own breathing, sit up straight and breathe from your belly. Close your mouth and inhale through your nose to the count of four. Hold your breath for a count of seven, then exhale, forcing out the air for a count of eight. Repeat four times.

3. **Protect your peepers.** If your contact lenses are ever going to irritate your eyes, you can bet it'll be on an adventure trip. That's when most men take hygiene shortcuts and damage their contacts, says Paul Donzis, M.D., an ophthalmologist at the University of California, Los Angeles. Never ignore redness, pain, or light sensitivity in either of your eyes. Other tips:

- Take your specs. Avoid wearing contacts in dusty, rugged locations. A dirty lens can damage your eye and cause an infection.
- Wear sunglasses. They'll protect your contacts from fine dust.
- Use lubricating eyedrops. A few daily droplets of Refresh ($9) can help prevent scratches.
- Carry plenty of saline solution. Never wash your lenses (or carrying case) at a faucet. That's trouble.
- Pack prescription drops. Ask your doctor for antibiotic eyedrops before you leave on a trip. They'll fight infection better than over-the-counter drops.
- Don't sleep with your lenses. Even remove the extended-wear type designed to stay in for a month. Sleeping with your contacts in will increase the chances that they'll irritate your eyes.

4. **Spread around the honey.** The next time you suffer a minor cut and find that you're out of antibiotic ointment, check your kitchen cabinet. A dab of honey on a cut can help prevent infection and speed healing. "Honey starves bacteria so they stop growing. It also serves as a protective barrier against new bacteria," explains Manfred Kroger, Ph.D., professor of food science at Pennsylvania State University in University Park. First wash the area, then smooth on pasteurized honey (the grocery-store variety) and cover with a bandage. Repeat three times a day.

5. **Relieve the itch.** To soothe the agony caused by poison ivy, make a paste of baking soda and water and carefully dab it on the rash. Don't rub the area, or you'll irritate it even more, says Rosemarie Young, M.D., an allergist.

6. **Ease sunburn's heat.** Fill a sock with uncooked oatmeal (not the instant kind), tie the end shut, and drop it into your bath. The oat protein will help repair your damaged skin.

7. **Switch toothpaste to end chapped lips.** Some toothpastes can dry out your lips. Tartar-control products are the most common irritants to your lips. Switching to a baking soda formula can solve the problem, says John E. Wolf, M.D., chairman of the department of dermatology at Baylor College of Medicine in Houston.

8. **Trick your brain.** For itchy skin under a cast, try scratching the same place on the other arm or foot, says James Dolezal, M.D., a dermatologist. Your brain may think you're scratching the real itch.

9. **Take an antacid for your hives.** If you have a case of hives that laughs at most antihistamines, take this tip. Heartburn medication may relieve a stubborn case of hives, says Stanley Goldstein, M.D., governor of the northeast region of the American Academy of Allergy, Asthma, and Immunology. Try a regular antihistamine first. But if the hives don't disappear after a day or two, Dr. Goldstein says, "take your regular medication again and combine it with an H2-blocker, such as Zantac 75 or Pepcid AC." See your doctor if the hives don't go away within 6 weeks.

10. **Eat a cherry.** Cherries may fight pain better than a regular dose of aspirin does, according to research published by the American Chemical Society. Muraleedharan G. Nair, Ph.D., a researcher at Michigan State University in East Lansing, found that the chemical that gives tart red cherries their color contains large concentrations of an antioxidant called anthocyanin, which has pain-relieving effects. "It could be just as good as aspirin or ibuprofen," says Dr. Nair. He believes that eating 20 cherries a day has the potential to reduce muscle pain; it may even slow the development of arthritis and gout.

11. **Opt for the older types.** Older antibiotics treat sinus infections just as effectively as newer antibiotics, according to a review done by researchers at New England Medical Center in Boston that examined 27 studies of 2,717 people with acute bacterial sinusitis. Older medications, such as amoxicillin, cost only $10 to $15 for a 10-day supply, but cefixime, a newer drug, can cost as much as $100. "Doctors are influenced by sales reps who push newer drugs and by patients who think bacteria are resistant to the older antibiotics," says Joseph Lau, M.D., the lead researcher. If you think you have acute sinusitis—symptoms include congestion, runny nose, and pain or pressure around the face—see your doctor to find out if treatment with one of the older antibiotics is right for you.

12. **Munch on magnesium.** In a study of 60 people with hypertension, researchers at the National Cardiovascular Center in Osaka, Japan, found that a daily magnesium supplement can lower blood pressure. The subjects took 480 milligrams of magnesium every day for 8 weeks. At the end of that period, their average systolic pressures (the top number) had dropped by 5.3 millimeters of mercury (mmHg), and their diastolic pressures had dropped by 2.7 mmHg. "We observed a significant decrease in blood pressure that supports the value of magnesium in the treatment of hypertension," says Yuhei Kawano, M.D., the lead author of the study. Green vegetables, baked potatoes, bananas, tuna, salmon, and whole-wheat bread are all good sources of magnesium.

13. **Heal a blister with milk.** A milk compress can relieve the pain of a blister. Simply saturate a washcloth with cool milk and apply it to the blister for 15 minutes, repeating as often as needed. "Applying a cool milk compress to a blister within the first 24 hours reduces the inflammation that causes pain," says Kathy Fields, M.D., clinical instructor of dermatology at the University of California, San Francisco. "Plus, the protein in milk may promote healing."

14. **Save your schnozz.** In addition to holding up your specs, your nose is a bodyguard for your face—it has first dibs on hostile elbows, fists, and doors. Here are three tips for nursing a smashed proboscis.

- If your nose is bleeding, lean forward. "Leaning back can cause you to choke on your blood," says Daniel G. Becker, M.D., director of facial plastic and reconstruction surgery for the University of Pennsylvania Health System in Philadelphia. Lean forward and pinch your nostrils closed. The bleeding should stop within 5 minutes.
- Test for a fracture. If the tip sounds squishy when you press it, it's broken, says Larry A. Bedard, M.D., former president of the American College of Emergency Physicians. See a doctor within 5 days. The doc will reset it or have you ice it for a week.
- Check your breathing. If the tenderness subsides within 3 days, you're probably okay. But a nasty shot can damage your septum, the partition of bone

and cartilage between your nostrils. If it's hard to breathe, see a doctor fast—a damaged septum can cause your schnozz to sink, resulting in a Joe Palooka look. The doctor will reset it.

15. **Have a ball.** To relieve troublesome neck pain, place two tennis balls in the toes of a sock and knot the sock so that they don't move. Then lie down with your neck between the balls. The pressure should help the muscles in your neck relax.

16. **Beat wrist pain while you sleep.** Men who snooze in fetal positions with their hands under their heads, or on their stomachs with their arms curled under their chests, seem to be at a greater risk of nighttime pain from carpal tunnel syndrome.

"These positions narrow the space through which the nerve passes. That's what wakes you up in the middle of the night with a tingling and dead feeling in your fingers," says Terry Whipple, M.D., clinical associate professor of orthopedics and rehabilitation at the University of Virginia School of Medicine in Charlottesville and an orthopedic surgeon with Tuckahoe Orthopaedic Associates in Richmond, Virginia.

To avoid the pain, try training yourself to sleep on your back, with your hands at your sides.

17. **Stop slurping to end burping.** Drinking hot or cold liquids too fast or through a straw causes you to swallow air. Instead, drink slowly and lose the straw, says Malcolm Robinson, M.D., founder and director of the Oklahoma Foundation for Digestive Research and clinical professor of medicine at the University of Oklahoma College of Medicine in Oklahoma City.

18. **Ask for the real thing.** Defizzed Coke works so well for nausea that there's an over-the-counter product called Emetrol that's made of essentially the same thing. You can make your own by simply opening a Coke and stirring it for a few minutes until it's flat.

19. **Rinse away bad breath.** If you discover that you've been afflicted with a malodorous mouth moments before an important meeting with the boss, swish some water vigorously and then spit it out, to wash away food and crank up your saliva production. Even simply drinking water will help to keep smelly bacteria on the move, says Cherilyn G. Sheets, D.D.S., of the Academy of General Dentistry and a dentist in Newport Beach, California.

20. **Know how to treat a heart attack.** The pain comes from nowhere, hits you smack in the chest, and maybe even spreads to your neck, shoulders, or arms.

Or maybe you can't catch your breath, your skin feels clammy, and you're on the verge of either throwing up or passing out. Don't ignore these signs, tough guy. You could be having a heart attack.

What should you do about it? Seek medical attention right away. The sooner doctors bust up the clot that's stifling the flow of blood through your oxygen-starved heart, the less likely it is you'll sustain any permanent damage. Call for an ambulance right away or, if it's faster, have someone take you to a hospital. In the meantime, here are some ways you can help yourself.

- Stay away from aspirin if you're allergic to it or if you have a history of ulcers.
- Cough if you feel faint. Severe light-headedness is a sign your brain isn't getting enough blood and oxygen. If you think you're about to pass out, start coughing as hard as you can—one cough every second—and don't stop until help arrives. This delivers a CPR-like push to the chest, says Richard O'Brien, M.D., a spokesman for the American College of Emergency Physicians.
- The coupling of the erection booster sildenafil (Viagra) with nitroglycerin or any other nitrate-containing heart drug can produce a deadly drop in blood pressure. Come clean with the paramedics and the hospital staff if you're taking Viagra or any other drug. Better yet, keep a list of your medications in your wallet.
- Emergency physicians can pull you through any immediate crisis, but once they finish their job, insist that a cardiologist oversee your care the rest of the way. Studies suggest that patients fare best under their care.

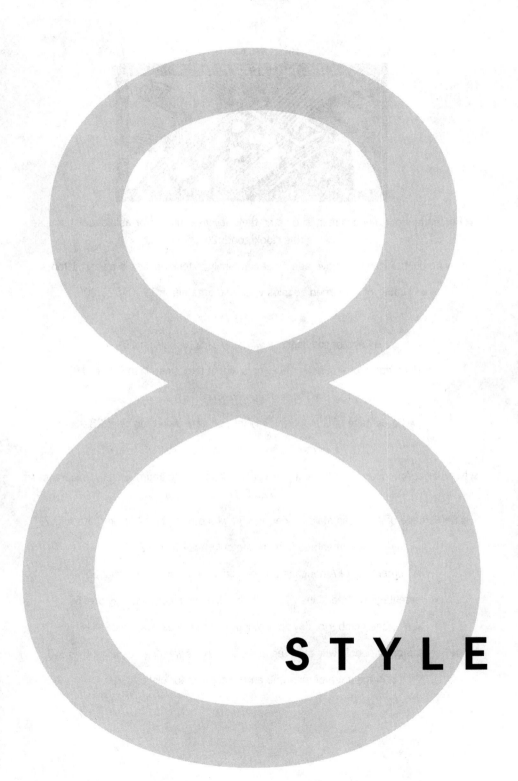

STYLE

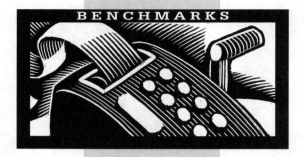

■ Percentage of American men who admit that they wear uncomfortable shoes because they look good: 20

■ Amount of laundry an average American family of four washes in a year: 1 ton

■ Number of unmarried couples who lived together in 1970: 523,000

■ In 1997: 4.1 million

■ Pairs of sunglasses owned by Jack Nicholson: 15

■ Percentage of American men who say that they sleep in the nude: 19

■ Percentage of women: 6

■ Percentage of liberals who say they've gone skinny-dipping: 28

■ Percentage of conservatives: 15

■ Number of Americans who have surgery each year solely to improve their appearances: 720,000

■ Percentage of American males under age 50 who own a pair of Dockers Khakis: 72

■ Percentage of men who color their hair: 12

■ Percentage of Americans who consider themselves romantic: 65

■ Percentage of Americans who think they look younger than they are: 57

■ Average number of days per month that men wear fragrance: 21

■ Percentage of people who show up at job interviews wearing casual clothes: 40

■ Percentage of men who enjoy shopping for clothes: 29

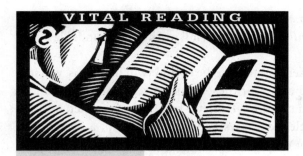

Back to Basics

These 10 fundamentals will spruce up your wardrobe.

To understand anything, you must first grasp the basics. This is especially true of complicated things, such as higher math, boccie, and assembling a wardrobe. Following are the 10 must-have, absolute, fundamental items that every man should keep on hand (and on the rest of his body).

1. Navy blue sport coat. Choose a medium-weight worsted wool coat, which you can wear all year. Keep it simple: no fancy cuts, no double-breasted or four-button styles. Select a classic two-button jacket and, to avoid looking like a yachting yahoo, skip the brass buttons in favor of something that matches the jacket.

2. White shirt. Your white dress shirts should be 100 percent cotton. They shouldn't, however, have button-down collars. Shirts with regular straight or spread collars are more versatile. "I'd feel very comfortable wearing a non-button-down with jeans, but I'd feel uncomfortable wearing a button-down with a double-breasted suit," says Djordje Stefanovic, fashion director for Ermenegildo Zegna. For a fresh look with a suit, try basket-weave fabric and French cuffs.

3. Turtleneck or mock turtleneck. The best yarns for keeping warm are extra-fine merino wool and cashmere. Choose solids; they combine with a wider range of top layers.

4. V-neck sweater. Choose a sweater with ribbed cuffs, collar, and bottom. "Make sure it's large enough to go over a collared shirt comfortably, but small enough to look great over a T-shirt," says Patty McGrath of Pendleton. You'll need a wool one for cool weather and a cotton one for warm.

5. Dark gray suit. Two- or three-button, single-breasted suits look good on nearly every body type, and they look equally fine with a shirt and tie or a

turtleneck. If Cary Grant could outrun an airplane in this kind of suit and look good (*North by Northwest*), odds are, it'll work for you under less perilous conditions.

6. Gray worsted wool trousers. Similar to the cotton twill in chinos, worsted wool is lightweight. You can wear these trousers year-round and on almost any occasion. "You can dress them up by wearing a jacket, or dress them down with a turtleneck," says Salvatore Cesarani, a designer of men's apparel from New York City.

7. Khaki chinos. Khaki-colored chinos are virtually seasonless, and they wear and travel well. Go with 100-percent cotton twill: It breathes in the heat and keeps you warm in the cold.

8. Brown loafers. "Keep them simple," says Jody Gietl, vice president of product management and merchandising at Bally. "The less ornamentation (such as tassels and buckles), the wider the variety of clothes you'll be able to wear them with." Why brown? It's more versatile than maroon.

9. Black lace-up shoes. Black matches most suits (except brown ones), and you can't go wrong with the lace-up look. "Buy a quality pair, and they could literally last you a decade," says Warren Christopher, *Men's Health* magazine's style editor. The shoes should be 100 percent leather, including soles and heels; leather breathes and molds to your foot. The upper should be sewn directly to the sole—no glue.

10. All-weather coat. This type of topper is appropriate over anything from suits to jeans. A zip-out lining makes it a four-season investment. A longer cut (more than 48 inches) may not be trendy, but it's always stylish—and it protects your clothes while keeping you warm. Look for diagonal-seamed (raglan) shoulders, which are sleeker and fit everyone well. Choose a dark or neutral color.

Be Invited Back

Follow these simple etiquette rules to shine by.

When the teacher busted us for our darkest classroom crimes, she would recite a special fifth-grade edition of the Miranda rights, ending with the knee-buckler: "This goes on your permanent record, mister." We'd quake in our Keds until a slightly older delinquent reassured us, "There's no such thing as a permanent record."

Ah, but that seventh-grader was wrong. There is indeed such a thing as a permanent record. It's made up of all the praise and scorn people utter after we've departed as guests from their presence. When we walk out the door, what people say about us becomes the permanent record of our life in this world.

So how can you ensure that your record includes terms such as "charming" and "delightful" rather than "clod" and "reminds me of Pauly Shore"? The key is to understand that each guest situation is unique and that you must employ different strategies and skills to master each one.

To help you understand just what these strategies and skills are, we asked etiquette professionals, psychologists, and veteran partyers what makes a charming guest. From the right attire to the right way to suck up to your host, here's how to be a gracious and graceful guy in these situations.

Your Neighbor's Dinner Party on Saturday Night

What to wear: The safest strategy is to call the host and ask what's appropriate. If you can't do that, err on the side of formality—in this case a blazer, a tie, and slacks. "If the affair is casual and you're overdressed, it's okay to remove your tie when you get there," says Hilka Klinkenberg, managing director of Etiquette International, a New York City–based organization that helps people polish their social skills.

What to bring: A wrapped bottle of chardonnay or merlot still defines graciousness. "But it should be something a little special," says Klinkenberg. In other words, hold the bottle of Thunderbird. And make it clear that the wine is a gift for the host, not your personal stash for the evening. "Say something like, 'Here's something for your wine collection,'" advises Klinkenberg.

The challenge: Small dinner parties test your ability to hold extended conversations, so come prepared with things to talk about. "My best advice is just to interview people," says Sally Quinn, a Washington, D.C., journalist and author of *The Party*, a book on socializing. "Ask people questions about what they like to do, where they've traveled, what they're reading."

How to endear yourself to your host: "Be the person who breaks the ice with other guests," advises Lillian Brown, a professional image consultant in Washington, D.C. "Draw the shy guest out, and get her involved. If you can do that, you'll always be invited back." (Just be careful with that shy blonde in the tube top.)

Your exit strategy: Once coffee is served, stay 30 to 60 more minutes.

How to say thank you: "There's no substitute for a handwritten thank-you note," says Dorothea Johnson, of the private Protocol School of Washington, D.C., which trains etiquette consultants to industry and government. It doesn't have to be elaborate. "Thanks for your hospitality" is enough. Write it within 24 hours.

An Acquaintance's Annual Holiday Bash

What to wear: The trick at a large cocktail party is to look nice without looking like every other guy in the room. (At some parties, you'll see enough blue blazers and gray slacks to outfit a pep band.) To stand out in a good way, try a slight variation on the classics, such as a blazer with a subtle pattern, suggests Salvatore Cesarani, a designer of men's apparel from New York City.

What to bring: No wine this time. If it's a big party, your hosts will end up with 50 bottles. Try another kind of gift. "A book is fitting; it shows you respect the person's intelligence," says Johnson.

The challenge: You'll have to hold short conversations with lots of different people, many of whom you may have just met. So brush up on your introduction skills. Graciously interrupt the conversation you're having, using the name of the person you're talking to. ("Excuse me, Bill.") Introduce the newcomer by first and last name, and add some personal details. ("This is Mark Smith. He's an accountant.") Then do the same for the person you were talking with. ("Mark, this is Dr. Bill Wilson. He's a cardiologist.")

Close your conversations when they've run their course. "Use a phrase like, 'I've enjoyed talking with you,' then move on," says Klinkenberg.

How to endear yourself to your host: Since your hosts may be too busy to do it themselves, ask whether there are any guests you can introduce to each other, suggests Brown. And don't be shy about introducing yourself to strangers.

Your exit strategy: No need to turn it into a Broadway musical; just say thanks for a wonderful time and head for the door. If you'll be leaving early, inform the host at the beginning with an apology. That way, no one will worry that you didn't enjoy yourself.

How to say thank you: Send a note, then reciprocate. If the Kowalskis have had you at their Christmas party for the past 3 years but you've never invited them, don't expect an invitation next year.

Your First Trip to Your In-Laws' House

What to wear: Anything but your Marilyn Manson T-shirt.

What to bring: A houseplant.

The challenge: To win the family's acceptance without looking like an overbearing suck up. To accomplish this, avoid seeking lifelong approval in one visit, advises Robert Pasick, Ph.D., a clinical psychologist in Ann Arbor, Michigan, and author of *Men in Therapy*. "Don't go into this kind of situation and try to be the center of attention," he says. "The family has its own dynamic. It has to find a role for you within that dynamic."

Ask questions about the photos, trophies, and other bric-a-brac on display in the house. And don't forget to make frequent eye contact with the family member who brought you. "Your mate is the one who's really on the spot," says Dr. Pasick. "She's the only bridge between two elements."

How to endear yourself to your host: Subtly float the idea that you're a trustworthy, upright guy. (Don't worry, you're allowed to fake it.) This is not the time to mention that you maxed out your credit cards making an independent film about body lice.

Your exit strategy: When your mate says go, go.

How to say thank you: Do the dishes.

A Business Dinner at a Fancy Downtown Restaurant

What to wear: The suit you wore to work is fine, but you'll look better if you put on a fresh shirt and tie.

What to bring: Leave the briefcase at the office, and stick with a pocket notebook or a slim portfolio. "The more formal the setting, the fewer flip charts you can haul out," says Elizabeth Craig, a business consultant and author of *Don't Slurp Your Soup: A Basic Guide to Business Etiquette.*

The challenge: You'll have to mix business with pleasure. "When you're invited to a relatively small business gathering, you're expected to bring useful ideas regarding the business and to contribute to the social atmosphere," says David Sandford, a business manager with the wireless communications firm Nortel. "If you don't have the business part covered, you probably won't feel relaxed enough to show your people skills." So read over the relevant materials beforehand and commit important statistics to memory.

As for the social part of the evening, Craig suggests keeping away from potentially sensitive topics (family, politics, religion). Focus instead on current bestsellers, news events, or sports.

How to endear yourself to your host: Say "please" and "thank you" to the waiters and waitresses. "If your dinner companions are wondering how you'd get along with lower-level staff members at their company, they'll pay attention to how you behave toward the restaurant staff," says Craig.

Your exit strategy: Your host should indicate when the evening is winding down.

How to say thank you: Send handwritten notes. "If the meeting included six people from your company and six people from their company, you can be strategic about who receives the thank-you notes," says Craig. Start with the host.

Your Kid's Dorm Room

What to wear: "Anything except what you think is really cool," says Dr. Pasick. Trust us, it probably isn't.

What to bring: Something that your son or daughter can eat after you've left.

The challenge: To accept your role as guest and recognize who has invited whom. "It's especially hard to grasp this reversal of roles if you're the one paying the tuition to the college bursar," says Dr. Pasick. You can instantly destroy the dynamic of this new situation by offering parental pointers. "Make sure you don't give any unwanted advice," he says. Such as? "Well, any advice."

Dr. Pasick also warns fathers to be ready for the appearance of a love interest on the scene, including evidence of cohabitation. This is to be greeted with pleasant, nonjudgmental patter. No whiff of disapproval—this isn't the time for it—and absolutely no nods or winks.

How to endear yourself to your host: If you're taking your kid out for a meal, offer to treat one or two of his friends as well. And slip him a couple of twenties before you head home.

Your exit strategy: Stay shorter rather than longer. "Don't hang out on a college campus," says Dr. Pasick.

How to say thank you: Treat it like a visit to a friend's house. Call afterward and say something like, "Thanks for the invitation; it was great to see where you live and meet your friends."

A Friend's Beach House for the Weekend

What to wear: Your nicest casual stuff—good shorts, sport shirts, khakis or jeans. And since you probably won't have a private bath, do everyone a favor and pack a decent bathrobe.

What to bring: Be aggressive and specific. Call your hosts and tell them you want to provide Sunday-morning bagels and muffins from a great bakery you know. Or name an hors d'oeuvre you can make. (Cheese curls don't count.)

The challenge: If you're spending the weekend, your charm has to have staying power. Follow these three rules.

1. Be a team player. Go along with whatever your hosts have planned—even if that antique-figurine show doesn't quite rival NASCAR in excitement, says Klinkenberg.
2. Don't expect your hosts to entertain you the entire time you're visiting. If they're pooped, busy, or sleeping late, go out and do something by yourself.
3. Show off your talents. "If someone invites you to his house for the weekend and you play the guitar, for heaven's sake bring it," says Ann LaGravenese,

who with her husband, Richard, frequently entertains on weekends. "If you're not going to play it then, when are you?"

How to endear yourself to your host: Wait on your hosts while they're waiting on you. LaGravenese's favorite guest is "the one who comes into the kitchen and offers to make the cook a cocktail."

Your exit strategy: When you're invited, find out how long your hosts are expecting you to stay. Say, "I'd like to make travel plans. What time would it be convenient for me to leave?"

How to say thank you: Send a note and a small gift. Peruse their CD collection, then give them something they don't have but would probably like.

An Excursion on Your Buddy's New Boat

What to wear: Footwear with white rubber soles. Black-soled shoes mark up the decks, says Rob Johnson, a Connecticut-based sailor and boat owner who has crewed on racing yachts since childhood.

What to bring: Warm layers and waterproof or water-resistant outerwear, all packed in a soft duffel bag. "There's no good place to stow a suitcase," says Johnson. Don't even think about bringing an umbrella—it's bad luck on a boat.

The challenge: To be as charming and helpful as possible, without vomiting. If you don't know anything about sailing, admit it. Then be ready for specific instructions about where to stand or sit and whose way to get out of. You can't become a seaman in one day, but listening and asking questions are expected.

Limit your time below: The air is stale, and the sense of instability is more intense. Also, take note if you yawn—it's a warning sign of nausea when you're at sea. If you do feel queasy, Johnson suggests, eat Triscuits and drink Coca-Cola.

How to endear yourself to your host: Help clean up the boat once you've docked. Chores include removing all trash, furling and covering (or stowing) the sails, and washing your vomit off the decks.

How to say thank you: Send a note, then reciprocate. (You don't have to buy a boat. Just ask your yachtsman friend over for cocktails. Make him drink a lot so he can vomit, too.)

Your Cousin Gino's Wedding

What to wear: All men should consider purchasing a tuxedo, says Dorothea Johnson. It will pay for itself if you're already renting one once a year. If the invitation says "formal," out comes your tux.

If the invitation reads "informal," wear a dark suit and a suitable tie instead.

"Then there are dress instructions like 'dressy casual,' which are very hard to interpret," she says. When in doubt, ask your host.

What to bring: A securely wrapped gift, with the card taped in place or tucked into the gift box. "For your own convenience, send your gift in advance if the wedding requires you to travel by air," recommends Johnson.

The challenge: "At events such as banquets and large weddings, you're not much more than a spectator," says Brown. But the fact that it would take extreme misbehavior to create embarrassment doesn't mean that you can't pull it off. Spill a glass of burgundy on a white tablecloth, or shout "You the man!" after the best man's touching toast, and you've fed the grapevine a big helping of gossip.

How to endear yourself to your host: "Do the few things that are expected. Compliment the bride, admire the decorations, and applaud at the right times," says Dorothea Johnson.

Tieless Tactics

Look sharp in today's casual world.

For as long as almost any man alive can remember, if you wanted to be taken seriously, you had to wear a tie. Then one day the rules changed, and a tie was no longer required for respect. When and why they changed are irrelevant. You need to know what to do about it.

Know before you go. Some occasions still demand a tie: funerals, weddings, appointments in traffic court. Elsewhere, common sense will usually provide an answer. For examples of lapses in common sense, check out the actors who show up at the Academy Awards in "alternative" tuxedos and neckwear.

If you're uncertain, wear a tie. If anybody asks if you forgot your tie, you've guessed wrong.

Wear the right T. Don't attempt to wear a basic white undershirt alone with a suit or sport coat. Some T-shirts are dressy enough to wear solo with a suit. The white ones that come in three-packs are not. Your rule: "If you want to wear a stand-alone T-shirt under a jacket, buy one with a ribbed knit," says Richard Bowes, fashion director of Bergdorf Goodman. Neutral or dark colors work under most jackets. Avoid pastels and bright colors. If you want to try this look, wear a sport coat and slacks or a dark suit—no double-breasted jackets.

No "replacement" ties. Ascots, bolo ties, and the like will make people think you're a character, as in, "Oh, he's a character." The world has never known a more backhanded compliment.

Buy strategically. "When you buy a suit or sport coat, you should purchase a few things that work with it," says Leon Hall, cohost of the E! Channel's *Fashion Emergency.* "First on the list are a white shirt and a perfect tie. Pick another shirt that has a bold color, an interesting stripe, or a tattersall check." A solid shirt that's darker than your suit can also work.

"A dark blue, dark brown, or black shirt looks great under a suit," says Bowes. "In the summer, a linen shirt under a suit also works well." Consider buying a black sport coat made of tropical-weight wool—it's comfortable in warm temperatures, and you can wear it with everything. Another option: a sport coat in a subtle plaid or neutral pattern, such as houndstooth.

Be a polo player. In the spring and summer, try a polo shirt made of silk, linen, cotton, rayon, or some blend thereof. A classic cotton piqué polo shirt is fine with a sport coat and khakis or linen pants after a round of golf. (Piqué has a raised, wafflelike appearance.) But at the office, piqué will look too casual, so wear a finer-grade cotton polo, such as one made from pima or Sea Island cotton (check the label). Richly colored polos in shades such as burgundy and deep purple complement navy, gray, and black suits. "Choose one with a collar that lies nicely, and never pull the collar of your polo shirt over your jacket lapels," says Hall.

Avoid mixing fabrics from different seasons. Summer polos aren't meant to be worn with winter-weight tweed blazers and heavy woolen trousers. But it's fine to pair them with linen or silk.

Add distractions. "A solid-color crew- or V-neck sweater over a white or black T-shirt looks great under a patterned sport coat," says Ron Chereskin, a New York sportswear designer. Even if you wear the crew, a little bit of the T-shirt will probably peek out, which is fine. Wear a silk or cotton sweater under a lightweight jacket during the warmer months, and switch to a lightweight wool or cashmere sweater in the fall.

See this in September. Come fall, wear lightweight wool or silk knit turtlenecks, or mock turtles in neutral shades, such as tan, gray, and black. Avoid a superbulky turtleneck under a jacket, though. And don't wear the cotton turtles you picked up at the end-of-winter sales. They're best worn under sweaters.

Keep trousers simple. For an uncomplicated look, pair a sport coat with pants in neutral colors, such as khaki and black. Never try to pass off your navy suit pants with a different jacket—nobody will be fooled.

Before you step out, do a shoe review. The black lace-ups you'd wear with a conservative suit and tie may be too dressy. So try a monk-strap (a shoe with a cross-over strap, not laces) or a more casual lace-up with a slightly square toe. When wearing khakis, a polo shirt, and a sport coat, you can go with lug-soled oxfords or boots.

Going Up?

Overcome these career obstacles and move on up.

Here's a list of the people who will be impressed when you're promoted: your banker (who becomes your "financial advisor" after the big raise); your mom (she needs bragging ammo for Ladies' Auxiliary meetings); your wife (she says, "cha-ching!" and rips your pants off); if you have one, your mother-in-law ("I always said you'd do well"); and your buddies ("Woo-hoo! Yeah, baby! More cabbage, more time off, more golf vacations!"). Damn, you're loving this promotion thing, aren't you? The only hang-up is that no one will be impressed until you actually receive the promotion.

"Although it varies from company to company, most young employees on the corporate fast track can expect to receive a promotion roughly every 2 years," says Michael Mercer, Ph.D., industrial psychologist and author of *How Winners Do It: High-Impact People Skills for Your Career Success.* Any significant delays in this timetable (you're 41 and you know how to fix the copier when it jams) suggest that you're getting in your own way.

With the help of workplace experts, we've identified the most common ways up-and-comers sabotage themselves before they reach the corner office.

1. You dress like Fred Sanford or Jerry Garcia. If you're one of those guys who think they should be judged only on performance, get a grip. No boss in his right mind will promote someone who dresses like a pizza delivery boy, says Neal Lenarsky, president of Strategic Transitions, an executive-coaching and career-management agency in Los Angeles. "You have to dress the part," he says. "Take cues from your boss and the people one level above you in deciding how to dress. You don't have to match them exactly, but at least be somewhat compatible."

   This usually means dressing up a notch or two, but you should also take the cue if your supervisors dress casually. "Being overdressed can be just as damaging as being underdressed," warns Lenarsky.

2. You're developing a taste for shoe polish. Nobody likes a bootlicking toady, which means it's hard to be good at sucking up. "You can flatter your boss, but do it sparingly," says Alan R. Schonberg, author of *169 Ways to Score Points with Your Boss* and chairman of Management Recruiters International, an executive-search firm based in Cleveland. "Give compliments too often, and you'll come across as a phony."

   Another thing to beware of is kissing up at the wrong time and place. Excessively praising your boss in front of a large group of coworkers will permanently brand you a brownnoser, says Lenarsky. Be subtle. It doesn't hurt to pay a compliment when the boss is being recognized for a major accomplishment, he says, but deliver your praise in private, not via loudspeaker to everyone within earshot.

3. Your delivery system is stuck in the silo. Here's the very short screen-play version of this problem: You have a great idea. You tell your boss. The end. The point is that you can't just deliver a great idea to your boss and expect it to translate automatically into favorable talk about you throughout the company. For starters, Dr. Mercer says, your boss may steal the credit. "Even if he doesn't, you need to impress other executives besides your boss if you want to move up in rank." Then again, sending a memo directly to your company's big dogs will make you seem like a bootlicker (see above) and piss off your boss. So here's Dr. Mercer's strategy: "Tell your boss about the idea, and then follow up with copies of the idea to other people who would logically be involved with it, such as technical support or the manager of the department you'd be working with." Because your name is attached to the memo, it'll be obvious that the idea is yours.

4. You're invisible, man. You've heard countless times that you need to be "your own P.R. agent," but what does this mean? Well, it doesn't mean bragging about yourself at every opportunity. "Before long, you'll make so many enemies that you'll have to leave the company," says Lenarsky.

   The key is to be visible within the organization but, once again, in a subtle way. If you're working on a big project, offer to give a presentation on it, or conduct a meeting where you brief the top brass on how it's going, Dr. Mercer suggests.

   Cultivating a mentor a few levels above you is also a great way to raise your visibility, says Lenarsky. How do you find one? Look for someone successful and likable, and simply ask him to help you. You'll be amazed at how willing people will be to help when you tell them you think you could learn a lot from them. When you've led or participated in a successful project, take your mentor out for dinner or a drink to celebrate. He'll find out about your latest accomplishments, and that's a direct plug-in to the grapevine.

5. The only game you play is Duke Nukem. We're not talking about Machiavellian political maneuvers, but some game-playing is necessary to rise through the ranks, our experts agree. "The rules of any game vary from organization to organization," says Lenarsky. "But an easy way to learn the rules that apply in your company is to emulate the behavior of people who were recently promoted." The key may be coming up with radical ideas,

working 19-hour days, or putting a double coat of wax on every V.P.'s Lexus. It doesn't matter: What worked before is likely to work again, Lenarsky says.

Another important part of game-playing is taking part in the activities that are important symbolically, even if they don't actually amount to any substance. Take company mission statements, for example. Although they're filled with phrases like "delivering unrivaled customer service and the best frankfurter west of the Pecos," they typically have as much effect on the company's operating procedure as e-mails to the President's dog have on U.S. foreign policy. Nonetheless, if you have the opportunity to help with drafting or redrafting your company's mission statement, jump at it, says Schonberg. It keeps you in tune with the priorities of your supervisors and gives you a chance to become acquainted with some of your company's top executives.

6. You report to Satan, Prince of Darkness and V.P. of Marketing. Sometimes the reason you can't get a promotion is simple: Your boss is a jerk. "There are bosses out there who operate on the principle, 'I don't give promotions,'" says Lenarsky. The worst tactic you can follow with a boss like this is to confront him or argue with him in front of others, Lenarsky says. "It'll just make him more determined to squelch your career." Bringing up your concerns in private and being a model employee may improve the environment, but there's no guarantee this will work either.

Ideally, you would catch these traits in a prospective boss at the interview stage and simply decline the job. Of course, "ideally" rarely happens. "But if you've been in a job for 2 years and the attitude of your boss has become a factor, you have to ask yourself whether that's really where you want to be," says Lenarsky. If you can't stand your boss, try to transfer within the company, he suggests. And if the company seems to encourage this kind of behavior in managers, take your services elsewhere.

7. You work for a company that sells eight-track tapes. If you're in the wrong industry, your chances of swiftly ascending to the big payoff are weak. There's not enough money and energy going around to boost anyone's career. So look toward technology- and computer-related companies, telecommunications, consumer products, entertainment, and the cable industry, which are growing so quickly that executive positions are plentiful. This isn't to say you should drop your current job to pursue a career selling bagels over the World Wide Web. But by changing companies or transferring to a department that is growing, you'll improve your odds of promotion, Lenarsky says.

8. You've never actually popped the question. Hard work and inner beauty may conceivably win you praise from loved ones and certain talk-show hosts, but our experts emphasize that this isn't enough to win over the big guy. You have to ask for the promotion. "If you don't, it's possible your boss may think you don't want the extra responsibility, or he may not even consider you in that light at all," Lenarsky explains.

Timing is everything when it comes to this request, Lenarsky says. You'll want to make sure that you're not asking too soon. "Find out what the practice is in your company. It may be that you're expecting the new title 18 months too early, which makes you look bad." If you've established that you're not rushing things, you'll want to ask fairly soon after completing a successful project. "Of course, you have to have a track record of accomplishments," he says. "But after a major achievement, your value to the company has ratcheted up."

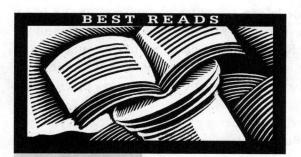

BEST READS

Clothes You Could Wear for the Rest of Your Life

One great thing about a man's wardrobe is that it doesn't have to be extensive to be complete. This excerpt from Beyond Soap, Water, and Comb: A Man's Guide to Good Grooming and Fitness *(Abbeville Press, 1998) by Ed Marquand shows how to assemble a great-looking wardrobe without dipping into your 401(k).*

Women, in general, build a fashion whole from many pieces. If you have the money, time, and talent, you can become a full-fledged clotheshorse, and for some men in some professions, it's even expected. But most of us aren't, and that's what makes dressing so simple for men. We can look great with a few standard items of good quality that fit well and are flattering. With a few accessories—ties being the most common—we can spruce up those basic items with a little more polish. Or not. That's the beauty: Men can get away with a basic, practical, and handsome set of uniforms and look great! So take advantage of this.

Ralph Lauren proved in his ads that you can look terrific in a blazer, a blue cotton work shirt, and a pair of worn jeans. To be fair, though, Ralph is rarely in an office setting in those photos, so you will probably need a few more items. But not many. Make sure you have the basics covered first.

Studies have consistently shown that women are more attuned than men to clothes their peers are wearing; take a lesson from them, and notice the clothes of friends, men you work with, or guys you pass on the street. Observe general "looks"—combinations of jackets, shirts, ties, slacks, and shoes. Notice what good-looking men of comparable builds, age, coloring, and profession wear well. Chances are, they are wearing some classic basics. Recreational and underclothes aside, you could make a short list of clothes that would serve you well to your grave. They would probably need to be replaced occasionally, but let's see just how simple it can be.

The blazer: Nothing is more versatile and good-looking than a well-cut, well-made navy blue wool blazer. Unless you live in the tropics, you'll need one in felt wool for winter and one in serge wool for the summer. Try on many from different stores before buying one; you will know when you've found the right one for you by the way it fits and looks. A blazer is more versatile without the gold buttons; if the blazer of your dreams has them, have the buttons replaced with dark ones, or go live on a boat. Single vents are most practical and versatile.

The sport jacket: Sport jackets come in many colors, types of cloths, and cuts. Buy a navy blazer first, but if you want more variety, a nice wool, silk and wool, or linen sport jacket is a good investment. If you like a pattern, make it subtle. As for cut, make it classic single vent with medium-width lapels if you plan to keep it for more than 5 years.

The suit: In many offices, the look is strictly casual all week, not just on Fridays. But even if you are fresh out of college, you need a suit. If you have only one, make it a good, conservative but comfortably cut model, in a medium-weight wool. Gray is the most versatile, but navy is a good second choice. (You can wear the gray slacks with your navy blazer, too, but navy slacks with the navy blazer is a mistake.) If you work in an office that expects more formal attire, you should add more suits in a variety of styles—but start with the gray.

How many suits do you need? Unless you are flat broke, buy enough suits to allow you to rotate them. Clothes last much longer if you give them at least a day or two to air out and dry, and of course, to go to the cleaners.

Slacks, chinos, and jeans: Again, you can't beat the classics. Gray flannel in two seasonal weights will serve you well. Since you wear your pants all day, and probably take your jacket off for most of it, consider buying two pairs of slacks for each blazer. Some men who have their suits tailored, in fact, regularly order a double pair for their workhorse suits.

Chinos. Ah, chinos, also known as khakis for their most common color—all cotton, comfortable, relatively cheap, easy to clean, lots of sizes to choose from, in safe, conservative colors. You can never have too many, but make sure they fit. Given the countless size, color, brand, and style variations available today, you have no excuse for not finding a pair that flatters your body.

And everyone's favorite, jeans. It should be easier to look good in jeans than most men do. But men often don't look very good in jeans for some basic reasons: They are the wrong size, they are the wrong cut, or they are worn with tops that make them look cheap and sloppy. Jeans look great when they are contrasted with something special. A pair of jeans with a good pair of leather shoes and a clean, white, pressed oxford shirt to set them off. Or another American classic: jeans and a T-shirt, perhaps with a pair of tennis shoes. The T-shirt should be really clean and very white without any logo emblazoned on it; a classic look should not turn you into a billboard. Black jeans can create a slightly more formal look than classic blue. For other colors, stick to chinos.

Shirts: Polo shirts are always smart, but knits do reveal the general countours of the body. So long as you are trim enough, wear them. Otherwise, stick to button-down shirts, which drape better. Stay with solids, and you can wear strong colors without looking goofy. Stripes and funny patterns should be reserved for the golf course.

Dress shirts don't need to be any more complicated than good-quality cotton, in white, off-white, and blue. Oxford cloth is durable and ages well. Finer cottons feel great, but they are more vulnerable to stains and signs of wear. Classic collars should be selected to suit your face shape. Button-down collars are slightly less formal and go better with the blazer than the suit—although it is no crime to wear them together during the business day. Wear a regular collar with a suit at a more formal dinner.

Classic collars can be worn with or without ties. Fasten the top button. Classic collars with longer points are best for normal to round faces. Shorter points are best for normal to long faces.

Button-downs are preppier than classic collars. They also hold their shape nicely. Wear button-downs with a tie or not.

Sweaters: Light wool or cotton sweaters in the summer. Heavier wool in the winter. Keep them simple, not too tight, in darker colors. Fold them carefully after each use—no hangers. Sweaters are classic and easy; it's hard to go wrong.

Ties: For many men, buying ties might as well be rocket science, but you can't go wrong when you follow these pointers.

- A guy can get away with 5 to 10 ties—if the variety is wide enough, if they suit the clothes they are worn with, and if they are handsome enough.
- Buy silk ties, although cotton ties can work in the summer on the hottest days.
- The more subtle the pattern and color, the longer you can wear a tie.
- Ties with black, brown, and other dark colors are more versatile because they can be worn with black or brown shoes.
- Learn to tie a tie carefully and properly.
- Wear your ties at the right length. The point should not extend beyond your belt.
- Thick ties make big, fat knots, so beware.
- Properly selected and cared for, ties will last several years.
- In the morning, choose a tie based on the clothes you are wearing it with. If you are wearing a gray suit, black shoes and belt, and a white or blue shirt, select one that has a deep color, with at least a little blue, and a black field or background in the pattern. Don't select a pale gray. A brown jacket will work better with a tie that has some browns or neutral tones in the background, but the primary color should provide a solid contrast to the jacket fabric.
- Don't buy a goofball tie unless you have the personality and chutzpah to pull it off.
- Bow ties can and do work on some men. Try one if you are tempted, but make sure it is a tied one and not a clip-on.

Shoes: Shoes give a guy away, so go for quality. Athletic shoes are fine in the gym, but it is hard to imagine classic men—say Cary Grant or Gary Cooper—bounding around in them. Sure, times have changed, but if you are old enough to buy a drink, you are old enough to wear good shoes. Yes, even when you aren't at work. Get used to it.

Shoes are expensive. As with most clothes, shoes need to rest between wearings, so invest in four or five pairs to get you started. You need a black pair, a dark brown or oxblood pair, and nicer casual shoes that fit your activities and climate. Wear loafers in the city; boots in the rougher country. Deck shoes are nice classics, as are good-quality suede oxfords. Watch for shoe sales, and you can save a bundle. A good pair of shoes can run over $200, but half-price sales at the end of a season can allow you to double your daily shoe options quickly.

If you really can't afford to invest in expensive shoes, there are some handsome alternatives. Look for the most conservative, simplest knockoffs of the real thing. Make sure they really fit before you buy them. Cut off any labels or tags the manufacturer may have sewn into a seam. They can pass until you can afford the higher grades.

To maintain your good leather shoes, wear them no more frequently than every other day. You will have them around for several years longer if you keep cedar shoe trees inside them when they are not in use. The wood soaks up perspiration, keeps the leather from molding, and maintains the shoes' proper shape and profile. Well-made soles, whether leather or rubber, can be replaced as they age, and if you maintain the tops with regular polishing, you'll get many, many fine miles out of them.

Belts should match your shoes in color and texture. Replace them before they look as if they pulled a Conestoga wagon across the prairie.

Jewelry: Generally, less is more, and a little is way too much.

Get Great Service

The next time you're in a restaurant and the service is lousy, do something about it instead of complaining to your guests. What to do? First, try to head off some potential problems, and if that isn't enough, then follow the tips provided in this excerpt from Guy Knowledge: Skills, Tricks, and Techniques That Your Father Meant to Teach You—But Probably Didn't *(Rodale Press, 1999) by Larry Keller, Christian Millman, and the editors of* Men's Health *Books.*

You can spend a lot of money on dinner in an elegant restaurant, only to have it ruined by a surly, inattentive serving staff that seems to regard you with more contempt than a cockroach adorning a baked potato. Or you might spoil the evening all by yourself acting boorish and superior to those waiting on you.

"There are people working in this business who have no business working in it, and there are guests who go out who really shouldn't," says Paul Paz, a professional career waiter for 18 years and president of the Waiters Association in Tigard, Oregon. "Both certainly are in the minority."

There are things you can do to make sure that your dinner out is an experience to savor. And they start before you get to the restaurant.

Make a reservation. By reserving a table, you ensure that you get one, and you avoid disappointment and embarrassment, Paz says. Reservations are especially helpful when there is a special occasion, such as a wedding party or the closing of a big business deal. "Depending on your event, the restaurant may have some extra features that they will offer," such as birthday cake or a special bottle of wine or champagne, Paz says.

If it's a popular spot in an urban area, figure on booking a week in advance, advises Eleanor Widmer, Ph.D., a restaurant reviewer for the San Diego *Reader* for more than 2 decades, a public radio and public television commentator, and author of *The New Smart Dining in San Diego and Tijuana*.

Be flexible. If you call for a reservation at the trendiest restaurant in town on the busiest night of the week, you may not be able to reserve a table exactly when you wish, Paz says. Be prepared to accept a less desirable time.

Fridays and Saturdays are busiest, especially from 7:00 to 9:00 P.M., Dr. Widmer says. Your best bet is Tuesday through Thursday. Consider dining shortly after the restaurant opens—say around 6:00 P.M. Forget about Monday—some restaurants are closed, and those that are open may be more inclined to serve leftovers from the weekend, she warns.

Be patient. If your reservation is at, say, 8:00 P.M. and your table isn't ready immediately, don't sweat it, Paz advises. Sometimes diners who have preceded you linger longer than expected. "That goes with the process of dining out," Paz says. "We can't just throw out those guests preceding you."

If your table isn't ready within 15 minutes of your reservation, though, consider leaving, Dr. Widmer suggests. You can complain to the manager, but chances are that this will get you nowhere, especially on a busy weekend, she says.

Give your waiter clues. If you and your fellow diners have perused the menu and decided what you want to order, don't continue to sit there with your menus open in front of you. Instead, stack them. "You're sending a message," Paz says. "If you're really in a hurry, take the stacked menus and place them on the edge of the table. I train people to look for those indicators."

Be specific. "A lot of times, guests just don't make enough of what I call customer noise," Paz says. If you like your steak cooked until it looks as black and crispy as a smoker's lungs, tell your waiter. If you'd rather eat monkey brains than taste even a dollop of mayonnaise on your sandwich, speak up. The more information you provide the person serving you, the more likely the meal will be to your liking.

Consider the specials. Some diners think a restaurant's daily specials are old dishes the chef is trying to get rid of, or discounted, inferior fare, Paz says. It does happen, but more often the specials are dishes about which the chef is particularly proud. "There is some feature item the chef has discovered, or he has created a new recipe, or there may be a new product on the market he wants to present to his customers," he says. So if you want to order a meal that's likely to be top-notch, try one of the specials.

Give your waiter a second chance. If there is a relatively minor problem with the service—say, you had to wait too long for a coffee refill—don't suffer silently, and don't seek out the manager, Paz says. If you bring the matter to your server's attention, odds are, it will be promptly addressed.

But if your server has been repeatedly remiss—no water refills, no bread, no checking back with you after you've begun your meal—talking to the waiter may be useless, Dr. Widmer says. They're either oblivious or they don't care, she says. Then the manager is your only recourse.

Don't make threats. One way to annoy your server and jeopardize service is to make negative references to the tip. It's rude to say things such as, "If this doesn't go right, you're not going to get a tip," or to tell the server that forgetting to bring a spoon with your coffee is going to affect the gratuity. "It's just tacky," Paz says.

Separate yourself early. A lot of servers—but not Paz—get irritated when customers ask for separate checks. Some computerized systems don't allow splitting checks after the data has been entered. "Where guests can help themselves is if they announce this at the beginning of the meal," Paz says. "When servers know in advance that there are separate checks to deal with, it's much easier for them to take care of it."

Passing the Bar

Good service isn't reserved only for fancy restaurants. You should expect it in your favorite bar as well. That means a bartender who is quick with a smile, attentive to your drink needs, and a good listener, says Bill Bade, who for 30 years has served as owner and director of the Midwest Bartender's School in Omaha, Nebraska.

If you're a regular, he will remember what drink you usually order. He also will place a napkin under your beverage, and he won't carelessly slap your drink down on the bar, Bade says. Nor will he allow a crowded bar to slow his service much.

"If he's a good bartender, he'll run a 20- to 30-foot bar and keep up on everything," Bade says.

The same way you appreciate friendly bartenders, they appreciate friendly customers, notes Bade. Here's how you can show your appreciation.

Tip him. If a bartender is giving good service, tip him at least 15 percent. Much of their income is derived from tips, Bade says.

If you're having more than one drink, tip when you leave rather than after each drink, says Dr. Widmer.

That still leaves the question of how to ensure your bartender's attention, since he won't know that you're a generous tipper until you leave the bar. Dr. Widmer suggests sliding a couple of dollars to him before you order your first drink and saying something like, "I want you to take care of me."

Be polite. Don't rattle your glass on the bar to get the bartender's attention, Bade says. If he's occupied at the opposite end of the bar, walk over and ask if you can get service at your end.

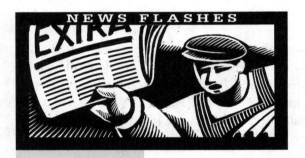

NEWS FLASHES

Nasal Sprays Effective on Cuts

BEVERLY HILLS, Calif.—Here's another use for nasal sprays: Those that contain the compound phenylephrine hydrochloride (Neo-Synephrine) can stop the bleeding of razor cuts, according to Robert Kotler, M.D., clinical instructor of surgery at the University of California, Los Angeles, and a facial cosmetic surgeon in Beverly Hills. Just wipe the nicked area and immediately apply a piece of cotton or tissue that's wet with the nasal spray. Within 5 minutes, the bleeding will stop.

"It makes sense," says Michael Caldwell, M.D., professor of surgery and biochemistry at the University of Minnesota in Minneapolis–St. Paul. "Phenylephrine hydrochloride constricts blood vessels, so it should be handy as a topical treatment to stop cuts from bleeding."

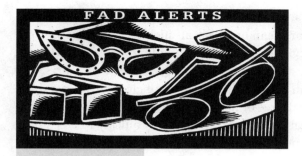

Triple-Blade Razor

The Gillette Mach 3 razor has the same undeniable appeal as breast implants: More is usually better. In this case, the company claims that the three blades shave progressively closer, annihilating stubborn whiskers in one swipe. At about $7 per razor—and nearly that much for four replacement blades—it had better deliver one damn good shave.

It does. One Mach 3 gave our editor about six work-ready shaves. And he used only downward strokes; he didn't have to shave "against the grain" to remove stubble. What's better, just one pass did the job. "That's important," says Jerald L. Sklar, M.D., a dermatologist at Baylor University Medical Center in Dallas. "Making a second or third pass can cause razor burn or ingrown hairs." The blade's swivel is a bit too loose, though. You'll need a stiffer razor to carve your sideburns, mustache, or goatee.

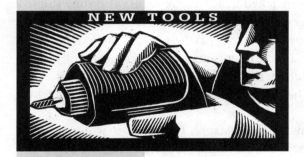

More Flexible Glasses

Flexon Frames

Flexon frames can supposedly twist into pretzels without snapping. They're made by Marchon and retail for $299. They look and feel like fragile, expensive glasses, but they're made with a titanium-and-nickel alloy that was invented by the U.S. Naval Ordnance Lab for use in missile heat shields. "This alloy was specially made to return to its original position after bending," says Philip Clapp, Ph.D., professor of metallurgy at the University of Connecticut in Storrs. "Although severe overstressing can deform the metal, these glasses will snap back into shape after any reasonable degree of flexing." To test Dr. Clapp's prediction, we crumpled the Flexons several times. Sure enough, they quickly wormed back to their pristine shape every time. For more information, call (800) 235-3966.

Handier Gadget

Swiss Tech Gold Tool

At $40, the Swiss Tech Gold Tool seemed like an overpriced Cracker Jack toy. But the hardened-steel gizmo packs a strong Phillips head and a flat screwdriver, plus a pair of compact pliers that'll bite any bolt that irks you. Fold the tool into an L, and you can apply white-knuckle torque to the screwdrivers without fear of bending them. Best of all, the 1-ounce device folds down smaller than a box of Tic Tacs, to fit easily into your pocket. Call (800) 414-8799 to order.

Smarter Watch Buying

Wristwatches

Your wristwatch tells more than just the time. It tells about you. Sporting a $5.99 calculator job with a mismatched band? You're telling everyone you're a dweeb. Wearing a diamond-encrusted gold chronograph that weighs half a pound? You're letting them know you're a very rich dweeb. What you want your watch to say is that you appreciate the finer things, perhaps that you fly antique biplanes or dive reefs in the Solomon Islands. To make sure yours makes the right comments about you, buy the best watch you can afford, maybe even stretching the budget a little.

1. Quartz watches are the lowest maintenance. They need no winding and no special attention. And they're also extremely accurate, varying only about 1 minute per year.
2. For the lover of craftsmanship and all things mechanical, a manual- or automatic-wind mechanical timepiece produced by Swiss craftsmen typically is the way to go. Generally speaking, mechanical timepieces cost more than quartz ones, and they require lubrication every few years.

3. Most watches are offered in gold plate, stainless steel, titanium, 18-karat gold, or a combination thereof. When purchasing a gold-plated watch, find out how thick the plating is. It's measured in microns: The higher the number (for instance, 10 or 5 microns versus 2 microns), the sturdier the finish. If you spend much time outdoors, you may prefer a stainless-steel or titanium finish; it won't scratch when you smash your wrist against your ice axe.

4. Water-resistant watches earn that designation by being tested under water pressure equivalent to 100 feet down. Watches that are water resistant at extreme depths (more than 300 meters) tend to be more expensive. If you're a jogger, mountain climber, or some other kind of rough-and-tumble guy, consider buying a shock-resistant watch.

5. Chronographs allow you to time a race or other event. Some chronographs offer telemeters (to determine distance), tachometers (to gauge speed), or pulsimeters (to tell your pulse rate). Chronometers are tested under stringent conditions in various positions, pressures, and temperatures.

6. Nearly every watch company offers at least a 1-year warranty on its timepieces. Some offer extended warranties that cover the case or bracelet as well as the movement. Ask for details before you buy.

7. Be sure you're buying your timepiece from an authorized dealer for that brand. With some higher-end luxury watches, the watch may not be covered if the dealer isn't authorized by the manufacturer.

8. Think ahead. If you can't find a repair center, visit www.fhusa.com, the Web site for the U.S. division of the Federation for the Swiss Watch Industry. It lists at least 50 brands, their U.S. headquarters, service locations, and phone numbers.

Smoother Shaving

Fog-Free Shower Mirror

"If you keep your face wet, you'll get a much closer shave," says Jerome Z. Litt, M.D., dermatologist at Case Western Reserve University School of Medicine in Cleveland. That's why shaving in the shower is smart. The best mirror we've found for the job is the Shower Tek Fog-Free Mirror. This heavy chrome job has a hollow, flexible arm that attaches to the shower pipe; the circulating water keeps the glass clear. One side is magnified for close work. $100. Call (800) 776-6364.

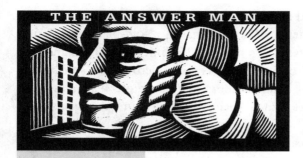

Uncertain Salesman

I'm a salesman, and when I call on clients on Fridays, they're all wearing casual clothes. Should I start dressing down, too?
—P. C., Conyers, Ga.

It depends on how many of your Friday clients have a casual dress code, says Judith Rasband, chief executive officer and director of the Conselle Institute of Image Management in Provo, Utah. If they're all showing up in sweaters and khakis, it's okay to dress a bit more casually than usual. "In that case, you can't go wrong with a sport coat, a tie, and a pair of coordinated pants," says Rasband. "It's less formal than the full suit, but you still look authoritative." On the other hand, if even one of your clients wears standard business clothing on Fridays, you should stick with your suit.

Knotty Problems

How can I get my tie ends to come out right the first time I tie my tie? And what's the proper length for it once it's knotted?
—V. K., Fayetteville, Ark.

While it may be a "Euro" look to have your tie hang down beyond the waistband of your pants, it's not a look you should copy, says Alan Flusser, a designer and the author of *Style and the Man*. The tip of your tie should reach the top of your belt.

To get the ends to come out evenly—or as close to even as possible—use a standard four-in-hand knot, and start with the wide end of the tie hanging 1 foot lower than the narrow end. (This will work only if you are tying a quality, full-length tie. It probably won't work on the one that plays Christmas music.)

Single Is Better

Is a double-breasted jacket the best way to camouflage my gut?
—J. S., Fresno, Calif.

No. A single-breasted jacket is generally a better choice for diverting attention away from your stomach, according to Hugh Belflower, manager of Lew's International Menswear in Hilton Head Island, South Carolina. Most double-breasted jackets look boxy, and the crossover buttoning attracts attention to your midsection. The goals here are to make you look more vertical and to divert an observer's eyes from your midsection. Wearing dark, solid colors also helps you look slimmer.

White in Winter

My dad told me never to wear light-colored trousers, including khakis, between Labor Day and Memorial Day. But I see people wearing khakis all year. Who's right?
—B. L., Boston

"Khakis are perfectly acceptable year-round—especially weightier khakis in earth tones," says Marcia Samuelson, of Samuelsohn, a Montreal-based clothier. As far as whites are concerned, you don't want to wear them in Baltimore in February.

If you're in Palm Beach or any other warm wintertime clime, however, the rules are different. "In that case, the standard is more a sense of fabric than a sense of color," says Jack Madda, sales associate at Kilgore-Trout, a top men's store in Cleveland. "Cream or tan flannels are acceptable where it's warm in wintertime."

Off with Their Hats

I see a lot of guys wearing baseball caps in restaurants these days. Are they total slobs, or am I just stuck in the Truman administration?
—D. D., San Diego

Regardless of whether you consider baseball caps the height of fashion or merely street hip, our experts concur that wearing a hat indoors—to breakfast, lunch, or dinner—is a faux pas. "It's simply inappropriate to keep a hat on in a restaurant," says Norman Usiak, co-owner of Camouflage, one of New York's most eclectic fashion stores. "The function of any hat is to protect the head in extreme weather. You don't get much extreme weather inside a building."

Flood Avoidance

Once and for all, what's the proper length for a pair of trousers? And what does "break" mean in terms of the length?
—C. B., Tulsa, Okla.

To answer, we'll start at the top—of your pants, that is. Except for jeans, your trousers should be worn around the waist, not down on your hips. Your pant waist should fall slightly above your navel and stay parallel to the ground all the way around you, says John T. Molloy, author of *New Dress for Success*. (In other words, the waist should not be lower in the front than in the back.)

From your waist, your pants should fall to within about 1 inch of the top of your shoe heel. The front of your trouser leg should rest on the top of your shoe; the touching of fabric to shoe will form a slight fold. That fold is called the break—it refers to the break that's created in the neat line of a crease.

Where to Dab

Where's the best place on my body to apply cologne?
—B. W., Miami

"If you're going to use cologne, avoid splashing it on your face," says Dennis Keogh, marketing vice president worldwide for Ralph Lauren Fragrances. "Cologne is simply too strong and your face is too sensitive." Instead, Keogh recommends dabbing it on your upper chest and lower neck. Note that the key word is "dab"—not "pour," "splash," or "dump."

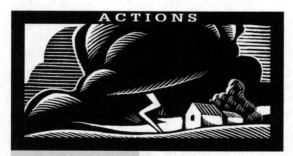

ACTIONS

There are two fundamental truths about style. The first is that style is about demeanor. A man of style carries himself with dignity, with strength, with purpose, with confidence. The second truth is that style is about being yourself. It is about knowing exactly who you are and then crafting a look that projects that, without compromise or bending to the winds of fashion or peer pressure. These tips will help you on your quest to become a man of style.

1. **Degunk a pocketknife.** You use your knife to scrape crud off your boots, slice cheese, stir coffee, and clean your fingernails—maybe even in that order. Pull it out and give it a good cleaning. Start with a pan of warm, sudsy water. Open up all the tools in your knife and drop it in. Let the knife soak for a few minutes, then reach in (carefully!) and open and close the blades; an old toothbrush will help you remove all the softened crud. Let the knife dry, then coat it lightly with a layer of cooking oil, rubbing off the excess with a paper towel. Voila! You're ready to scrape more crud, slice more cheese, stir the coffee, and pick at your fingernails.

2. **Be kind to the help.** "The way you deal with waiters and the staff says a lot about how you deal with people in general," says Jeff Livingston, Ph.D., past director of the National Association of Business Consultants in Raleigh, North Carolina, and an information analyst for Cisco Systems in Research Triangle Park, North Carolina. Be polite and professional, not condescending or overbearing. Also, understand that there is an art and science to waiting a table properly. A good waiter observes how the meal is progressing from a distance and silently, efficiently, takes care of your needs, be it providing an extra knife, removing dishes, refilling water glasses, or presenting the check.

3. **Gracefully handle poor service.** If your service at a restaurant is in need of a tune-up, discreetly excuse yourself mid-meal and ask to speak to the manager. Then politely have your say. Don't wait until you're done eating and your outing is ruined. And never argue, be rude, or condescend.

4. **See a tailor for a perfect fit.** The nice thing about being fitted for a suit by an expert tailor is that you don't have to bother sucking in your gut. "Just be yourself and relax," says Mimmo Spano, a tailor with 27 years of experience working at Bergdorf Goodman in New York City. "He doesn't want to change you, and he's not going to tell you to lose weight. He will tell you whether you stand hunched or erect, or whether your shoulders are square or rounded. He'll also let you know if one arm or leg is longer than the other, and he'll adjust the suit accordingly. His job is to make your suit look great on the body you have, not the body you want."

Spano's number one rule: Don't try to fit yourself into a cut that isn't right for your body shape. "You'll know it's wrong when the salesman says, 'You look great. All the tailor will have to do is take it in here and let it out there and you'll be in business,'" Spano says. You'll also know that you're in the wrong store.

Here's what Spano looks for when you try on a suit for him.
- If he sees horizontal ripples in the fabric running down the center of your back, it means your shoulders are broader than the jacket will accommodate.
- Vertical lines running down the back mean that the jacket is meant for broader shoulders.

- If the jacket bunches at the waist on one side, one shoulder is higher than the other, so the shoulder pads need adjusting.
- If the front of the jacket hangs lower than the back, you're a "stooper." The tailor should let some fabric out of the rear hem and take it up in the front.
- Spano will ask you whether the pants fit. "If the pants aren't comfortable as soon as you try them on," he says, "they never will be, no matter how much work the tailor does." When buying a suit, he suggests, buy the trousers first, then the jacket. Trousers provide the least amount of leeway for alterations—there's not a lot of extra fabric down there.

5. **Pick your shoes' texture.** The texture of your suit fabric should help determine the texture of your shoes, says Gregg Andrews, central states fashion coordinator for Nordstrom. "Smooth, sleek leathers tend to look best with smooth, finer wools. If the trouser is of a heavier, textured fabric, such as tweed or corduroy, shoes in pebble-grained leather or textured suede are a nice complement."

Tom Julian, trend analyst with the Fallon McElligott advertising agency in New York City, agrees. "A heavier-weight suit should be worn with heavier-weight footwear," he says. "Textured trousers look sportiest with a lug-sole or monk-strap shoe. With gabardine or crepe fabric, though, try a loafer for a sportier influence."

6. **Dream away wrinkles.** Sleep on your back. Eight hours with your face pressed against a pillow wrinkles your skin and causes permanent creases over time.

7. **Dab the grease.** To treat oily skin, dab a few drops of vinegar on a tissue and then dab it on your skin. Rinse with water. That should kill the shine.

8. **Reach for the oil.** If you realize, as you grope around in the morning, that you forgot to replace the empty can of shaving cream, here's a way out: Go for a few drops of olive oil. The next-best option is petroleum jelly.

9. **Don't dis robes.** Hugh Hefner you're not, and maybe you never want to be. But the old playboy is on to something when it comes to loungewear. Robes are comfortable. Any woman will tell you that the thin, discount-store robe that you wore as a kid won't cut it. Nothing cuts it short of thick, luxurious, warm, and full-length. Good robes can cost $40 or more, but they'll last and are worth every penny. (And they'll look great on her, too.)

10. **Get rid of stains for good.** It's a law of nature: If it flies off your fork, it lands on your shirt. Here are some tips to get rid of the nastiest stains.

- Faster is better. Your best chance of removing a stain is just after impact, before it has time to penetrate the fabric and set.
- Blot, don't scrub. Scrubbing at a stain will damage fabric fibers and drive the stain into the fabric.
- Use hot water on a grease stain. That will help the stain dissolve. Cold water will only solidify a grease stain.
- Use cold water on a wet stain. That's any spot that contains water or is water-based, such as grape juice.
- Spit on your tie. The enzymes in saliva can help break down protein-based food stains. Since your tie is (we hope) silk, don't scrub at it with soap and water. Gently rub in the saliva with a cloth. Take the tie to the cleaner if spit doesn't work.
- Suck it up. A liquid stain is going to spread, so put a cloth napkin under the stained section of fabric to absorb the liquid before your shirt does.
- Go easy on the club soda. The moment anything lands on their clothes, most people start spraying themselves with more club soda than Krusty the Clown ever used. Club soda can work as a substitute for tap water, but it's not a miracle potion.

11. **Condition your hair.** A good-quality conditioner will thicken and smooth your hair, giving it shine and bounce and character. After shampooing, rub conditioner in and leave it on for a minute before rinsing.

12. **Cut your fingernails the right way.** When clipping, use several small clips per nail. "Turn your hand around so that it's facing you and the tips of your nails are pointing down," advises Firozé, a manicurist and pedicurist in New York City.

13. **Buy clothes for feeling, not for status.** Buying clothes to impress other people "is the wrong reason," says Murray Pearlstein, owner of Louis, Boston, an upscale men's and women's clothier. "The right reason is to feel good—to feel special. You work better and you think better when you're feeling good about yourself." And clothes can go a long way to getting you into that frame of mind.

14. **Go for the good stuff.** Or, as Carolyn Gustafson, a New York City–based image consultant who has appeared on numerous television programs, including *The Oprah Winfrey Show*, puts it: "Buy quality, buy quality, buy quality." Her rationale for breaking open the piggy bank on a few expensive articles of clothing as opposed to a lot of inexpensive rags is that "it's more important to look good every day than different every day." If you're a penny-pincher, she suggests that rather than having a heart attack when you get a gander at the price tag of an expensive item, convert it via the cost-per-wear formula. Divide the cost by the number of times that you'll wear it during the life of the garment. And remember, she adds, the better the quality of the garment, the larger the number of wears and the cheaper the cost to wear it each time.

15. **Clean 'em up.** A pair of glasses takes more abuse than a scab at a Teamsters picnic. And since spectacles provide you with your view of the world, you should know how to keep them clean and healthy.

Wet them before you clean them. When your lenses are dirty, your first instinct is to use a tissue or your shirttail to wipe the smudges off. Bad move, according to Anne Sumers, M.D., of the American Academy of Ophthalmology. "Don't wipe your glasses while they are dry," she cautions. "Once you wet them, use terry cloth or soft tissue to clean them. Don't use paper towels—they scratch lenses." Also stay away from scented tissues (they leave smears) and soap. Regular old tap water will do just fine. Don't use detergent or dishwashing soap, which may damage any anti-reflective or UV coating on your lenses. "Detergents cause a Michelangelo effect on your lenses, creating tiny cracks in the sheen of the tint," says Dr. Sumers.

According to Dr. Sumers, you can expect to get 2 years out of everyday glasses, and less out of sunglasses and reading glasses, which tend to get tossed around more. To maximize the life of your glasses, buy a case for them, and use it. Make sure it's strong enough to save your glasses even if you sit on them.

Credits

"Dayhiking: Wonderful Walking" on page 18 is reprinted from *The Ragged Mountain Press Guide to Outdoor Sports* by Jonathan and Roseann Hanson. © 1997 by Jonathan and Roseann Hanson. Reprinted by permission of the McGraw-Hill Companies.

"The SAD Diet" on page 59 is reprinted from *The Complete Idiot's Guide to Living Longer and Healthier* by Allan Magaziner, D.O. Published by Alpha Books, an imprint of Macmillan USA. © 1999 by Allan Magaziner, D.O. Reprinted by permission of the publisher.

"Discovering Viagra" on page 93 is reprinted with permission of Simon and Schuster, Inc., from *The Virility Solution: Everything You Need to Know about the FDA-Approved Potency Pill That Can Restore and Enhance Male Sexuality* by Steven Lamm, M.D., and Gerald Secor Couzens. © 1998 by Steven Lamm, M.D., and Gerald Secor Couzens.

"Sex and the Middle-Age Male" on page 97 is reprinted from *Midlife Man* by Art Hister, M.D. © 1998 by Art Hister, M.D. Published in Canada by Greystone Books, a division of Douglas & McIntyre. Reprinted by permission of the publisher.

"The Secret to Permanent Weight Control" on page 132 is reprinted from *Let My Heart Attack Save Your Life: A Simple, Sound, Workable Weight Management Plan* by Joseph Mason. © 1998 by Joseph Mason. Reprinted by permission of John Wiley & Sons, Inc.

"Why Most Men Are Emotionally Impotent" on page 202 is reprinted from *Thriving: The Complete Mind-Body Guide for Optimal Health and Fitness for Men* by Robert S. Ivker and Edward Zorensky. © 1997 by Robert S. Ivker and Edward Zorensky. Reprinted by permission of Crown Publishing, Inc.

"Relaxation Therapies" on page 207 is reprinted with the permission of Macmillan General Reference, a wholly owned subsidiary of IDG Books Worldwide, Inc. from *The People's Medical Society Men's Health and Wellness Encyclopedia* by Charles Inlander. © 1998 by the People's Medical Society.

"A Menopause for Men" on page 236 is reprinted from *The Testosterone Syndrome: Thr Critical Factor for Energy, Health, and Sexuality—Reversing the Male Menopause* by Eugene Shippen, M.D., and William Fryer. © 1998 by Eugene Shippen, M.D., and William Fryer. Published by M. Evans and Company, New York. Reprinted by permission of the publisher.

"10 Common Surgeries and Procedures" on page 242 is reprinted from *Men's Health for Dummies*® by Charles Inlander and the People's Medical Society. © 1999 by IDG Books Worldwide, Inc. All rights reserved. Reproduced here by permission of IDG Books Worldwide, Inc. For Dummies is a registered trademark of IDG Books Worldwide, Inc.

"Clothes You Could Wear for the Rest of Your Life" on page 279 is reprinted from *Beyond Soap, Water, and Comb: A Man's Guide to Good Grooming and Fitness* by Ed Marquand. © 1998 by Ed Marquand. Courtesy of Abbeville Press.

Index

Boldface references indicate illustrations.